W9-CFV-602

Arthritis

SOURCEBOOK

Fifth Edition

Health Reference Series

Fifth Edition

Arthritis
SOURCEBOOK

*Basic Consumer Health Information about the Risk
Factors, Symptoms, Diagnosis, and Treatment of
Osteoarthritis, Rheumatoid Arthritis, Juvenile Arthritis,
Gout, Infectious Arthritis, and Autoimmune Disorders
Associated with Arthritis*

*Along with Facts about Medications, Surgeries, and
Self-Care Techniques to Manage Pain and Disability,
Tips on Living with Arthritis, a Glossary of Related
Terms, and Resources for Additional Help and
Information*

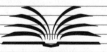

OMNIGRAPHICS
615 Griswold, Ste. 901, Detroit, MI 48226

Bibliographic Note
Because this page cannot legibly accommodate all the copyright notices, the Bibliographic Note portion of the Preface constitutes an extension of the copyright notice.

* * *

OMNIGRAPHICS
Angela L. Williams, *Managing Editor*
***

Copyright © 2018 Omnigraphics

ISBN 978-0-7808-1626-8
E-ISBN 978-0-7808-1627-5

Library of Congress Cataloging-in-Publication Data

Names: Omnigraphics, Inc., issuing body.

Title: Arthritis sourcebook: basic consumer health information about the risk factors, symptoms, diagnosis, and treatment of osteoarthritis, rheumatoid arthritis, juvenile arthritis, gout, infectious arthritis, and autoimmune disorders associated with arthritis; along with facts about medications, surgeries, and self-care techniques to manage pain and disability, tips on living with arthritis, a glossary of related terms, and resources for additional help and information.

Description: Detroit, MI: Omnigraphics, [2018] | Series: Health reference series | Includes bibliographical references and index.

Identifiers: LCCN 2018009370 (print) | LCCN 2018009720 (ebook) | ISBN 9780780816275 (eBook) | ISBN 9780780816268 (hardcover: alk. paper)

Subjects: LCSH: Arthritis--Popular works.

Classification: LCC RC933 (ebook) | LCC RC933.A665257 2018 (print) | DDC 616.7/22--dc23

LC record available at https://lccn.loc.gov/2018009370

Table of Contents

Preface xiii

Part I: Introduction to Arthritis

Chapter 1 — Understanding the Bones, Muscles,
and Joints 3

    Section 1.1 — What Are Bones, Muscles,
and Joints? 4

    Section 1.2 — Importance of Healthy
Bones 9

Chapter 2 — Overview of Arthritis and Rheumatic
Diseases 23

Chapter 3 — Statistics on Arthritis in the United
States 29

Chapter 4 — Risk Factors for Arthritis 35

    Section 4.1 — Modifiable and
Nonmodifiable Risk
Factors for Arthritis 36

    Section 4.2 — Genetics as Risk Factor for
Arthritis 37

Chapter 5 — Joints Affected by Arthritis 41

    Section 5.1 — Arthritis of the Shoulder 42

    Section 5.2 — Arthritis of the Wrist 44

    Section 5.3 — Arthritis of the Hip 48

Section 5.4 — Arthritis of the Knee.................. 52

Section 5.5 — Arthritis of the Foot and
Ankle 56

Part II: Types of Arthritis, Related Rheumatic Diseases, and Other Associated Medical Conditions

Chapter 6 — Osteoarthritis (OA).. 63

Section 6.1 — Understanding
Osteoarthritis............................. 64

Section 6.2 — Spinal Stenosis Can Be
Caused by OA............................. 68

Chapter 7 — Rheumatoid Arthritis (RA)................................. 71

Section 7.1 — Understanding
Rheumatoid Arthritis (RA)......... 72

Section 7.2 — Painful Joints? Early
Treatment for Rheumatoid
Arthritis Is Key.......................... 77

Section 7.3 — Arthritis Mechanisms
May Vary by Joint 79

Chapter 8 — Childhood Arthritis (Juvenile Arthritis) 81

Section 8.1 — Kids and Their Bone Health 82

Section 8.2 — What Is Childhood Arthritis?..... 85

Section 8.3 — Juvenile Rheumatoid
Arthritis and Vision Loss 94

Section 8.4 — Juvenile Idiopathic Arthritis 99

Section 8.5 — Biologics: New Treatments
for Juvenile Arthritis................ 101

Chapter 9 — Ankylosing Spondylitis.. 105

Chapter 10 — Behçet Disease 109

Chapter 11 — Bone Spurs, Bursitis, and Tendonitis.................. 113

Section 11.1 — Bone Spurs 114

Section 11.2 — Bursitis..................................... 118

Section 11.3 — Tendonitis 121

Chapter 12 — Carpal Tunnel Syndrome (CTS) 125

Chapter 13—Fibromyalgia 131

    Section 13.1—Understanding
               Fibromyalgia 132

    Section 13.2—Drugs Approved to
               Manage Pain 137

    Section 13.3—Mind and Body Therapy
               for Fibromyalgia 141

Chapter 14—Gout and Chondrocalcinosis 2 145

    Section 14.1—Understanding Gout 146

    Section 14.2—Chondrocalcinosis 2 149

Chapter 15—Infectious Forms of Arthritis 153

    Section 15.1—Arthritis Associated with
               Lyme Disease 154

    Section 15.2—Reactive Arthritis 159

    Section 15.3—Septic Arthritis
               (Infectious Arthritis) 161

Chapter 16—Lupus 163

    Section 16.1—Systemic Lupus
               Erythematosus 164

    Section 16.2—Lupus and Osteoporosis 168

    Section 16.3—Lupus and Women 171

Chapter 17—Myositis 181

Chapter 18—Osteoporosis 185

    Section 18.1—Understanding
               Osteoporosis 186

    Section 18.2—Osteoporosis and Arthritis:
               Two Common But Different
               Conditions 204

    Section 18.3—What People with RA
               Need to Know about
               Osteoporosis 207

    Section 18.4—Osteoporosis in Women 210

    Section 18.5—Osteoporosis in Men 220

    Section 18.6—Osteoporosis in Aging 227

Chapter 19—Paget Disease of Bone 231

    Section 19.1—What Is Paget Disease
          of Bone? 232

    Section 19.2—Paget Disease of Bone and
          Osteoarthritis: Different
          Yet Related................................ 236

    Section 19.3—Pain and Paget Disease of
          Bone... 239

    Section 19.4—FAQs on Paget Disease of
          Bone... 241

Chapter 20—Polymyalgia Rheumatica and Giant
    Cell Arteritis 245

Chapter 21—Psoriasis and Psoriatic Arthritis 249

    Section 21.1—Psoriasis 250

    Section 21.2—Psoriatic Arthritis..................... 253

Chapter 22—Scleroderma 257

Chapter 23—Sjögren Syndrome... 263

Chapter 24—Work-Related Arthritis and Ergonomics............. 271

Chapter 25—Arthritis-Related to Other Disorders 275

    Section 25.1—Comorbidities............................ 276

    Section 25.2—Arthritis and Human
          Immunodeficiency Virus........... 280

    Section 25.3—Arthritis and Inflammatory
          Bowel Disease 282

Part III: Medical and Surgical Treatments for Arthritis

Chapter 26—Your Arthritis Healthcare Provider...................... 289

    Section 26.1—Choosing a Doctor...................... 290

    Section 26.2—Talking with Medical
          Specialists: Tips for
          Patients 293

    Section 26.3—For People with
          Osteoporosis: How to
          Find a Doctor 295

Chapter 27—Diagnosing and Treating Rheumatoid
    Arthritis... 299

Chapter 28—Osteoarthritis Medicines..................................... 307

Chapter 29—Rheumatoid Arthritis Medicines 315

Chapter 30—Help Your Arthritis Treatment Work.................. 321

    Section 30.1—Treating and Managing
        Arthritis................................... 322

    Section 30.2—Heat and Cold Therapies
        for Arthritis.............................. 324

    Section 30.3—Long-Term Benefit of
        Steroid Injections for
        Knee Osteoarthritis
        Challenged 326

Chapter 31—Surgical Procedures Used to Treat
    Arthritis... 329

    Section 31.1—Arthroscopic Surgery............... 330

    Section 31.2—Bone Fusion Surgery 333

Chapter 32—Understanding Joint Replacement
    Surgery... 341

Chapter 33—Knee Replacement 345

Chapter 34—Other Types of Joint Surgery............................. 349

    Section 34.1—Hip Replacement 350

    Section 34.2—Shoulder Replacement............. 356

    Section 34.3—Joint Fusion Surgery
        (Arthrodesis) 363

Part IV: Arthritis Self-Management: Strategies to Reduce Pain and Inflammation

Chapter 35—Managing Arthritis... 371

Chapter 36—Chronic Pain Management 375

Chapter 37—Arthritis and Sleep Deprivation 381

Chapter 38—Weight Management and Arthritis 385

Chapter 39—Exercise and Arthritis 395

    Section 39.1—Physical Activity for
                          Arthritis.................................... 396

    Section 39.2—Yoga Promotes Physical
                          Fitness and Joint Health.......... 399

    Section 39.3—Tai Chi and Qi Gong for
                          Knee Osteoarthritis 403

    Section 39.4—Water Aerobics Can
                          Benefit People with
                          Arthritis.................................... 406

Chapter 40—Herbs, Dietary Supplements, and
    Arthritis.. 409

    Section 40.1—Glucosamine and
                          Chondroitin 410

    Section 40.2—Cat's Claw 413

    Section 40.3—Evening Primrose Oil 415

    Section 40.4—Flaxseed and Flaxseed Oil 417

    Section 40.5—Ginger.. 419

    Section 40.6—Thunder God Vine 421

    Section 40.7—Turmeric.................................... 423

    Section 40.8—Dietary Supplements for
                          Osteoarthritis........................... 425

    Section 40.9—Omega-3 Fatty Acids 427

Chapter 41—Complementary and Alternative
    Medicine for Arthritis.. 431

    Section 41.1—What Is Complementary
                          and Alternative
                          Medicine?.................................. 432

    Section 41.2—Complementary Health
                          Approaches for Chronic
                          Pain... 435

    Section 41.3—Acupuncture.............................. 437

    Section 41.4—Magnets..................................... 439

    Section 41.5—Research on Massage
                          Therapy and Arthritis 440

Part V: Living with Arthritis

Chapter 42—Living with Arthritis and Other
     Rheumatic Diseases............................... 445

Chapter 43—Healthy Eating and Arthritis............................... 449

Chapter 44—Arthritis and Mental Health............................... 455

Chapter 45—Maintaining Independence 459

    Section 45.1—Modifying Your Home for
         Independence 460

    Section 45.2—Avoiding Falls and
         Fractures.................................. 464

    Section 45.3—Assistive Devices Can
         Make Life with Arthritis
         Easier 470

    Section 45.4—Driving When You Have
         Arthritis.................................... 473

Chapter 46—Arthritis and Sexuality 477

Chapter 47—Starting a Family: Pregnancy and
     Arthritis... 481

    Section 47.1—Pregnancy, Breastfeeding,
         and Bone Health 482

    Section 47.2—Rheumatic Disease
         Management in Pregnant
         Women...................................... 485

Part VI: Additional Help and Information

Chapter 48—Glossary of Terms Related to
     Arthritis and Rheumatic Diseases...................... 493

Chapter 49—Directory of Organizations That Help
     People with Arthritis and Their
     Families... 503

Index... 521

Preface

About This Book

Arthritis affects 54.4 million U.S. adults, more than 1 of 4. Studies reveal arthritis as a leading cause of work disability in the United States. It is one of the most common chronic conditions in the nation. Symptoms like joint pain, stiffness, and inflammation associated with arthritis and related rheumatic diseases can interfere with activities of daily life, school, and employment. Fatigue and emotional consequences of the disease can negatively impact relationships and mental well-being. On a positive note, medications, surgery, appropriate physical exercise, proper nutrition, and complementary and alternative therapies often offer pain and symptom relief. Although a cure remains elusive, these types of care strategies enable many people to experience significant improvements in daily functioning and overall quality of life.

Arthritis Sourcebook, Fifth Edition provides updated information about diagnosing, treating, and managing degenerative, inflammatory, and other specific forms of arthritis. It also explains the symptoms and treatments of related diseases that affect the joints, tendons, ligaments, bones, and muscles. Details about currently used medical, surgical, and self-care management strategies are included along with tips for reducing joint pain and inflammation and managing arthritis-related disability. The book concludes with a glossary of terms and directory of resources for additional help and information.

How to Use This Book

This book is divided into parts and chapters. Parts focus on broad areas of interest. Chapters are devoted to single topics within a part.

Part I: Introduction to Arthritis provides general information about the types, prevalence, risk factors, and causes of arthritis and related rheumatic diseases. Information about how arthritis affects specific joints in different parts of the body—the shoulder, wrist, hip, knee, ankle, and foot—is also included.

Part II: Types of Arthritis, Related Rheumatic Diseases, and Other Associated Medical Conditions discusses the symptoms, diagnosis, and treatments for common forms of arthritis, including osteoarthritis, rheumatoid arthritis, and juvenile rheumatoid arthritis. Separate individual chapters focus on rheumatic diseases caused by or related to arthritis. These disorders, such as ankylosing Behçet disease, fibromyalgia, gout, lupus, psoriasis, Sjögren syndrome, and scleroderma, may also cause chronic joint pain, stiffness, and inflammation.

Part III: Medical and Surgical Treatments for Arthritis begins with information about how arthritis patients can find and communicate with appropriate healthcare providers. It provides information about over-the-counter and prescription medications used for arthritis-related pain and inflammation. Surgical procedures, including arthroscopic, bone fusion, and joint replacement surgery, are also described.

Part IV: Arthritis Self-Management: Strategies to Reduce Pain and Inflammation highlights various ways arthritis patients can cope with pain, sleep deprivation, and other symptoms that may accompany arthritis. Weight management tips, exercise programs, and diet-related information are discussed, and facts about the use of herbs and other complementary and alternative therapies are provided.

Part V: Living with Arthritis describes some of the emotional concerns and daily challenges encountered by people who are coping with the effects and limitations of joint disease. These include handling depression, managing stress, maintaining independence, and preserving healthy relationships. Tips are also provided for arthritis patients who have questions about starting a family and other related issues.

Part VI: Additional Help and Information offers a glossary of important terms related to arthritis and rheumatic diseases. A directory of resources contains a list of organizations able to help people with arthritis.

Bibliographic Note

This volume contains documents and excerpts from publications issued by the following government agencies: Agency for Healthcare Research and Quality (AHRQ); Centers for Disease Control and Prevention (CDC); Genetic and Rare Diseases Information Center (GARD); Genetics Home Reference (GHR); National Center for Complementary and Integrative Health (NCCIH); National Heart, Lung, and Blood Institute (NHLBI); National Heart, Lung, and Blood Institute (NHLBI); National Institute of Allergy and Infectious Diseases (NIAID); National Institute of Arthritis and Musculoskeletal and Skin Diseases (NIAMS); National Institute of Diabetes and Digestive and Kidney Diseases (NIDDK); National Institute of Mental Health (NIMH); National Institute of Neurological Disorders and Stroke (NINDS); National Institute on Aging (NIA); National Institutes of Health (NIH); *NIH News in Health*; Office of Dietary Supplements (ODS); Office on Women's Health (OWH); U.S. Department of Agriculture (USDA); and U.S. Food and Drug Administration (FDA).

It may also contain original material produced by Omnigraphics and reviewed by medical consultants.

About the Health Reference Series

The *Health Reference Series* is designed to provide basic medical information for patients, families, caregivers, and the general public. Each volume takes a particular topic and provides comprehensive coverage. This is especially important for people who may be dealing with a newly diagnosed disease or a chronic disorder in themselves or in a family member. People looking for preventive guidance, information about disease warning signs, medical statistics, and risk factors for health problems will also find answers to their questions in the *Health Reference Series*. The *Series*, however, is not intended to serve as a tool for diagnosing illness, in prescribing treatments, or as a substitute for the physician/patient relationship. All people concerned about medical symptoms or the possibility of disease are encouraged to seek professional care from an appropriate healthcare provider.

A Note about Spelling and Style

Health Reference Series editors use *Stedman's Medical Dictionary* as an authority for questions related to the spelling of medical terms and the *Chicago Manual of Style* for questions related to grammatical structures, punctuation, and other editorial concerns. Consistent adherence is not always possible, however, because the individual volumes within the *Series* include many documents from a wide variety of different producers, and the editor's primary goal is to present material from each source as accurately as is possible. This sometimes means that information in different chapters or sections may follow other guidelines and alternate spelling authorities. For example, occasionally a copyright holder may require that eponymous terms be shown in possessive forms (Crohn's disease vs. Crohn disease) or that British spelling norms be retained (leukaemia vs. leukemia).

Medical Review

Omnigraphics contracts with a team of qualified, senior medical professionals who serve as medical consultants for the *Health Reference Series*. As necessary, medical consultants review reprinted and originally written material for currency and accuracy. Citations including the phrase, "Reviewed (month, year)" indicate material reviewed by this team. Medical consultation services are provided to the *Health Reference Series* editors by:

Dr. Vijayalakshmi, MBBS, DGO, MD
Dr. Senthil Selvan, MBBS, DCH, MD
Dr. K. Sivanandham, MBBS, DCH, MS (Research), PhD

Our Advisory Board

We would like to thank the following board members for providing initial guidance on the development of this series:

- Dr. Lynda Baker, Associate Professor of Library and Information Science, Wayne State University, Detroit, MI

- Nancy Bulgarelli, William Beaumont Hospital Library, Royal Oak, MI

- Karen Imarisio, Bloomfield Township Public Library, Bloomfield Township, MI

- Karen Morgan, Mardigian Library, University of Michigan-Dearborn, Dearborn, MI

- Rosemary Orlando, St. Clair Shores Public Library, St. Clair Shores, MI

Health Reference Series *Update Policy*

The inaugural book in the *Health Reference Series* was the first edition of *Cancer Sourcebook* published in 1989. Since then, the *Series* has been enthusiastically received by librarians and in the medical community. In order to maintain the standard of providing high-quality health information for the layperson the editorial staff at Omnigraphics felt it was necessary to implement a policy of updating volumes when warranted.

Medical researchers have been making tremendous strides, and it is the purpose of the *Health Reference Series* to stay current with the most recent advances. Each decision to update a volume is made on an individual basis. Some of the considerations include how much new information is available and the feedback we receive from people who use the books. If there is a topic you would like to see added to the update list, or an area of medical concern you feel has not been adequately addressed, please write to:

Managing Editor
Health Reference Series
Omnigraphics
615 Griswold, Ste. 901
Detroit, MI 48226

Part One

Introduction to Arthritis

Chapter 1

Understanding the Bones, Muscles, and Joints

Chapter Contents

Section 1.1—What Are Bones, Muscles, and Joints?................... 4

Section 1.2—Importance of Healthy Bones 9

Section 1.1

What Are Bones, Muscles, and Joints?

This section contains text excerpted from the following sources: Text
under the heading "What to Know about Your Bones" is excerpted
from "Healthy Bones Matter," National Institute of Arthritis and
Musculoskeletal and Skin Diseases (NIAMS), April 12, 2017;
Text under the heading "Basic Facts about Muscles" is excerpted
from "Healthy Muscles Matter," National Institute of Arthritis
and Musculoskeletal and Skin Diseases (NIAMS), March 9, 2017;
Text under the heading "What Exactly Is a Joint?" is excerpted
from "Healthy Joints Matter," National Institute of Arthritis and
Musculoskeletal and Skin Diseases (NIAMS), April 12, 2017.

What to Know about Your Bones

Bones support your body and allow you to move. They protect your
brain, heart, and other organs from injury.

Bone is a living, growing tissue. It is made mostly of two materials: collagen, a protein that provides a soft framework, and calcium,
a mineral that adds strength and hardness. This combination makes
bone strong and flexible enough to hold up under stress.

Bone releases calcium and other minerals into the body when you
need them for other uses.

How Bones Grow

Think of your bones as a "bank" where you "deposit" and "withdraw"
bone tissue. During your childhood and teenage years, new bone is
added (or deposited) to the skeleton faster than old bone is removed
(or withdrawn). As a result, your bones become larger, heavier, and
denser.

For most people, bone formation continues at a faster pace than
removal until sometime after age 20. After age 30, bone withdrawals
can begin to go faster than deposits. If your bone deposits don't keep
up with withdrawals, you can get osteoporosis when you get older.
Osteoporosis is a disease in which the bones become weak and more
likely to break (fracture). People with osteoporosis most often break
bones in the hip, spine, and wrist.

What Can Go Wrong?

What You Need to Do Now—and Why

If you want to be able to make "deposits" of bone tissue and reach your greatest possible peak bone mass, you need to get enough calcium, vitamin D, and physical activity—important factors in building bone. If you want the strongest bones possible, the best time to build up your "account" is right now and especially during your childhood and teenage years.

Why Should I Care about This Now?

You may know some older people who worry about their bones getting weak. You might even know someone who has trouble getting around because they have broken a bone because of osteoporosis. You might think that this is something that only older people need to worry about.

But you can take action right now to help make sure that as you get older your bones are as healthy as they can be. Eating a balanced diet that includes calcium and vitamin D, getting plenty of physical activity, and having good health habits now can help keep your bones healthy for your whole life.

Basic Facts about Muscles

Did you know you have more than 600 muscles in your body? These muscles help you move, lift things, pump blood through your body, and even help you breathe.

When you think about your muscles, you probably think most about the ones you can control. These are your voluntary muscles, which means you can control their movements. They are also called skeletal muscles, because they attach to your bones and work together with your bones to help you walk, run, pick up things, play an instrument, throw a baseball, kick a soccer ball, push a lawnmower, or ride a bicycle. The muscles of your mouth and throat even help you talk!

Keeping your muscles healthy will help you to be able to walk, run, jump, lift things, play sports, and do all the other things you love to do. Exercising, getting enough rest, and eating a balanced diet will help to keep your muscles healthy for life.

Why Healthy Muscles Matter to You

Healthy muscles let you move freely and keep your body strong. They help you to enjoy playing sports, dancing, walking the dog, swimming, and other fun activities. And they help you do those other (not so fun) things that you have to do, like making the bed, vacuuming the carpet, or mowing the lawn.

Strong muscles also help to keep your joints in good shape. If the muscles around your knee, for example, get weak, you may be more likely to injure that knee. Strong muscles also help you keep your balance, so you are less likely to slip or fall.

And remember—the activities that make your skeletal muscles strong will also help to keep your heart muscle strong!

Different Kinds of Muscles Have Different Jobs

Skeletal muscles are connected to your bones by tough cords of tissue called tendons. As the muscle contracts, it pulls on the tendon, which moves the bone. Bones are connected to other bones by ligaments, which are like tendons and help hold your skeleton together.

Smooth muscles are also called involuntary muscles since you have no control over them. Smooth muscles work in your digestive system to move food along and push waste out of your body. They also help keep your eyes focused without your having to think about it.

Cardiac muscle. Did you know your heart is also a muscle? It is a specialized type of involuntary muscle. It pumps blood through your body, changing its speed to keep up with the demands you put on it. It pumps more slowly when you're sitting or lying down, and faster when you're running or playing sports and your skeletal muscles need more blood to help them do their work.

What Can Go Wrong?

Injuries

Almost everyone has had sore muscles after exercising or working too much. Some soreness can be a normal part of a healthy exercise. But, in other cases, muscles can become strained. Muscle strain can be mild (the muscle has just been stretched too much) to severe (the muscle actually tears). Maybe you lifted something that was too heavy and the muscles in your arms were stretched too far. Lifting heavy things in the wrong way can also strain the muscles in your back. This can be very painful and can even cause an injury that will last a long time and make it hard to do everyday things.

The tendons that connect the muscles to the bones can also be strained if they are pulled or stretched too much. If ligaments (remember, they connect bones to bones) are stretched or pulled too much, the injury is called a sprain. Most people are familiar with the pain of a sprained ankle.

Contact sports like soccer, football, hockey, and wrestling can often cause strains. Sports in which you grip something (like gymnastics or tennis) can lead to strains in your hand or forearm.

What Exactly Is a Joint?

A joint is where two or more bones are joined together. Joints can be rigid, like the joints between the bones in your skull, or movable, like knees, hips, and shoulders. Many joints have cartilage on the ends of the bones where they come together. Healthy cartilage helps you move by allowing bones to glide over one another. It also protects bones by preventing them from rubbing against each other.

Keeping your joints healthy will allow you to run, walk, jump, play sports, and do the other things you like to do. Physical activity, a balanced diet, avoiding injuries, and getting plenty of sleep will help you stay healthy and keep your joints healthy too.

What Can Go Wrong?

Some people get arthritis. The term arthritis is often used to refer to any disorder that affects the joints. Although you might think arthritis affects only older people, it can affect young people, too. There are many different forms of arthritis:

- **Osteoarthritis (OA)** is the most common type of arthritis and is seen especially among older people. In osteoarthritis, the surface cartilage in the joints breaks down and wears away, allowing the bones to rub together. This causes pain, swelling, and loss of motion in the joint. Sometimes, it can be triggered by an injury to a joint, such as a knee injury that damages the cartilage.

- **Rheumatoid arthritis (RA)** is known as an autoimmune disease, because the immune system attacks the tissues of the joints as if they were disease-causing germs. This results in pain, swelling, stiffness, and loss of function in the joints. People with rheumatoid arthritis may also feel tired and sick, and they sometimes get fevers. It can cause permanent damage to the joints and sometimes affects the heart, lungs, or other organs.

- **Gout** is a form of arthritis that is caused by a buildup of uric acid crystals in the joints, most commonly in the big toe. It can be extremely painful. There are several effective treatments for gout that can reduce disability and pain.

- **Juvenile arthritis (JA)** is a term often used to describe arthritis in children. Children can develop almost all types of arthritis that affect adults, but the most common type that affects children is juvenile idiopathic arthritis.

- **Other forms of arthritis** may be associated with diseases like lupus, fibromyalgia, psoriasis, or certain infections. In addition, other diseases might affect the bones or muscles around a joint, causing problems in that joint.

How Do I Keep My Joints More Healthy?

Physical Activity

Being physically active is one of the most important things you can do to keep your joints healthy. Regular activity helps keep the muscles around your joints strong and working the way they should. Even people who already have arthritis can benefit from regular physical activity, which will help reduce disability and keep the joints working well. Children and teenagers should get 60 minutes or more of physical activity each day. Adults should get at least 30 minutes of physical activity each day. When exercising or playing sports, be sure to wear the proper protective equipment to avoid injuring your joints. Remember that injuries to your knee early in life can lead to osteoarthritis, later on, so be sure to wear protective pads and shoes that fit well. It's also important to warm up and stretch before exercise. If you have any concerns about your health, talk to your doctor or a physical therapist to find out what kinds of activities are right for you.

Eat a Healthy Diet

Physical activity, along with a balanced diet, will help you manage your weight. Excess weight puts stress on your joints, especially in your knees, hips, and feet. Avoiding excess weight can help reduce the wear and tear that may lead to arthritis later in life.

Speaking of diet, no specific diet will prevent or cure arthritis. However, eating a balanced diet will help manage your weight and provide a variety of nutrients for overall health. A balanced diet:

- Emphasizes fruits, vegetables, whole grains, and fat-free or low-fat dairy products like milk, cheese, and yogurt

- Includes protein from lean meats, poultry, seafood, beans, eggs, and nuts

- Is low in solid fats, saturated fats, cholesterol, salt (sodium), added sugars, and refined grains

- Is as low as possible in trans fats

- Balances calories taken in through food with calories burned in physical activity to help maintain a healthy weight

What about Dietary Supplements

Many people take dietary supplements such as glucosamine and chondroitin for joint health. Current research shows that these supplements may not have much benefit for people with osteoarthritis. However, they do seem to reduce moderate or severe osteoarthritis pain in some, but not all, people. There is no evidence that they can prevent any form of arthritis.

Scientists are also researching the effects of other dietary supplements, such as green tea and various vitamins, to see if they can keep your joints healthy. Check with your doctor before taking dietary supplements.

Section 1.2

Importance of Healthy Bones

This section includes text excerpted from "The Surgeon General's Report on Bone Health and Osteoporosis: What It Means to You," National Institutes of Health (NIH), February 2017.

Strong bones begin in childhood. With good habits and medical attention when needed, we can have strong bones throughout our lives. People who have weak bones are at higher risk for fractures.

You can improve your bone health by getting enough calcium, vitamin D, and physical activity. If you have osteoporosis or another bone disease, your doctor can detect and treat it. This can help prevent painful fractures.

Broken bones are very painful at any age. For older people, weak bones can be deadly. 1 in 5 people with a hip fracture dies within a year of their injury. One in three adults who lived independently before their hip fracture remains in a nursing home for at least a year after their injury. Many others become isolated, depressed, or frightened to leave home because they fear they will fall.

Why Healthy Bones Are Important to You

Strong bones support us and allow us to move. They protect our heart, lungs, and brain from injury. Our bones are also a storehouse for vital minerals we need to live. Weak bones break easily, causing terrible pain. You might lose your ability to stand or walk. And as bones weaken, you might lose height.

Silently and without warning, bones may begin to weaken early in life if you do not have a healthy diet and the right kinds of physical activity. Many people already have weak bones and don't know it. Others are making choices that will weaken their bones later.

There are several kinds of bone disease. The most common is osteoporosis. In this disease, bones lose minerals like calcium. They become fragile and break easily. With osteoporosis, your body's frame becomes like the frame of a house damaged by termites. Termites weaken your house like osteoporosis weakens your bones. If you have severe fractures from osteoporosis, you risk never walking again. Weak bones can break easily. This can be fatal.

Fragile bones are not painful at first. Unfortunately, most people don't realize they have weakened bones until one breaks. By that time, it is hard to make your bones strong again.

The good news is that you are never too old or too young to improve your bone health. There are many things you can do to keep bones strong and prevent fractures. At all ages, a diet with enough calcium and vitamin D, together with weight-bearing physical activity every day, can prevent problems later. You can work with your doctor to check out warning signs or risk factors. When you are older, you can have your bones tested and take medicine to strengthen them.

Don't Risk Your Bones

Many things weaken bones. Some are outside your control. If you have a family member who has bone problems, you could also be at risk. Some medical conditions can also make you prone to bone disease.

There are some things you can control:

- **Get enough calcium and vitamin D** in your diet at every age
- **Be physically active**
- **Reduce hazards** in your home that could increase your risk of falling and breaking bones
- **Talk with your doctor about medicines** you are taking that could weaken bones, like medicine for thyroid problems or arthritis. Also talk about ways to take medicines that are safe for bones. Discuss ways to protect bones while treating other problems.
- **Maintain a healthy weight:** Being underweight raises the risk of fracture and bone loss
- **Don't smoke.** Smoking can reduce bone mass and increase your risk for a broken bone
- **Limit alcohol use.** Heavy alcohol use reduces bone mass and increases your risk for broken bones

Bones Are Not What You Think They Are

When you think of bones, you might imagine a hard, brittle skeleton. In reality, your bones are living organs. They are alive with cells and flowing body fluids. Bones are constantly renewed and grow stronger with a good diet and physical activity.

The amount of calcium that makes up your bones is the measure of how strong they are. But your muscles and nerves must also have calcium and phosphorus to work. If these are in short supply from foods you eat, your body simply takes them from your bones.

Each day calcium is deposited and withdrawn from your bones. If you don't get enough calcium, you could be withdrawing more than you're depositing. As mentioned previously, our bodies build up calcium in our bones efficiently until we are about 30 years old. Then our bodies stop adding new bone. But healthy habits can help us keep the bone we have.

When Bones Break

There is some natural bone loss as women and men age. As we grow older, bones can break or weaken if we don't take steps to keep them strong. The most common breaks in weak bones are in the wrist, spine, and hip.

Broken bones in your spine are painful and very slow to heal. People with weak bones in their spine gradually lose height and their posture becomes hunched over. Over time a bent spine can make it hard to walk or even sit up.

Broken hips are a very serious problem as we age. They greatly increase the risk of death, especially during the year after they break. People who break a hip might not recover for months or even years. Because they often cannot care for themselves, they are more likely to have to live in a nursing home.

Tips for Keeping Bones Strong

- Calcium is found in foods like milk, leafy green vegetables, and soybeans. Enjoy snacks of yogurt and cheese to increase your calcium. You can also take calcium supplements or eat food specially fortified with calcium.

- Your body needs vitamin D to absorb calcium. Make sure you get enough vitamin D from your diet, sunshine, or supplements.

- Even simple activities like walking and stair climbing will strengthen your bones. Get at least 30 minutes of physical activity a day, even if it's only 10 minutes at a time. (Children should get at least 60 minutes a day.)

You Could Be at Risk

Too many of us assume we are not at risk for bone loss or fractures. We believe that if we haven't had any signs of bone damage, then our bones are strong. Because there are no obvious warning signs, even doctors often miss signs of the problem. Most of us have our blood pressure and cholesterol checked for heart health. Testing bone density is an important way to check for bone health.

The risk of osteoporosis is highest among women. It is also higher for whites and Asians than other groups. However, it's important to remember that it is a real risk for older men and women of all backgrounds.

Here are some clues that you are at risk:

- Your older relatives have had fractures

- You have had illnesses or have been on medications that might weaken bones

- You are underweight

That's why it is important to know the risks for poor bone health at all ages. There are many "red flags" that are signs that you are at risk for weak bones. In addition, your calcium and vitamin D intake, level of physical activity, and medications should all be evaluated.

Why Being Active Makes Your Bones Strong

When you jump, run, or lift a weight, it puts stress on your bones. This sends a signal to your body that your bones need to be made stronger. New cells are added to strengthen your bones. If you are right-handed, the bones in your right arm are slightly larger and stronger from the extra use.

Bone Up on Your Diet

Calcium

To keep your bones strong, eat foods rich in calcium. Some people have trouble digesting the lactose found in milk and other dairy foods, including cheese and yogurt. Most supermarkets sell lactose-reduced dairy foods. Many nondairy foods are also calcium rich.

Table 1.1. Calcium-Rich Foods

Food	Calcium (mg)
Fortified oatmeal, 1 packet	350
Sardines, canned in oil, with edible bones, 3 oz.	324
Cheddar cheese, 1½ oz. shredded	306
Milk, nonfat, 1 cup	302
Milkshake, 1 cup	300
Yogurt, plain, low-fat, 1 cup	300
Soybeans, cooked, 1 cup	261
Tofu, firm, with calcium, ½ cup	204
Orange juice, fortified with calcium, 6 oz.	200–260 (varies)
Salmon, canned, with edible bones, 3 oz.	181
Pudding, instant (chocolate, banana, etc.) made with 2 percent milk, ½ cup	153
Baked beans, 1 cup	142
Cottage cheese, 1 percent milk fat, 1 cup	138

Table 1.1. Continued

Food	Calcium (mg)
Spaghetti or lasagna, 1 cup	125
Frozen yogurt, vanilla, soft-serve, ½ cup	103
Ready-to-eat cereal, fortified with calcium, 1 cup	100–1000 (varies)
Cheese pizza, 1 slice	100
Fortified waffles (2)	100
Turnip greens, boiled, ½ cup	99
Broccoli, raw, 1 cup	90
Ice cream, vanilla, ½ cup	85
Soy or rice milk, fortified with calcium, 1 cup	80–500 (varies)

Vitamin D

Vitamin D helps your body absorb calcium. As you grow older, your need for vitamin D goes up. Vitamin D is made by your skin when you are in the sun. For many, especially seniors, getting enough vitamin D from sunlight is not practical. Almost all milk and some other foods are fortified with vitamin D. If you are not getting enough calcium and vitamin D in your diet, supplements can be bone savers.

Table 1.2. Need of Calcium and Vitamin D

Calcium Requirement	Calcium (mg)	Vitamin D (IU)
Infants 0–6 months	200	400
Infants 6–12 months	260	400
1–3 years	700	600
4–8 years	1,000	600
9–13 years	1,300	600
14–18 years	1,300	600
19–30 years	1,000	600
31–50 years	1,000	600
51-70-year-old males	1,000	600
51-70-year-old females	1,200	600
>70 years	1,200	800
14–18 years, pregnant/lactating	1,300	600
19–50 years, pregnant/lactating	1,000	600

Protect Your Bones at Every Age

People of all ages need to know what they can do to have strong bones. You are never too old or too young to improve your bone health.

Babies

Bone growth starts before babies are born. Premature and low birth weight infants often need extra calcium, phosphorus, and protein to help them catch up on the nutrients they need for strong bones. Breastfed babies get the calcium and nutrients they need for good bone health from their mothers. That's why mothers who breastfeed need extra vitamin D. Most baby formula contains calcium and vitamin D.

What If Your Toddler Doesn't Like to Drink Milk?

- Include some low-fat cheese chunks or yogurt for snacks
- Make a cheesy sauce for vegetables or for a dip
- Offer strawberry or chocolate milk as an afternoon treat

Children

Good bone health starts early in life with good habits. While children and young adults rarely get bone diseases, kids can develop habits that endanger their health and bones. Parents can help by encouraging kids to eat healthful food and get at least an hour of physical activity every day. Jumping rope, running, and sports are fun activities that are great for building strong bones. Children need the amount of calcium equal to 3 servings of low-fat milk each day. If your child doesn't drink enough milk, try low-fat cheese, yogurt, or other foods that are high in calcium. If your child is allergic to milk or lactose intolerant, talk to your pediatrician about milk substitutes.

Teens

Teens are especially at risk for not developing strong bones because their bones are growing so rapidly. Boys and girls from ages 9–18 need 1,300 milligrams of calcium each day, more than any other age group. Parents can help teens by making sure they eat 4 servings of calcium-rich and vitamin D fortified foods a day. At least 1 hour a day of physical activities—like running, skateboarding, sports, and dance—is also critical. But take note: extreme physical exercise, when combined with under eating, can weaken teens' bones. In young women, this situation can lead to a damaging lack of menstrual periods. Teens who miss adding bone to their skeletons during these critical years never make it up.

Adults

Adulthood is a time when we need to look carefully at our bone health. As adults, we need 1,000–1,200 milligrams of calcium, depending on our age, and at least 30 minutes of moderate physical activity every day. Activity that puts some stress on your bones is very important.

Adults: Keep Your Bones Strong with Physical Activity

- Physical activity at least 30 minutes every day
- Strength training 2–3 times a week
- Balance training once a week

Many women over age 50 are at risk for bone disease, but few know it. At menopause, which usually happens in women over age 50, a woman's hormone production drops sharply. Because hormones help protect bones, menopause can lead to bone loss. Hormone therapy was widely used to prevent this loss, but now it is known to increase other risks. Your doctor can help advise you on protecting bone health around menopause.

Seniors

Seniors can take steps to help prevent bone problems. Physical activity and diet are vital to bone health in older adults. Calcium, together with vitamin D, helps reduce bone loss. Activities that put stress on bones keep them strong. Find time for activities like walking, dancing, and gardening. Strengthening your body helps prevent falls. Protecting yourself against falls is key to avoiding a broken hip or wrist. All women over age 65 should have a bone density test.

Seniors should also know that studies have concluded that anyone over age 50 should increase his or her vitamin D intake to 600 International Units (IU) per day. After age 70, 800 IU per day is needed.

Falls Break Bones

You Can Prevent Most Falls

Falls are not just the result of getting older. But as you age, falls become more dangerous. Most falls can be prevented. By changing some of the things listed here, you can lower the chances of falling for you or someone you love.

1. **Begin a regular exercise program.** Exercise is one of the most important ways to reduce your chances of falling. It makes you stronger and helps you feel better. Exercises that improve balance and coordination, like dancing, and tai chi, are the most helpful. Consider joining an organized program at your local community center or gym.

2. **Make your home safer.**

   - Remove things you can trip over from stairs and places where you walk

   - Remove all small rugs

   - Don't use step stools. Keep items you need within easy reach.

   - Have grab bars put in next to your toilet and in the bathtub or shower

   - Use nonslip mats in the bathtub and shower

   - Use brighter light bulbs in your home

   - Add handrails and light in all staircases

   - Wear shoes that give good support and have nonslip soles

3. **Ask a healthcare professional to review your medicines.** Ask your doctor, nurse, pharmacist, or other healthcare professional to review all the medicines you are taking.

   Make sure to mention over-the-counter (OTC) medicine, such as cold medicine. As you get older, the way some medicines work in your body can change. Some medicines, or combinations of medicines, can make you drowsy or light-headed, which can lead to a fall.

4. **Have your vision checked.** Poor vision increases your risk of falling. You could be wearing the wrong glasses or have a condition such as glaucoma or cataracts that limits your vision.

Live Well, Live Strong, Live Long

The average American eats too little calcium. And nearly half of us do not get enough physical activity to strengthen our bones.

The same healthy lifestyle that strengthens your bones strengthens your whole body. You might not hear as much about bone health as other health concerns. But healthy habits are good for all your organs, including your bones.

- **Be physically active every day**—at least 60 minutes for children, 30 minutes for adults. Do strength building and weight-bearing activities to build strong bones.

- **Eat a healthy diet.** Educate yourself on proper nutrition. Be aware that certain foods are naturally rich in calcium and vitamin D. Get the recommended amounts of calcium and vitamin D daily.

- **Reduce your risks of falling.** Check your home for loose rugs, poor lighting, etc. Take classes that increase balance and strength—like tai chi or yoga. Make stretching a part of your workout.

Even people who know better don't always do what's good for their bones. Make yourself an exception. Be aware of your risks and work to reduce them. Get help from your family and friends and your doctor, nurse, pharmacist, or other healthcare professional. Building healthy bones begins at birth and lasts your whole life.

Your Doctor Can Help Protect Your Bones

Talk to your doctor about bone health. Together you can evaluate your risks. Some things to discuss include your current health, your diet and physical activity levels, and your family background.

Your doctor can look at your age, weight, height, and medical history. From that he or she can determine if you need a bone density test. Broken bones are a "red flag" for your doctor. If you break a bone after the age of 50, talk to your doctor about measuring your bone density. Even if you broke a bone in an accident, you might have weak bones. It is worth checking.

Your doctor might recommend a medical test called a bone mineral density (BMD) test. Bone density tests use X-rays or sound waves to measure how strong your bones are. These tests are quick (5–10 minutes), safe, and painless. They will give you and your doctor an idea of how healthy your bones are. All women over age 65 should have a bone density test. Women who are younger than age 65 and at high risk for fractures should also have a bone density test.

Your doctor might also want to do a blood test to check for a vitamin D deficiency or abnormal calcium levels.

If your doctor finds that your bones are becoming weaker, there are things you can do to make them stronger. You can be more physically active, change your diet, and take calcium and vitamin D supplements. If your bones are already weak, there are medicines that stop bone loss. They can even build new bone and make it less likely that you will suffer a broken bone.

Your doctor might suggest medications to help you build stronger bones. To reduce the chance that you might fall, have your vision checked. When you speak to your doctor, be prepared with a list of questions and concerns.

See Your Doctor

Although osteoporosis is the most common disease that harms bones, certain other conditions can also be harmful. Your doctor can help you learn if you are at risk and can help you treat these conditions.

- **Rickets and osteomalacia.** Too little vitamin D causes these diseases in children and adults. They can lead to bone deformities and fractures.

- **Kidney disease.** Renal osteodystrophy (ROD) can cause fractures.

- **Paget disease of bone.** Bones become deformed and weak, which can be caused by genetic and environmental factors.

- **Genetic abnormalities.** Disorders like osteogenesis imperfecta (OI) cause bones to grow abnormally and break easily.

- **Endocrine disorders.** Overactive glands can cause bone disease.

What to Discuss with Your Doctor

Talk with your doctor, nurse, or other healthcare professional about your bone health. Use this checklist to start your discussion.

- Ask to check your risk for bone disease

- Discuss your need for a bone density test

- Talk about any fall, even ones in which you were not hurt. Tell him or her about any broken bones you've had.

- If you have fallen, ask about the need for a full evaluation. Tests include vision, balance, walking, muscle strength, heart function, and blood pressure.

- Go over all the medications you are taking (including OTC ones). Do this at least once a year. This helps avoid dangerous drug interactions and taking higher doses of drugs than you need, which can lead to falls.

- Ask if your doctor checks vision. Annual vision checks can help eliminate bone-breaking falls.

- Know your calcium and vitamin D intake. Report your totals to your doctor.

- If you would like to try a new physical activity, ask about the best choices for you

Are You at Risk for Weak Bones?

Check any of these that apply to you.

- I'm older than 65
- I've broken a bone after age 50
- My close relative has osteoporosis or has broken a bone
- My health is "fair" or "poor"
- I smoke
- I am underweight for my height
- I started menopause before age 45
- I've never gotten enough calcium
- I have more than two drinks of alcohol several times a week
- I have poor vision, even with glasses
- I sometimes fall
- I'm not active

I have one of these medical conditions:

- Hyperthyroidism

- Chronic lung disease (CLD)
- Cancer
- Inflammatory bowel disease (IBD)
- Chronic hepatic or renal disease
- Hyperparathyroidism
- Vitamin D deficiency
- Cushing disease
- Multiple sclerosis (MS)
- Rheumatoid arthritis (RA)

I take one of these medicines:

- Oral glucocorticoids (steroids)
- Cancer treatments (radiation, chemotherapy)
- Thyroid medicine
- Antiepileptic medications
- Gonadal hormone suppression
- Immunosuppressive agents

If you have any of these "red flags," you could be at high risk for weak bones. Talk to your doctor, nurse, pharmacist, or other healthcare professional.

Chapter 2

Overview of Arthritis and Rheumatic Diseases

The term "arthritis" is often used to refer to any disorder that affects the joints. These disorders fall within the broader category of rheumatic diseases. There are more than 100 rheumatic diseases that together affect millions of Americans.

"Arthritis" literally means joint inflammation, which is a symptom of the disease.

Symptoms of rheumatic diseases include inflammation (redness or heat, swelling, pain) and loss of function of one or more of the body's support structures. They especially affect joints, tendons, ligaments, bones, and muscles. Some rheumatic diseases can also involve internal organs.

Who Gets Arthritis and Rheumatic Diseases

Rheumatic diseases affect millions of people of all races and ages in the United States. Some rheumatic diseases are more common among certain populations. For example:

- Rheumatoid arthritis (RA), scleroderma, fibromyalgia, and lupus mostly affect women

This chapter includes text excerpted from "Arthritis and Rheumatic Diseases," National Institute of Arthritis and Musculoskeletal and Skin Diseases (NIAMS), April 14, 2017.

- The spondyloarthropathies and gout are more common in men. However, after menopause, the incidence of gout in women begins to rise.

- Lupus is more common and more severe in African Americans and Hispanics than Caucasians

Types of Arthritis and Rheumatic Diseases

There are numerous types of arthritis and other rheumatic diseases, including:

- **Osteoarthritis (OA)** is the most common type of arthritis, damages both the cartilage (the tissue that cushions the ends of bones within the joint) and the underlying bone. OA can cause joint pain and stiffness. Disability results most often when the disease affects the spine, knees, and hips.

- **RA** is a less common type of arthritis that occurs when the immune system attacks the lining of the joint (synovium). This produces pain, swelling, and loss of joint function. The most commonly affected joints are those in the hands and feet.

- **Gout** is a type of arthritis caused by needle-like crystals of uric acid that gather in the joints, usually beginning in the big toe. Symptoms may come and go and include inflammation, swelling, and pain in the affected joint(s).

- **Infectious arthritis** is caused by infectious agents such as bacteria or viruses. Parvovirus arthritis and gonococcal arthritis are examples of infectious arthritis, as is arthritis that occurs with Lyme disease, a bacterial infection caused by the bite of infected ticks.

- **Juvenile idiopathic arthritis (JIA)** is the most common form of arthritis in childhood. Symptoms include pain, stiffness, swelling, and loss of joint function. It may be associated with rashes or fevers and may affect various parts of the body.

- **Spondyloarthropathies** is a group of rheumatic diseases that usually affect the spine.

- **Ankylosing spondylitis** may also affect the hips, shoulders, and knees.

- **Reactive arthritis** is caused by infection of the lower urinary tract, bowel, or other organ. It is commonly associated with eye problems, skin rashes, and mouth sores.

- **Psoriatic arthritis** is a form of arthritis that occurs in some patients with the skin disorder psoriasis. Psoriatic arthritis often affects the joints at the ends of the fingers and toes and is accompanied by changes in the fingernails and toenails. Back pain may occur if the spine is involved.

- **Bursitis** occurs due to inflammation of the bursae (small, fluid-filled sacs that help reduce friction within the joint). Symptoms include pain and tenderness. Movement of nearby joints may also be affected.

- **Fibromyalgia** symptoms include widespread muscle pain and tender points—areas on the body that are painful when pushed. Many people also experience fatigue and sleep disturbances.

- **Polymyalgia rheumatica** involves tendons, muscles, ligaments, and tissues around the joint. Symptoms include pain, aching, and morning stiffness in the shoulders, hips, neck, and lower back. It is sometimes the first sign of giant cell arteritis, a disease of the arteries characterized by headaches, inflammation, weakness, weight loss, and fever.

- **Polymyositis** causes inflammation and weakness in the muscles. The disease may affect the whole body and cause disability.

- **Scleroderma** is also known as systemic sclerosis. The disease is caused by excessive production of collagen (a fiber-like protein), leading to thickening of and damage to the skin, blood vessels, joints, and sometimes internal organs such as the lungs and kidneys.

- **Systemic lupus erythematosus** is also known as lupus or SLE. This disease is caused when the immune system attacks the body's own healthy cells, resulting in inflammation of and damage to the joints, skin, kidneys, heart, lungs, blood vessels, and brain.

- **Tendonitis** is the inflammation of tendons (tough cords of tissue that connect muscle to bone). This is caused by overuse, injury, or a rheumatic condition and may restrict movement of nearby joints.

Symptoms of Arthritis and Rheumatic Diseases

Different types of arthritis and rheumatic diseases have different signs and symptoms. In general, people who have arthritis feel pain and stiffness in one or more joints. There may also be tenderness, warmth, redness in a joint, and/or difficulty using or moving a joint normally.

Causes of Arthritis and Rheumatic Diseases

There are probably many genes that make people more likely to have rheumatic diseases. Some genes have been identified in certain diseases, such as rheumatoid arthritis, juvenile arthritis, and lupus. People with osteoarthritis may have inherited cartilage weakness.

If you have the disease gene, something in your environment may trigger the disease. For example, scientists have found a connection between Epstein-Barr virus and lupus. In addition, repeated joint injury may lead to osteoarthritis.

Diagnosis of Arthritis and Rheumatic Diseases

To diagnose you with arthritis or another rheumatic disease, your doctor may:

- Ask you about your medical history
- Give you a physical exam
- Take samples of blood, urine, or synovial fluid (lubricating fluid in the joint) for a laboratory test
- Take X-rays

Treatment of Arthritis and Rheumatic Diseases

Although there is no cure for arthritis and rheumatic diseases, medications may slow the course of the disease and prevent further damage to joints or other parts of the body. Exercise and diet changes may also help. Surgery may be recommended in some cases.

Common **medications** include:

- **Pain relievers** that are taken by mouth. Examples include over-the-counter (OTC) acetaminophen or prescription opioid medications such as oxycodone or hydrocodone for severe pain.

- **Creams or ointments** that are rubbed into the skin over sore muscles or joints to relieve pain.

- **Nonsteroidal anti-inflammatory drugs (NSAIDs)** are used to treat pain and inflammation. Ibuprofen and naproxen sodium are available over the counter, whereas other NSAIDs are available by prescription only.

- **Disease-modifying antirheumatic drugs (DMARDs)** slow or stop the immune system from attacking the joints and causing damage.

- **Biologic response modifiers** block specific immune pathways that are involved in the inflammatory process.

- **Janus kinase** inhibitors are a new class of medications that block specific pathways that are involved in the body's immune response.

- **Corticosteroids** are strong inflammation-fighting drugs that are given by mouth, in creams applied to the skin, intravenously, or by injection directly into the affected joint(s).

- **Surgery** may be required to repair damage to a joint after an injury or to restore function or relieve pain in a joint damaged by arthritis. Many types of surgery are performed for arthritis, such as:

  - Outpatient procedures performed arthroscopically (through small incisions over the joints)

  - Total joint replacement, or replacement of a damaged joint with an artificial joint

- **Exercise and diet.** Physical activity can reduce joint pain and stiffness and increase flexibility, muscle strength, and endurance. Although there is not a specific diet that helps arthritis, a well-balanced diet, along with exercise, helps people manage their body weight and stay healthy.

Chapter 3

Statistics on Arthritis in the United States

General Statistics

Prevalence of Arthritis in the United States

- From 2013–2015, an estimated 54.4 million U.S. adults (22.7%) annually had been told by a doctor that they had some form of arthritis, rheumatoid arthritis (RA), gout, lupus, or fibromyalgia.

- The percentage of adults with arthritis varies by state, ranging from 17.2 percent in Hawaii to 33.6 percent in West Virginia in 2015.

- The most common form of arthritis is osteoarthritis (OA). Other common rheumatic conditions include gout, fibromyalgia, and RA.

Projected Prevalence

- By 2040, an estimated 78 million (26%) U.S. adults ages 18 years or older are projected to have doctor-diagnosed arthritis.

This chapter includes text excerpted from "Arthritis—National Statistics," Centers for Disease Control and Prevention (CDC), March 6, 2017.

Prevalence of Arthritis by Age / Race / Gender

- The risk of arthritis increases with age and arthritis is more common among women than men
- From 2013–2015 in the United States:
  - Of persons ages 18–44, 7.1 percent reported doctor-diagnosed arthritis
  - Of persons ages 45–64, 29.3 percent reported doctor-diagnosed arthritis
  - Of persons ages 65 or older, 49.6 percent reported doctor-diagnosed arthritis
  - Twenty-six percent of women and 19.1 percent men reported doctor-diagnosed arthritis
  - 4.4 million Hispanic adults reported doctor-diagnosed arthritis
  - 41.3 million Non-Hispanic Whites reported doctor-diagnosed arthritis
  - 6.1 million Non-Hispanic Blacks reported doctor-diagnosed arthritis
  - 1.5 million Non-Hispanic Asians reported doctor-diagnosed arthritis

Overweight / Obesity and Arthritis

- Adults 18 or older who are overweight or obese report doctor-diagnosed arthritis more often than adults with a lower body mass index (BMI).
- More than 16 percent of under/normal weight adults report doctor-diagnosed arthritis
- Almost 23 percent of overweight and 31 percent of obese U.S. adults report doctor-diagnosed arthritis

Health Disparity Statistics

Health disparities are differences in health outcomes and their causes among different groups of people. Reducing health disparities is a major goal of public health.

White, Non-Hispanic

- Prevalence of doctor-diagnosed arthritis: 22.6 percent
- Prevalence of arthritis-attributable activity limitations among adults with arthritis: 40.1 percent

African American/Black, Non-Hispanic

- Prevalence of arthritis: 22.2 percent
- Prevalence of activity limitations among adults with arthritis: 48.6 percent

Hispanic/Latino

- Prevalence of arthritis: 15.4 percent
- Prevalence of activity limitations among adults with arthritis: 44.3 percent

Asian, Non-Hispanic

- Prevalence of arthritis: 11.8 percent
- Prevalence of activity limitations among adults with arthritis: 37.6 percent

Multi Race, Non-Hispanic

- Prevalence of arthritis: 25.2 percent
- Prevalence of activity limitations among adults with arthritis: 50.5 percent

American Indian/Alaska Native

- Prevalence of arthritis: 24.4 percent
- Prevalence of activity limitations among adults with arthritis: 51.6 percent

Cost Statistics

The Cost of Arthritis in U.S. Adults

Arthritis has a profound economic, personal, and societal impact in the United States. In 2013, the total national arthritis-attributable medical care costs and earnings losses among adults with arthritis were $303.5 billion or 1 percent of the 2013 U.S. Gross Domestic Product (GDP).

Medical Costs

- In 2013, the national arthritis-attributable medical costs were $140 billion.

- That's $2,117 in extra medical costs per adult with arthritis

- Ambulatory care medical care costs accounted for nearly half of arthritis-attributable medical costs

- Medical care costs include prescriptions

Earnings Losses

- Total national arthritis-attributable lost wages were $164 billion in 2013.

- That's $4,040 less pay for an adult with arthritis compared with an adult without arthritis

- The high earnings losses were because of the substantially lower percentage of adults with arthritis working compared with adults without arthritis. This indicates the need for interventions that keep people with arthritis in the workforce.

Cost of OA

OA, the most common type of arthritis, affects more than 30 million adults in the United States. It is also among the most expensive conditions to treat when joint replacement surgery is required. In fact, OA was the second most costly health condition treated at U.S. hospitals in 2013. In that year, it accounted for $16.5 billion, or 4.3 percent, of the combined costs for all hospitalizations.

OA was also the most expensive condition for which privately insured patients were hospitalized, accounting for over $6.2 billion in hospital costs.

Disability and Limitation Statistics

Why Are Disabilities and Limitations Important for People with Arthritis?

Arthritis impacts function and mobility that can result in activity and other limitations, and is a leading cause of work disability among U.S. adults.

National Prevalence of Arthritis and Arthritis-Attributable Limitations

Based on 2013–2015 data from the National Health Interview Survey (NHIS), an estimated:

- 54.4 million (22.7%) of adults 18 years or older have self-reported doctor-diagnosed arthritis

- 23.7 million (43.5%) of adults with arthritis 18 years or older have arthritis-attributable activity limitation

Based on 2010–2012 data from the National Health Interview Survey (NHIS), a projected:

- 78 million (26%) adults aged 18 years or older will have doctor-diagnosed arthritis by the year 2040

- Of those with arthritis, an estimated 44 percent (35 million adults) will report arthritis-attributable activity limitations by the year 2040

Chapter 4

Risk Factors for Arthritis

Chapter Contents

Section 4.1—Modifiable and Nonmodifiable Risk
    Factors for Arthritis... 36
Section 4.2—Genetics as Risk Factor for Arthritis.................... 37

Section 4.1

Modifiable and Nonmodifiable Risk Factors for Arthritis

Text in this section begins with excerpts from
"Arthritis—At a Glance Reports," Centers for Disease
Control and Prevention (CDC), December 27, 2017; Text under the
heading "Risk Factors" is excerpted from "Arthritis—Risk Factor,"
Centers for Disease Control and Prevention (CDC), May 8, 2017.

In the United States, 23 percent of all adults, or over 54 million people, have arthritis. It is a leading cause of work-related disability. The annual direct medical costs are at least 81 billion.

The term arthritis refers to more than 100 diseases and conditions affecting the joints. The most common type of arthritis is osteoarthritis (OA). Other forms of arthritis are gout, lupus, and rheumatoid arthritis (RA).

Symptoms of arthritis are pain, aching, stiffness, and swelling in or around the joints. RA and lupus can affect multiple organs and cause widespread symptoms.

Arthritis commonly occurs with other chronic diseases. About half of U.S. adults with heart disease or diabetes and one-third of people who are obese also have arthritis. Having arthritis and other chronic conditions can reduce the quality of life and make disease management harder.

Risk Factors

Certain factors have been shown to be associated with a greater risk of arthritis. Some of these risk factors are modifiable while others are not.

Nonmodifiable Risk Factors

- **Age:** The risk of developing most types of arthritis increases with age

36

- **Gender:** Most types of arthritis are more common in women; 52 percent of all adults with arthritis are women. Gout is more common in men.

- **Genetic:** Specific genes are associated with a higher risk of certain types of arthritis, such as RA, systemic lupus erythematosus (SLE), and ankylosing spondylitis

Modifiable Risk Factors

- **Overweight and obesity:** Excess weight can contribute to both the onset and progression of knee OA.

- **Joint injuries:** Damage to a joint can contribute to the development of OA in that joint.

- **Infection:** Many microbial agents can infect joints and potentially cause the development of various forms of arthritis.

- **Occupation:** Certain occupations involving repetitive knee bending and squatting are associated with OA of the knee.

Section 4.2

Genetics as Risk Factor for Arthritis

This section contains text excerpted from the following sources: Text under the heading "Juvenile Idiopathic Arthritis (JIA)" is excerpted from "Juvenile Idiopathic Arthritis," Genetics Home Reference (GHR), National Institutes of Health (NIH), February 2015; Text under the heading "Psoriatic Arthritis" is excerpted from "Psoriatic Arthritis," Genetics Home Reference (GHR), National Institutes of Health (NIH), March 6, 2018; Text under the heading "Rheumatoid Arthritis (RA)" is excerpted from "Rheumatoid Arthritis," Genetics Home Reference (GHR), National Institutes of Health (NIH), March 6, 2018.

Juvenile Idiopathic Arthritis (JIA)

Juvenile idiopathic arthritis (JIA) is thought to arise from a combination of genetic and environmental factors. The term "idiopathic" indicates that the specific cause of the disorder is unknown. Its signs and symptoms result from excessive inflammation in and around the joints. Inflammation occurs when the immune system sends signaling molecules and white blood cells to a site of injury or disease to fight microbial invaders and facilitate tissue repair. Normally, the body stops the inflammatory response after healing is complete to prevent damage to its own cells and tissues. In people with JIA, the inflammatory response is prolonged, particularly during movement of the joints. The reasons for this excessive inflammatory response are unclear.

Researchers have identified changes in several genes that may influence the risk of developing JIA. Many of these genes belong to a family of genes that provide instructions for making a group of related proteins called the human leukocyte antigen (HLA) complex. The HLA complex helps the immune system distinguish the body's own proteins from proteins made by foreign invaders (such as viruses and bacteria). Each *HLA gene* has many different normal variations, allowing each person's immune system to react to a wide range of foreign proteins. Certain normal variations of several *HLA genes* seem to affect the risk of developing JIA, and the specific type of the condition that a person may have.

Normal variations in several other genes have also been associated with JIA. Many of these genes are thought to play roles in immune system function. Additional unknown genetic influences and environmental factors, such as infection and other issues that affect immune health, are also likely to influence a person's chances of developing this complex disorder.

Psoriatic Arthritis

The specific cause of psoriatic arthritis is unknown. Its signs and symptoms result from excessive inflammation in and around the joints. Inflammation occurs when the immune system sends signaling molecules and white blood cells to a site of injury or disease to fight microbial invaders and facilitate tissue repair. When this has been accomplished, the body ordinarily stops the inflammatory response to prevent damage to its own cells and tissues. Mechanical stress on the joints, such as occurs in movement, may result in an excessive inflammatory response in people with psoriatic arthritis. The reasons for this excessive inflammatory response are unclear. Researchers have identified changes in several genes that may influence the risk of developing psoriatic arthritis. The most well-studied of these genes belong to a family of genes called the HLA complex. The HLA complex helps the immune system distinguish the body's own proteins from proteins made by foreign invaders (such as viruses and bacteria). Each *HLA gene* has many different normal variations, allowing each person's immune system to react to a wide range of foreign proteins. Variations of several HLA genes seem to affect the risk of developing psoriatic arthritis, as well as the type, severity, and progression of the condition.

Variations in several other genes have also been associated with psoriatic arthritis. Many of these genes are thought to play roles in immune system function. However, variations in these genes probably make only a small contribution to the overall risk of developing psoriatic arthritis. Other genetic and environmental factors are also likely to influence a person's chances of developing this disorder.

Rheumatoid Arthritis (RA)

Rheumatoid arthritis (RA) probably results from a combination of genetic and environmental factors, many of which are unknown.

RA is classified as an autoimmune disorder, one of a large group of conditions that occur when the immune system attacks the body's own tissues and organs. In people with RA, the immune system triggers abnormal inflammation in the membrane that lines the joints (the synovium). When the synovium is inflamed, it causes pain, swelling, and stiffness of the joint. In severe cases, the inflammation also affects the bone, cartilage, and other tissues within the joint, causing more serious damage. Abnormal immune reactions also underlie the features of RA affecting other parts of the body.

Variations in dozens of genes have been studied as risk factors for RA. Most of these genes are known or suspected to be involved in immune system function. The most significant genetic risk factors for RA are variations in *HLA genes*, especially the *HLA-DRB1 gene*. The proteins produced from HLA genes help the immune system distinguish the body's own proteins from proteins made by foreign invaders (such as viruses and bacteria). Changes in other genes appear to have a smaller impact on a person's overall risk of developing the condition.

Other, nongenetic factors are also believed to play a role in RA. These factors may trigger the condition in people who are at risk, although the mechanism is unclear. Potential triggers include changes in sex hormones (particularly in women), occupational exposure to certain kinds of dust or fibers, and viral or bacterial infections. Long-term smoking is a well-established risk factor for developing RA; it is also associated with more severe signs and symptoms in people who have the disease.

Chapter 5

Joints Affected by Arthritis

Chapter Contents

Section 5.1—Arthritis of the Shoulder.. 42

Section 5.2—Arthritis of the Wrist 44

Section 5.3—Arthritis of the Hip 48

Section 5.4—Arthritis of the Knee.. 52

Section 5.5—Arthritis of the Foot and Ankle 56

Section 5.1

Arthritis of the Shoulder

This section contains text excerpted from the following
sources: Text under the heading "Shoulder and Shoulder Pain" is
excerpted from "Shoulder Problems," National Institute of Arthritis
and Musculoskeletal and Skin Diseases (NIAMS), April 30, 2014.
Reviewed April 2018; Text beginning with the heading "What Is
Arthritis of Shoulder?" is excerpted from "Questions and Answers
about Shoulder Problems," National Institute of Arthritis and
Musculoskeletal and Skin Diseases (NIAMS), 2006.
Reviewed April 2018.

Shoulder and Shoulder Pain

The shoulder is a ball-and-socket-type joint that helps the
shoulder:

- Move forward and backward

- Allow the arm to rotate in a circular motion

- Hinge out and up away from the body

Most shoulder problems happen when soft tissues in the joint and
shoulder region breakdown.

To better understand shoulder problems and how they occur,
figure 5.1 describes the bones, ligaments, and tendons that make up
the shoulder.

The bones of the shoulder are held in place by:

- **Muscles,** which help the shoulder move.

- **Tendons,** which are tough cords of tissue that attach the shoulder muscles to bone.

- **Ligaments,** which attach the shoulder bones

Rotator cuff, which is made up of tendons and muscles and holds the
ball at the top of the arm bone in the socket. It also provides mobility
and strength to the shoulder joint.

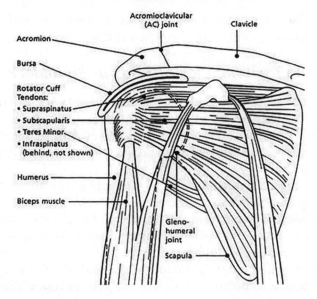

Figure 5.1. *Shoulder Joint*

What Is Arthritis of Shoulder?

Arthritis is a degenerative disease caused by either wear and tear of the cartilage (osteoarthritis (OA)) or an inflammation (rheumatoid arthritis (RA)) of one or more joints. Arthritis not only affects joints, but may also affect supporting structures such as muscles, tendons, and ligaments.

What Are the Signs and Symptoms of Arthritis of Shoulder?

The usual signs of arthritis of the shoulder are pain, particularly over the acromioclavicular joint, and a decrease in shoulder motion.

How Is Arthritis of Shoulder Diagnosed?

A doctor may suspect the patient has arthritis when there is both pain and swelling in the joint. The diagnosis may be confirmed by a physical examination and X-rays. Blood tests may be helpful for diagnosing RA, but other tests may be needed as well. Analysis of synovial fluid from the shoulder joint may be helpful in diagnosing some kinds of arthritis. Although arthroscopy permits direct visualization of damage to cartilage, tendons, and ligaments, and may confirm a diagnosis, it is usually done only if a repair procedure is to be performed.

What Is the Treatment for Arthritis of Shoulder?

Treatment of shoulder arthritis depends in part on the type of arthritis. Osteoarthritis of the shoulder is usually treated with nonsteroidal anti-inflammatory drugs, such as aspirin and ibuprofen. RA may require physical therapy and additional medications such as corticosteroids.

When nonoperative treatment of arthritis of the shoulder fails to relieve pain or improve function, or when severe wear and tear of the joint cause parts to loosen and move out of place, shoulder joint replacement (arthroplasty) may provide better results. In this operation, a surgeon replaces the shoulder joint with an artificial ball for the top of the humerus and a cap (glenoid) for the scapula. Passive shoulder exercises (where someone else moves the arm to rotate the shoulder joint) are started soon after surgery.

Patients begin exercising on their own about 3–6 weeks after surgery. Eventually, stretching and strengthening exercises become a major part of the rehabilitation program. The success of the operation often depends on the condition of rotator cuff muscles prior to surgery and the degree to which the patient follows the exercise program.

Section 5.2

Arthritis of the Wrist

"Arthritis of the Wrist," © 2015 Omnigraphics.
Reviewed April 2018.

Arthritis is a general term used to describe conditions involving inflammation of the joints. Arthritis often affects the joints between the twenty-nine small bones that make up the hand and wrist, and the pain and swelling associated with this condition can make it difficult for people to perform daily activities. Most cases of arthritis of the wrist derive from either osteoarthritis or rheumatoid arthritis. In fact, two-thirds of people with rheumatoid arthritis experience symptoms involving the hand and wrist.

Causes of Arthritis of the Wrist

Osteoarthritis (OA) is a progressive, degenerative condition that destroys the layer of smooth cartilage that covers the ends of healthy bones. When this protective cushion wears away, the bones rub together, causing pain, swelling, and impaired motion of the joint. Osteoarthritis of the wrist can result from normal, accumulated "wear and tear" or from a traumatic injury, such as a wrist sprain. It can also develop from Kienböck disease, a condition characterized by an interruption in blood flow to the lunate bone at the base of the hand.

Rheumatoid arthritis (RA) is a chronic, autoimmune disorder in which the body's immune system attacks the synovial fluid. This fluid plays a vital role in joint health by lubricating joints and nourishing bones and cartilage. Inflammation of the synovial fluid, known as synovitis, results in pain, swelling, and stiffness in the joints. As the disease progresses, the inflammation can stretch the supporting structures of the joints, including muscles, ligaments, and tendons. As a result, the joints become increasingly deformed and unstable, and eventually the underlying cartilage and bone wears away. Rheumatoid arthritis (RA) commonly affects the two bones of the forearm, the radius, and the ulna, causing deformity of the wrist joint and problems straightening the fingers.

Symptoms of Arthritis of the Wrist

The primary symptoms of arthritis of the wrist include swelling, pain, weakness, and impaired motion of the wrist joint. In cases caused by rheumatoid arthritis, the swelling and stiffness often extend to the knuckle joints of the hand, and the fingers may feel hot and appear red. Additional symptoms of RA in the hand and wrist may include firm bumps on the fingers or elbows; soft lumps on the back of the hands; abnormal bending or deformity of finger joints; and bones in the wrist that appear to stick out.

Diagnosis of Arthritis of the Wrist

Doctors use a combination of physical examination, patient and family medical history, blood tests, and imaging tests to diagnose arthritis of the wrist.

Laboratory Tests

- Rheumatoid factor test
- Anti-cyclic citrullinated peptide (anti-CCP) antibody test
- Complete blood count
- C-reactive protein
- Erythrocyte sedimentation rate
- Synovial fluid analysis

Imaging Tests

- Joint ultrasound or magnetic resonance imaging (MRI)
- Joint X-rays

Treatment of Arthritis of the Wrist

Nonsurgical Treatment

Although there is no cure for arthritis, various types of nonsurgical treatment can help relieve symptoms and slow the progression of the disease.

- **Modifying or limiting activities.** For many people with arthritis—especially in the early stages of the disease—changing the ways in which they use their hands and wrists can help maintain function and reduce pain and swelling. Doctors may recommend restricting some activities that aggravate the condition.

- **Immobilizing the wrist.** Supportive devices such as splints or braces can be worn to protect the wrist as well as relieve symptoms.

- **Using hot and cold packs.** Applying heat or cold (or a combination of the two) to joints can ease the symptoms of arthritis. Heat treatment reduces stiffness by increasing blood flow, while cold treatment reduces inflammation and pain by numbing the affected area.

- **Exercising.** Therapists often prescribe exercise to help maintain the range of motion in arthritis-affected joints as well as to strengthen the muscles that support them.

Medications

Nonsurgical options for treating arthritis of the wrist also include several different categories of drugs.

- **Nonsteroidal anti-inflammatory drugs (NSAIDs).** More than a dozen medications in this category are available in prescription or over-the-counter forms to help ease the pain and inflammation associated with arthritis.

- **Disease-modifying anti-rheumatic drugs (DMARDs).** DMARDs include a variety of prescription medicines that slow or stop the autoimmune response by which rheumatoid arthritis destroys the joints.

- **Biologic response modifiers.** Biologics are genetically engineered drugs that target the proteins and cells involved in rheumatoid arthritis and disrupt the cycle of events that causes inflammation and joint damage.

- **Steroids.** Steroids are synthetic, quick-acting drugs that reduce immune system response and help control inflammation. They may be taken orally or injected directly into the joint.

Surgical Treatment

In cases where nonsurgical treatment fails to relieve symptoms associated with arthritis of the wrist, or the loss of hand and wrist function is progressive and severe, surgical options may prove helpful.

- **Surgical removal of the carpal bones.** Removing the three carpal bones in the wrist is a well-established surgical technique that can help relieve pain and improve range of motion for people with severe arthritis.

- **Fusion of the carpal bones.** Partial or complete fusion of the carpal bones is a surgical alternative for people whose pain is aggravated by moving the wrist. Although both options help relieve pain, partial fusion allows patients to retain some degree of wrist motion, while total fusion eliminates wrist motion but preserves forearm rotation.

- **Joint replacement.** In this surgical procedure, the damaged wrist joint is replaced with a prosthetic device made of synthetic components. Replacing the worn-out bones can help patients retain or improve wrist movement.

References

1. American Academy of Orthopaedic Surgeons (AAOS). "Arthritis of the Wrist," OrthoInfo, 2013.

2. American Society for Surgery of the Hand (ASSH). "Conditions and Injuries: Arthritis-Osteoarthritis," 2015.

3. National Institute of Arthritis and Musculoskeletal and Skin Diseases (NIAMS). "Handout on Health: Rheumatoid Arthritis," NIH Publication No. 14-4179, August 2014.

Section 5.3

Arthritis of the Hip

"Arthritis of the Hip," © 2018 Omnigraphics.
Reviewed April 2018.

Anatomy of the Hip Joint

The hip is a ball-and-socket joint formed between the upper part of the femur (thigh bone) and the hip bones (ossa coxae) of the pelvis, the complex of bones that connects the axial skeleton (head and trunk) to the lower limbs. The cup-shaped cavity of the hip bones, known as the acetabulum, forms the socket into which the rounded head of the femur (ball) fits to form one of the most important weight-bearing surfaces of the human body in both static (standing) and dynamic (walking, running) postures.

In addition to providing a wide range of motion, the hip joint also contributes significantly to stability and balance of the body. Both the acetabulum and the head of the femur are lined by the hyaline cartilage, which allows friction-free motion of the articulating surfaces. In addition, the articulating surfaces of the joint comprise a joint capsule made of a thick outer fibrous tissue and an inner synovial membrane filled with synovial fluid. The ligamentous fibrous tissue is innervated and provides stability to the joint, while the synovial fluid nourishes the joint capsule and serves as a shock absorber.

Arthritic Conditions of the Hip Joint

As with any joint in the body, the hip joint can be affected by arthritis caused either by degenerative changes from wear and tear or by autoimmune disorders. Osteoarthritis (OA) is one of the leading causes of arthritis of the hip and affects a large number of people of both sexes every year, second only to osteoarthritis of the knee. Other types of arthritic conditions that affect the hip joint include rheumatoid arthritis (RA), psoriatic arthritis, and ankylosing spondylitis.

Osteoarthritis

Caused by the wearing away of the articular cartilage that lines the femoral head and the acetabulum, this type of arthritis is multifactorial in etiology. While the exact cause for the degenerative changes is still unclear, studies show that age, gender, and genes may contribute significantly to the articular degeneration associated with arthritis. Osteoarthritis affects more women than men, and age appears to be a risk factor for the development of degenerative changes in the joint. Other extrinsic factors that may increase the incidence and progression of hip osteoarthritis include an increase in body mass index (BMI), high levels of certain types of repetitive physical activity, and injury, all of which may contribute to joint load and microtrauma; instability; and structural damage of the joint. These, in turn, trigger a joint response that leads to inflammation of the subchondral bone (shock-absorbing bone beneath the cartilage) and the synovial membranes. The cartilage degeneration from the mechanical breakdown of the joint may also lead to the formation of osteophytes (bone spurs), bony overgrowths on the surface of the joint formed as a result of the body's compensatory mechanism to joint degeneration. Bone spurs may or may not produce any symptoms.

Symptoms

Arthritis of the hip is typically characterized by stiffness and pain around the hip, the pain being either a dull ache or a sharp stabbing one that may worsen with activity or prolonged rest. Often, the pain appears to be pronounced in the mornings and may also be aggravated by cold weather. In some cases, a grinding noise (crepitus) is experienced during movement. This is caused by loose fragments of cartilage and other tissues interfering with the smooth articulation of the hip. Pain caused by arthritis of the hip joint can sometimes radiate to the groin, knee, buttocks, or the front of the leg. Called referred pain (pain perception distant from the site of stimulus), this is usually caused by entrapment of the branch of the femoral nerve, which supplies the hip joint, and is sometimes the only sign of hip arthritis. In severe cases, a patient's gait may also be compromised and may range from a slight limp, or "waddle," to a severe gait impairment depending on the extent of degenerative changes.

Diagnosis

Physical examination and laboratory tests in conjunction with an imaging study are the usual protocol for diagnosing arthritis of the hip. The physical examination involves checking for range of motion (ROM). The doctor tests both active (without assistance) ROM and passive (assisted) ROM. Plain radiography is the most commonly used imaging tool for assessing hip osteoarthritis. While it does not offer visualization of soft tissue or cartilage, it is useful in assessing joint alignment, bone spurs, and joint space. The narrowing of joint space provides an indication of cartilage wear and the severity of arthritis. In some cases, a magnetic resonance imaging (MRI) scan or a computed tomography (CT) scan may be necessary to obtain 3-D images of the bone and soft tissues. Considered superior to conventional X-ray images, these tests can help assess damage to the soft tissues (muscles, tendons, or ligaments) surrounding the hip.

Treating Arthritis of Hip

Nonsurgical Treatment

Early treatment of hip arthritis primarily involves pain-relieving medications such as acetaminophen and NSAIDs (nonsteroidal anti-inflammatory drugs). Naproxen and ibuprofen are the most commonly used NSAIDs and are administered for a period of 10 days with a repeat course if needed. Topical anti-inflammatory gels or creams rubbed on the affected area may also help alleviate pain. Corticosteroids are powerful anti-inflammatories that are also usually used either orally or as intra-articular injections for pain relief in severe cases.

Physical therapy and exercise help strengthen the muscles, tendons, and ligaments around the joints and reduce the pressure on joints. Exercise regimens are typically tailored to meet the needs and lifestyles of patients.

Assistive devices may improve mobility and independence for people with chronic arthritis. Walking supports such as a cane, crutches, a walker, or a long-handled reacher can assist with activities associated with daily living and reduce pain associated with movement.

Surgical Treatment

When arthritis fails to respond to nonsurgical treatment and leads to disability, surgery may be recommended after taking into consideration factors such as the patient's anatomy, age, occupation, and lifestyle.

Femoral osteotomy, a once-commonly used surgical intervention for osteoarthritis of the hip, is currently used only in young patients who have femoral deformities or dysplasias that could typically lead to abnormal joint wear and arthritis over time. The procedure involves partial cutting of either the femoral head or the acetabulum to reshape or realign and thereby take pressure off the hip joint.

Total hip replacement (THR) is usually indicated when all types of conservative treatment have failed, particularly in the case of advanced arthritis accompanied by a high degree of functional loss. THR involves surgical removal of both the damaged acetabulum and the femoral head, and replacement of the joint surfaces with prosthetic implants made from metal, plastic, or ceramic components to help restore the function of the hip joint. Like most surgical procedures, THR is also associated with potential complications, the most common being hip dislocation. Other adverse events, such as infection, blood clots, and limb length discrepancy, may also follow a THR.

In recent years, hip resurfacing has emerged as an alternative to total hip replacement. Used mainly in noninflammatory degenerative joint disease, this type of surgery involves a metal-on-metal resurfacing system in which metal cups are placed over the femoral head and acetabulum to replace the articulating surfaces of the hip joint. A marked improvement in quality of life has been observed with hip resurfacing arthroplasty. Moreover, as a bone-preserving procedure, hip resurfacing offers the advantage of a subsequent THR revision surgery as there is an intact femoral head for insertion of the THR implant.

References

1. "Hip Osteoarthritis: Where Is the Pain?" The Royal College of Surgeons of England, 2004.

2. "Osteoarthritis of the Hip." American Academy of Orthopaedic Surgeons (AAOS), n.d.

3. "How Does the Hip Joint Work?" Arthritis Research UK., n.d.

4. "Hip Osteoarthritis: Etiopathogenesis and Implications for Management," U.S. National Library of Medicine (NLM), September 26, 2016.

5. "Hip Osteoarthritis and Work," U.S. National Library of Medicine (NLM), June 10, 2015.

Section 5.4

Arthritis of the Knee

This section contains text excerpted from the following sources: Text under the heading "Knee and Joint" is excerpted from "Knee Problems," National Institute of Arthritis and Musculoskeletal and Skin Diseases (NIAMS), March 30, 2016; Text beginning with the heading "What Is Arthritis of the Knee?" is excerpted from "Questions and Answers about Knee Problems," National Institute of Arthritis and Musculoskeletal and Skin Diseases (NIAMS), May 2014. Reviewed April 2018.

Knee and Joint

Your knee is the joint where the bones of the upper leg meet the bones of the lower leg, allowing hinge-like movement while providing stability and strength to support the weight of your body. Flexibility, strength, and stability are needed for standing and for motions like walking, running, crouching, jumping, and turning.

The point at which two or more bones are connected is called a joint. Several kinds of supporting and moving parts, including bones, cartilage, muscles, ligaments, and tendons, help the knees do their job.

In all joints your:

- Bones are kept from grinding against each other by a lining called cartilage.

- Bones are joined to bones by strong, elastic bands of tissue called ligaments.

- Muscles are connected to bones by tough cords of tissue called tendons. Muscles pull on tendons to move joints.

Although muscles are not technically part of a joint, they're important because strong muscles help support and protect your joints.

Each of these structures is subject to disease and injury. When a knee problem affects your ability to do things, it can have a big impact on your life. Knee problems can interfere with many things, from participation in sports to simply getting up from a chair and walking.

Parts of the Knee

Like any joint, the knee is composed of:

- Bones
- Cartilage
- Ligaments
- Tendons
- Muscles

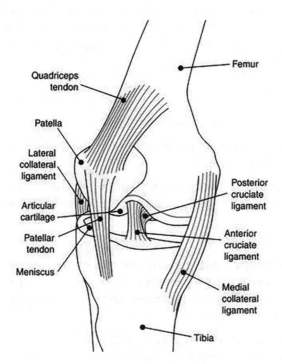

Figure 5.2. *Lateral View of the Knee*

Bones and Cartilage

The knee joint is the junction of three bones:

- The **femur,** also known as the thigh bone or upper leg bone.

- The **tibia,** also known as the shin bone or larger bone of the lower leg.

- The **patella** or kneecap. The patella is 2–3 inches wide and 3–4 inches long. It sits over the other bones at the front of the knee joint and slides when the knee moves. It protects the knee and gives leverage to muscles.

The cartilage in the knee joint includes:

- **Articular cartilage,** a tough elastic material that covers the ends of the three bones in the knee joint. Articular cartilage helps absorb shock and allows the knee joint to move smoothly.

- **Menisci,** two crescent-shaped discs of connective tissue that separate the bones of the knee. They are between the tibia and femur, on the outer and inner sides of each knee. The two menisci in each knee act as shock absorbers, cushioning the lower part of the leg from the weight of the rest of the body as well as enhancing stability.

Muscles

There are two groups of muscles at the knee.

- The four quadriceps muscles on the front of the thigh work to straighten the knee from a bent position.

- The hamstring muscles, which run along the back of the thigh from the hip to just below the knee, help to bend the knee.

Tendons and Ligaments

The quadriceps tendon connects the quadriceps muscle to the patella (the kneecap) and provides the power to straighten the knee. The following four ligaments connect the femur and tibia and give the joint strength and stability:

- The **medial collateral ligament,** which runs along the inside of the knee joint, provides stability to the inner (medial) part of the knee.

- The **lateral collateral ligament,** which runs along the outside of the knee joint, provides stability to the outer (lateral) part of the knee.

- The **anterior cruciate ligament,** in the center of the knee, limits rotation and the forward movement of the tibia.

- The **posterior cruciate ligament,** also in the center of the knee, limits backward movement of the tibia.

The knee capsule is a protective, fiber-like structure that wraps around the knee joint. Inside the capsule, the joint is lined with a thin, soft tissue called synovium.

What Is Arthritis of the Knee?

Arthritis of the knee is most often osteoarthritis (OA). In this disease, the cartilage in the joint gradually wears away. In rheumatoid arthritis (RA), which can also affect the knees, the joint becomes inflamed and cartilage may be destroyed. Arthritis not only affects joints; it can also affect supporting structures such as muscles, tendons, and ligaments.

OA may be caused by excess stress on the joint from deformity, repeated injury, or excess weight. It most often affects middle-aged and older people. A young person who develops OA may have an inherited form of the disease or may have experienced continuous irritation from an unrepaired torn meniscus or other injuries. RA often affects people at an earlier age than OA.

Signs and Diagnosis

Someone who has arthritis of the knee may experience pain, swelling, and a decrease in knee motion. A common symptom is morning stiffness that lessens as the person moves around. Sometimes the joint locks or clicks when the knee is bent and straightened, but these signs may occur in other knee disorders as well. The doctor may confirm the diagnosis by performing a physical examination and examining X-rays, which typically show a loss of joint space. Blood tests may be helpful for diagnosing RA, but other tests may be needed too. Analyzing fluid from the knee joint may be helpful in diagnosing some kinds of arthritis. The doctor may use arthroscopy to directly see damage to cartilage, tendons, and ligaments and to confirm a diagnosis, but arthroscopy is usually done only if a repair procedure is to be performed.

Treatment

Most often OA of the knee is treated with pain-reducing medicines, such as aspirin or acetaminophen (Tylenol*); nonsteroidal anti-inflammatory drugs (NSAIDs), such as ibuprofen (Motrin, Nuprin, Advil); and exercises to restore joint movement and strengthen the knee. Losing excess weight can also help people with OA.

RA of the knee may require physical therapy and more powerful medications. In people with arthritis of the knee, a seriously damaged joint may need to be replaced with an artificial one. (A new procedure designed to stimulate the growth of cartilage by using a patient's own cartilage cells is being used experimentally to repair cartilage injuries at the end of the femur at the knee. It is not, however, a treatment for arthritis.)

Brand names included in this section are provided as examples only, and their inclusion does not mean that these products are endorsed by the National Institutes of Health (NIH) or any other government agency. Also, if a particular brand name is not mentioned, this does not mean or imply that the product is unsatisfactory.

Section 5.5

Arthritis of the Foot and Ankle

The foot and ankle contain twenty-eight bones and thirty-three joints, which makes them particularly vulnerable to arthritis. Although the term "arthritis" covers a number of different conditions that affect the normal functioning of joints, all types of arthritis are characterized by inflammation and pain. When these symptoms affect the foot and ankle, patients may experience significant problems with standing and walking.

Causes of Arthritis of the Foot and Ankle

The main types of arthritis affecting the foot and ankle are osteoarthritis, posttraumatic arthritis, and rheumatoid arthritis.

Osteoarthritis is a progressive, degenerative condition that destroys the smooth, slippery cartilage that covers the ends of healthy bones. When this protective layer wears away, the bones can rub together, causing pain, swelling, and impaired motion of the joint. Osteoarthritis of the foot and ankle develops gradually over time as a result of normal, accumulated "wear and tear."

Posttraumatic arthritis develops as a result of a traumatic injury—such as a sprain, dislocation, or fracture—that causes damage to the surface of a joint. A person who has experienced an injury to the foot or ankle is seven times more likely to develop arthritis in that joint. Posttraumatic arthritis may develop several years after the joint has sustained damage, and it may occur even if the initial injury received proper medical treatment.

Rheumatoid arthritis is a chronic disease in which the body's immune system attacks the synovial fluid. This fluid plays a vital role in joint health by lubricating joints and nourishing bones and cartilage. Rheumatoid arthritis causes the synovium to become inflamed, resulting in pain, swelling, and stiffness in the joints. Although rheumatoid arthritis can affect any joint in the body, ninety percent of patients experience symptoms in the foot and ankle. As the disease progresses, the inflamed synovium may damage surrounding bones and ligaments, causing deformity of the joints and problems with mobility.

Symptoms of Arthritis of the Foot and Ankle

The most common symptoms associated with arthritis of the foot and ankle are pain, tenderness, inflammation, warmth and redness, and loss of mobility in the affected joint. People in the early stages of the disease may experience these symptoms only after prolonged activity. As the disease progresses, the symptoms may occur more frequently, and eventually, the pain and other problems may persist even during periods of inactivity.

Osteoarthritis of the foot or ankle often causes osteophytes (bone spurs) to form. As arthritis damages the cartilage in the joints, the body responds by trying to repair or regenerate the bone in that area. This natural process creates small, bony outgrowths around the arthritic joint. As the bony projections put pressure on the surrounding nerves and soft tissues, patients may experience considerable pain in the foot and ankle.

The pain, inflammation, and stiffness associated with rheumatoid arthritis often appear in several joints of both feet. The symptoms may begin with mild to moderate pain in the soles or balls of the feet. As the disease progresses, the tightening of tendons and connective tissue may lead to bone deformity and the collapse of the foot arch. This condition—commonly known as flat feet—affects the patient's gait, which in turn places strain on the joints of the legs, hips, and back as these structures try to compensate for the changes.

Other foot conditions that may be associated with arthritis include claw foot, in which the joint at the base of the toes bend upward and the other toe joints bend downward; hammertoe, in which one or more toes bend downward; and bunions, in which bony projections form at the base of the big toe.

Diagnosis of Arthritis of the Foot and Ankle

To diagnose arthritis of the foot or ankle, doctors will usually begin by taking a complete medical history and conducting a physical examination of the patient. During this process, the doctor will typically inquire about the person's symptoms, occupation, level of physical activity, past injuries, and previous conditions involving the foot and ankle. The doctor may also observe the patient's gait to assess the alignment, strength, and functioning of the joints. Finally, the doctor may examine the patient's shoes to check for uneven wear and sufficient foot and ankle support.

Following the initial examination, the doctor may order additional tests. These tests may include X-rays to gauge the extent of damage to the joints, and blood tests to check for the rheumatoid factor, an antibody that is often present in people with rheumatoid arthritis. Other tests commonly used to evaluate foot and ankle conditions include bone scans, computed tomography (CT) scans, or magnetic resonance imaging (MRI).

Treatment of Arthritis of the Foot and Ankle

Although there is no cure for arthritis, there are a number of treatment options available that can help reduce pain and inflammation and maintain functioning and mobility.

Nonsurgical Treatment Options

- Rest

- Diet and weight management to reduce stress on joints

- Physical therapy to increase strength and range of motion

- Exercise that does not place stress on the foot and ankle, such as swimming or cycling

- Cold packs to ease pain and inflammation

- Anti-inflammatory pain medication

- Steroid injections

- Orthotic devices, such as shoe inserts or ankle braces

- Assistive devices, such as a cane or braces, to support joints

Surgical Treatment Options

When nonsurgical treatment options fail to relieve a patient's symptoms or improve joint function, doctors may recommend surgery. There are numerous surgical options for the treatment of foot and ankle arthritis. The best choice depends on the location and type of arthritis and the extent to which the disease has progressed.

- **Arthroscopy.** This minimally invasive surgical technique allows surgeons to examine and repair tissues of the foot and ankle using a tiny camera called an arthroscope, which is inserted into the joint through a small incision. After evaluating the condition of the joint, the surgeons can insert instruments to remove damaged tissues, such as bone spurs and pieces of cartilage, or repair torn muscles, ligaments, or tendons. Recovery tends to be faster with this technique as compared to traditional open surgery.

- **Arthrodesis.** This traditional surgical procedure involves removing damaged cartilage and then fusing two or more bones together to create a continuous bone in place of a joint. The surgeon typically inserts pins, screws, or rods to hold the joint in a fixed position. Sometimes a bone graft from the leg or hip may be used to stimulate bone growth and help the bones fuse together. When used to treat ankle arthritis, arthrodesis often fuses the talus (ankle bone) and tibia (shin bone). To treat arthritis of the foot, arthrodesis may fuse two or more joints of the big toe, heel, and mid-foot. Although surgical fusion is generally successful in relieving pain, it results in a total loss of motion in the joint.

- **Arthroplasty.** In this procedure, commonly known as a joint replacement, arthritic joint surfaces are surgically removed and replaced with prosthetic components. This option is usually considered for patients who continue to experience severe pain and loss of joint function following more conservative methods of treatment. Total joint arthroplasty (TJA) may be the only option for retaining joint function in patients with debilitating end-stage arthritis. It not only preserves a high degree of joint movement, but it also helps protect the surrounding joints from excessive stress and wear. Arthroplasty of the joints in the toes or foot is mainly used to correct severe deformities. Ankle replacement surgery, on the other hand, is increasingly being considered for younger patients who want to preserve joint mobility and reduce pain during activity.

References

1. American Academy of Orthopaedic Surgeons. "Arthritis of the Foot and Ankle," OrthoInfo, 2015.

2. American Orthopaedic Foot and Ankle Society. "Treatments," FootCareMD, 2015.

3. Vann, Madeline. "Arch Nemesis: Rheumatoid Arthritis and Flat Feet," Everyday Health, 2015.

Part Two

Types of Arthritis, Related Rheumatic Diseases, and Other Associated Medical Conditions

Chapter 6

Osteoarthritis (OA)

Chapter Contents

Section 6.1—Understanding Osteoarthritis 64

Section 6.2—Spinal Stenosis Can Be Caused by OA 68

Section 6.1

Understanding Osteoarthritis

This section includes text excerpted
from documents published by two public domain sources.
Text under the headings marked 1 are excerpted from
"Osteoarthritis," National Institute on Aging (NIA), National
Institutes of Health (NIH), May 1, 2017; Text under headings
marked 2 are excerpted from "Arthritis—Osteoarthritis,"
Centers for Disease Control and Prevention (CDC),
September 6, 2017.

What is Osteoarthritis (OA)?[1]

Osteoarthritis (OA) is the most common form of arthritis among older people, and it is one of the most frequent causes of physical disability among older adults.

The disease affects both men and women. Before age 45, OA is more common in men than in women. After age 45, OA is more common in women.

OA occurs when cartilage, the tissue that cushions the ends of the bones within the joints, breaks down and wears away. In some cases, all of the cartilage may wear away, leaving bones that rub up against each other.

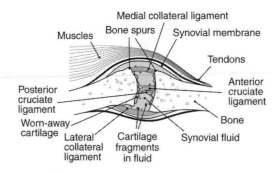

Figure 6.1. *A Joint with Severe Osteoarthritis (OA)* (Source: "Osteoarthritis," National Institute of Arthritis and Musculoskeletal and Skin Diseases (NIAMS).)

OA in the United States[2]

OA affects over 30 million U.S. adults.

Symptoms of OA[1]

Symptoms range from stiffness and mild pain that comes and goes to severe joint pain. Common signs include joint pain, swelling, and tenderness; stiffness after getting out of bed; and a crunching feeling or sound of bone rubbing on bone. Not everyone with OA feels pain.

OA most commonly affects the hands, lower back, neck, and weight-bearing joints such as knees, hips, and feet. OA affects just joints, not internal organs.

Hands

OA of the hands seems to run in families. If your mother or grandmother has or had OA in their hands, you're at greater-than-average risk of having it, too. Women are more likely than men to have OA in the hands. For most women, it develops after menopause.

When OA involves the hands, small, bony knobs may appear on the end joints (those closest to the nails) of the fingers. They are called Heberden nodes. Similar knobs, called Bouchard nodes, can appear on the middle joints of the fingers. Fingers can become enlarged and gnarled, and they may ache or be stiff and numb. The base of the thumb joint also is commonly affected by OA.

Knees

The knees are among the joints most commonly affected by OA. Symptoms of knee OA include stiffness, swelling, and pain, which make it hard to walk, climb, and get in and out of chairs and bathtubs. OA in the knees can lead to disability.

Hips

The hips are also a common site of OA. As with knee OA, symptoms of hip OA include pain and stiffness of the joint itself. But sometimes pain is felt in the groin, inner thigh, buttocks, or even the knees. OA of the hip may limit moving and bending, making daily activities such as dressing and putting on shoes a challenge.

Spine

OA of the spine may show up as stiffness and pain in the neck or lower back. In some cases, arthritis-related changes in the spine can cause pressure on the nerves where they exit the spinal column, resulting in weakness, tingling, or numbness of the arms and legs. In severe cases, this can even affect bladder and bowel function.

Complications of OA[2]

OA can cause severe joint pain, swelling, and stiffness. In some cases it also causes reduced function and disability; some people are no longer able to do daily tasks and, in some cases, are not able to work. Severe cases may require joint replacement surgery, particularly for knee or hip OA.

Causes and Risk Factors of OA[1]

Researchers suspect that OA is caused by a combination of factors in the body and the environment. The chance of developing OA increases with age.

Putting too much stress on a joint that has been previously injured, improper alignment of joints, and excess weight all may contribute to the development of OA.

Diagnosis of OA[1]

To make a diagnosis of OA, most doctors use a combination of methods and tests, including a medical history, a physical examination, X-rays, and laboratory tests.

Treatment Goals: Manage Pain and Improve Function[1]

OA treatment plans often include exercise, rest and joint care, pain relief, weight control, medicines, surgery, and complementary treatment approaches. Current treatments for OA can relieve symptoms such as pain and disability, but there are no treatments that can cure the condition.

Although healthcare professionals can prescribe or recommend treatments to help you manage your arthritis, the real key to living well with the disease is you. Research shows that people with OA who take part in their own care report less pain and make fewer doctor visits. They also enjoy a better quality of life.

How Can Someone with OA Improve Their Quality of Life?[2]

- **Get physically active.** Experts recommend that adults engage in 150 minutes per week of moderate physical activity, or 30 minutes a day for 5 days. Moderate, low impact activities recommended include walking, swimming, or biking. Regular physical activity can also reduce the risk of developing other chronic diseases such as heart disease, stroke, and diabetes.

- **Go to effective physical activity programs.** For those who worry about making OA worse or are unsure how to exercise safely, participation in physical activity programs can help reduce pain and disability-related to arthritis and improve mood and the ability to move. Classes take place at local Ys, parks, and community centers. These classes can help people with OA feel better.

- **Join a self-management education class,** which helps people with arthritis and other chronic conditions—including OA—understand how arthritis affects their lives and increase their confidence in controlling their symptoms and living well.

- **Lose weight.** For people who are overweight or obese, losing weight reduces pressure on joints, particularly weight-bearing joints like the hips and knees. Reaching or maintaining a healthy weight can relieve pain, improve function, and slow the progression of OA.

Section 6.2

Spinal Stenosis Can Be Caused by OA

This section includes text excerpted from "Spinal Stenosis,"
National Institute of Arthritis and Musculoskeletal and
Skin Diseases (NIAMS), August 30, 2016.

What Is Spinal Stenosis?

Spinal stenosis occurs when the spine is narrowed in one or more areas. This puts pressure on the spinal cord and nerves to cause pain.

In people with spinal stenosis, the spine is narrowed in one or more areas:

- The space at the center of the spine

- The canals where nerves branch out from the spine

- The space between the bones of the spine

This narrowing puts pressure on the spinal cord and nerves and can cause pain.

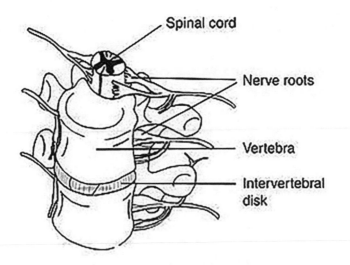

Figure 6.2. *Section of Spine*

Who Gets Spinal Stenosis

Spinal stenosis is most common in men and women over 50 years old. Younger people who were born with a narrow spinal canal or who hurt their spines may also get spinal stenosis.

What Are the Symptoms?

There may be no symptoms of spinal stenosis, or symptoms may appear slowly and get worse over time. Signs include:

- Pain in the neck or back
- Numbness, weakness, cramping, or pain in the arms or legs
- Pain going down the leg
- Foot problems

A serious type of spinal stenosis occurs when there is pressure on nerves in the lower back. You should call your doctor if you have any of these symptoms:

- Loss of control of the bowel or bladder
- Problems having sex
- Pain, weakness, or loss of feeling in one or both legs

What Causes It

Spinal stenosis could be caused by a number of things, including:

- Getting older, which can cause changes in the spine. This is the most common cause.
- Arthritis can affect the spine in some cases.
- Inherited conditions, which you are born with, can affect the spine. For example, you might have been born with a small spinal canal or a curved spine.
- Tumors of the spine
- Injuries
- Paget disease (a disease that affects the bones)
- Too much fluoride in the body
- Calcium deposits on ligaments that run along the spine

Is There a Test?

To diagnose spinal stenosis, your doctor may do the following:

- Ask you about your medical history
- Give you a physical exam
- Take pictures of your spine

How Is It Treated?

Spinal stenosis may be treated by:

- **Medications** to reduce swelling or pain
- **Braces** for your lower back
- **Alternative treatments,** such as chiropractic treatment and acupuncture. More research is needed on the value of these treatments.
- **Surgery,** if you have:
  - Symptoms that get in the way of walking
  - Problems with bowel or bladder function
  - Problems with your nervous system

Who Treats It

Because spinal stenosis has many causes and symptoms, you may require treatment from different doctors such as:

- **Rheumatologists,** who treat arthritis and other diseases of the bones, joints, and muscles.
- **Neurologists and neurosurgeons,** who treat diseases of the nervous system.
- **Orthopedic surgeons,** who treat problems with the bones, joints, and ligaments.
- **Physical therapists,** who help improve function.

Living with It

Your doctor may recommend the following to help you live with spinal stenosis:

- Limits on your activity
- Exercise and/or physical therapy. Talk to your doctor about an exercise program before beginning.

Chapter 7

Rheumatoid Arthritis (RA)

Chapter Contents

Section 7.1—Understanding Rheumatoid
Arthritis (RA) 72

Section 7.2—Painful Joints? Early Treatment for
Rheumatoid Arthritis Is Key 77

Section 7.3—Arthritis Mechanisms May Vary
by Joint 79

Section 7.1

Understanding Rheumatoid Arthritis (RA)

This section contains text excerpted from the following sources:
Text in this section begins with text excerpted from "Rheumatoid Arthritis," National Institute of Arthritis and Musculoskeletal and Skin Diseases (NIAMS), April 30, 2017; Text beginning with the heading "What Are the Complications of Rheumatoid Arthritis (RA)?" is excerpted from "Arthritis—Rheumatoid Arthritis," Centers for Disease Control and Prevention (CDC), March 8, 2017.

Rheumatoid arthritis (RA), sometimes referred to as RA, is an inflammatory disease that causes pain, swelling, stiffness, and loss of function in the joints. It occurs when the immune system, which normally helps protect the body from infection and disease, attacks the membrane lining the joints.

RA is different from other kinds of arthritis in several ways. For example:

- RA generally occurs in a symmetrical pattern, meaning that if one knee or hand is involved, the other one also is.

- RA often affects the wrist joints and the finger joints closest to the hand.

- RA can also affect other parts of the body besides the joints, such as the heart, lungs, blood, nerves, eyes, and skin.

- People with RA may have fatigue, occasional fevers, and a loss of appetite.

Fortunately, current treatments allow most people with the disease to lead active and productive lives. In recent years, research has led to a new understanding of RA, which may result in even better ways to treat the disease.

What Happens in RA?

RA is an autoimmune disease (auto means self). The immune system attacks joint tissues for unknown reasons. RA occurs when:

- White blood cells (WBCs) in the immune system travel to tissue that surrounds the joint, called synovium, and cause inflammation

- The normally thin synovium becomes thick, making the joint swollen, red, painful, and sometimes warm to the touch

- As RA progresses, the inflamed synovium invades and destroys the cartilage and bone within the joint

- The surrounding muscles, ligaments, and tendons that support and stabilize the joint become weak and don't work normally. This leads to pain and joint damage.

Researchers now believe that RA begins to damage the bones within the joint during the first year or two that a person has the disease. This is one reason why early diagnosis and treatment are so important.

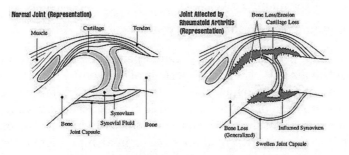

Figure 7.1. *Representation of Normal Joint versus Joint Affected by Rheumatoid Arthritis*

Who Gets RA

About 1.5 million people, or about 0.6 percent of the U.S. adult population, have RA. It is more common among certain groups:

- **Age:** The disease often begins in middle age and is more common in older adults. However, older teenagers and young adults may also get the disease. Children and younger teenagers may be diagnosed with juvenile idiopathic arthritis (JIA), a condition related to RA.

- **Sex:** Like some other forms of arthritis, RA is more common among women than men. About 2–3 times as many women as men have the disease.

- **Race/ethnicity:** RA occurs in all races and ethnic groups.

73

Symptoms of RA

Common signs and symptoms of RA include:

- Tender, warm, swollen joints

- Symmetrical pattern of affected joints

- Joint inflammation often affecting the wrist and finger joints closest to the hand

- Joint inflammation sometimes affecting other joints, including the neck, shoulders, elbows, hips, knees, ankles, and feet

- Fatigue or low energy

- Occasional fevers

- Pain and stiffness lasting for more than 30 minutes in the morning or after a long rest

- Symptoms that last for many years

RA affects people differently. Some people have mild or moderate forms of the disease. They have periods of worsening symptoms, called flares, and periods in which they feel better, called remissions. Others have a severe form of the disease that is active most of the time, last for many years or a lifetime and leads to serious joint damage and disability.

Some people with RA also have other health problems:

- Many people develop anemia which is a decrease in the production of red blood cells (RBCs)

- Less often, people have neck pain and dry eyes and mouth

- Rarely, inflammation of the blood vessels, the lining of the lungs, or the sac enclosing the heart

- Depression, anxiety, feelings of helplessness, and low self-esteem

Causes of RA

Scientists still do not know exactly what causes the immune system to turn against the body's own tissues in RA. Research over the last few years has begun to piece together the factors involved. These include:

Genetic (inherited) factors: Scientists have discovered that certain genes known to play a role in the immune system are associated with RA. However, some people who have these particular genes never develop the disease. This suggests that genes are not the only factor in the development of RA. What is clear, however, is that more than one gene is involved in determining whether a person develops RA and how severe the disease will become.

Environmental factors: Many scientists think that something must occur to trigger the disease process in people whose genetic makeup puts them at risk for RA. Many factors have been suggested, but a specific one has not been confirmed.

Other factors: Some scientists also think that hormonal factors, such as shortages or changes in certain sex hormones, may play a role when genetic and environmental factors also are involved. Scientists believe this because:

• Women are more likely to develop RA than men.

• The disease may improve during pregnancy and flare after pregnancy.

• Breastfeeding may worsen the disease.

We do not know all the answers, but we do know that RA develops from an interaction of many factors. Researchers are trying to understand these factors and how they work together.

What Are the Complications of RA?

Rheumatoid arthritis (RA) has many physical and social consequences and can lower quality of life. It can cause pain, disability, and premature death.

• **Premature heart disease.** People with RA are also at a higher risk for developing other chronic diseases such as heart disease and diabetes. To prevent people with RA from developing heart disease, treatment of RA also focuses on reducing heart disease risk factors. For example, doctors will advise patients with RA to stop smoking and lose weight.

• **Obesity.** People with RA who are obese have an increased risk of developing heart disease risk factors such as high blood pressure and high cholesterol. Being obese also increases risk of developing chronic conditions such as heart disease and diabetes. Finally, people with RA who are obese experience fewer benefits from their medical treatment compared with those with RA who are not obese.

- **Employment.** RA can make work difficult. Adults with RA are less likely to be employed than those who do not have RA. As the disease gets worse, many people with RA find they cannot do as much as they used to. Work loss among people with RA is highest among people whose jobs are physically demanding. Work loss is lower among those in jobs with few physical demands, or in jobs where they have influence over the job pace and activities.

How Can Someone with RA Improve Their Quality of Life?

RA affects many aspects of daily living including work, leisure, and social activities. Fortunately, there are multiple low-cost strategies in the community that are proven to increase the quality of life.

- **Get physically active.** Experts recommend that ideally, adults be moderately physically active for 150 minutes per week, like walking, swimming, or biking 30 minutes a day for five days a week. You can break these 30 minutes into three separate 10-minute sessions during the day. Regular physical activity can also reduce the risk of developing other chronic diseases such as heart disease, diabetes, and depression.

- **Go to effective physical activity programs.** If you are worried about making arthritis worse or unsure how to safely exercise, participation in physical activity programs can help reduce pain and disability related to RA and improve mood and the ability to move. Classes take place at local Ys, parks, and community centers. These classes can help people with RA feel better.

- **Join a self-management education class.** Participants with arthritis gain confidence in learning how to control their symptoms, how to live well with arthritis, and how arthritis affects their lives.

- **Stop smoking.** Cigarette smoking makes the disease worse and can cause other medical problems. Smoking can also make it more difficult to stay physically active, which is an important part of managing RA.

- **Maintain a healthy weight.** Obesity can cause numerous problems for people with RA and so it's important to maintain a healthy weight.

Section 7.2

Painful Joints? Early Treatment for Rheumatoid Arthritis Is Key

This section includes text excerpted from "Painful Joints?" *NIH News in Health*, National Institutes of Health (NIH), April 2017.

Arthritis is an inflammation of the joints. There are over 100 types of arthritis. While their symptoms can be similar, their underlying causes vary. Osteoarthritis (OA) is the most common type of arthritis. It's far more common than rheumatoid arthritis (RA). OA is caused by wear and tear on your joints. In RA, your immune system—which normally helps protect your body from infection and disease—starts attacking your joint tissues.

Anyone can get RA. The disease most often begins in middle age or later. But it can occur at any age. Even children sometimes get a similar form of arthritis. Some types of arthritis affect one joint at a time, but RA can affect your whole body.

It's important to get the correct diagnosis because each form of arthritis needs to be treated differently. To diagnose RA, doctors use medical history, physical exams, X-rays, and lab tests. There's no single test for the disease. It's not easy to diagnose.

"The joint swelling in RA is squishy and very different from the hard bony enlargement of the finger joints that is sometimes present in osteoarthritis," explains Dr. Michael M. Ward, who oversees RA research at National Institutes of Health (NIH).

Your joints may appear red and feel warm. Pain and stiffness may be worse after you wake up or have been resting for a long time. Over time, your immune system damages the tough, flexible tissue (cartilage) that lines joints. This damage can be severe and deform your joints.

Scientists don't know exactly what causes RA. It's likely a combination of genetics and environmental triggers, such as tobacco smoke or viruses. Hormones may also play a role. More women are diagnosed with RA than men. The disease sometimes improves during pregnancy or flares up after pregnancy.

What scientists do know is that the damage is caused by the immune system gone awry. The body's defense system mistakenly attacks the membrane that lines joints, such as in the wrists, fingers, and toes. Joints in the neck, knees, hips, ankles, and elsewhere can also be affected.

"The immune system is supposed to be something that does good things for you," says Dr. M. Kristen Demoruelle, an NIH-funded arthritis expert at the University of Colorado (CU) Anschutz Medical Campus. "It's supposed to help you fight infections. But in RA—for reasons that we don't yet understand—the immune system gets confused and then starts to attack your joints instead."

There's no cure for RA. But there are effective treatments. Treatment can relieve pain, reduce joint stiffness and swelling, and prevent further joint damage.

Research advances have improved patient outcomes in the past 10–20 years. Doctors no longer wait to start treating a person with RA. Now, they know to begin treatment right away—before joint damage worsens. Early detection is very important to increase the chance that treatment is successful.

"If we can get you into low disease activity by 6 months and remission [no signs of the disease] by 1 year, we've got an incredibly good chance of the disease having a very minimal impact on your life," says Dr. Vivian P. Bykerk, an NIH-funded arthritis researcher at the Hospital for Special Surgery in New York.

There are many different classes of drugs available. Many of the drugs, like Nonsteroidal anti-inflammatory drugs (NSAIDs) and steroids, work by reducing inflammation. Such drugs may be used in combination with others that have been shown to slow joint destruction.

NIH scientists helped develop a new class of drug for RA called Janus kinase (JAK) inhibitors. These drugs work by suppressing the body's immune response. Several years ago, the first drug in this new class was approved by U.S. Food and Drug Administration (FDA) for moderate to severe RA. Researchers continue to investigate new types of drugs and drug combinations.

"We really have to rely on our experience. We consider the combination of signs, symptoms, and blood tests to choose the right treatment," Bykerk explains. Once treatment for RA is underway, patients need frequent checkups. Doctors may need to try and adjust different drugs or drug combinations to find the best fit for each person. Treatments are usually required for the long-term to maintain control of the disease. For some people, symptoms go on for years, even a lifetime. Sometimes after months of mild disease, symptoms can flare up again.

Bykerk also works on an NIH-supported team of scientists who are searching for more effective treatment approaches. The team analyzes joint tissue and blood samples from people with RA to better understand the genes and proteins that trigger and drive the disease. The researchers aim to learn why some people respond differently to different treatments. They also hope to one day be able to tailor treatments to each person. Other studies are exploring how long people need to be treated once the disease is under control to prevent it from returning.

RA can affect virtually every area of your life, from work to relationships. If you have RA there are many things you can do to help maintain your lifestyle and keep a positive outlook. Exercise helps keep your muscles healthy and strong, preserve joint mobility, and maintain flexibility. Rest helps to reduce joint inflammation, pain, and fatigue. Ask your doctor how best to balance exercise and rest for your situation.

New research advances continue to help improve quality of life for people with RA. Talk with your doctor about how to treat your joint pain and stiffness so that you can lead a full, active, and independent life.

Section 7.3

Arthritis Mechanisms May Vary by Joint

This section includes text excerpted from "Arthritis Mechanisms May Vary by Joint," *NIH News in Health*, National Institutes of Health (NIH), August 2016.

Knee and hip joints with rheumatoid arthritis have different genetic markers linked to inflammation, suggesting that different joints may have varying disease mechanisms. These new findings may lead to more effective, personalized therapies for rheumatoid arthritis.

People with rheumatoid arthritis have swelling and pain in joints throughout the body. These problems arise when the immune system, which protects the body from germs and infections, mistakenly attacks the joints. For unknown reasons, different joints are affected differently in people with rheumatoid arthritis.

An NIH-funded research team previously found that certain cells in joints have unique patterns of chemical tags—called epigenetic markers—that differ between rheumatoid arthritis and osteoarthritis. Such tags can affect when genes turn on or off and can regulate immune function.

In the new study, the scientists examined epigenetic patterns in joint cells from 30 people with rheumatoid arthritis and 16 with osteoarthritis. Rheumatoid arthritis and osteoarthritis cells had differing patterns of epigenetic tags as expected. But unexpectedly, in patients with rheumatoid arthritis, the patterns in knee joint cells differed from cells in hip joints.

The scientists next assessed the affected biological pathways that distinguish different joints. Knee and hip joints with rheumatoid arthritis had differing activated genes and biological pathways. Many of these pathways were related to immune system function.

The team also found that new drugs for treating rheumatoid arthritis may affect some of these pathways. Their findings might offer an opportunity for developing more precise approaches to treating different arthritic joints.

"We showed that the epigenetic marks vary from joint to joint in rheumatoid arthritis," says study co-author Dr. Gary S. Firestein of the University of California, San Diego. "This might provide an explanation as to why some joints improve while others do not, even though they are exposed to the same drug."

Chapter 8

Childhood Arthritis (Juvenile Arthritis)

Chapter Contents

Section 8.1—Kids and Their Bone Health.................................. 82

Section 8.2—What Is Childhood Arthritis?.............................. 85

Section 8.3—Juvenile Rheumatoid Arthritis and
              Vision Loss.. 94

Section 8.4—Juvenile Idiopathic Arthritis............................. 99

Section 8.5—Biologics: New Treatments for
              Juvenile Arthritis.. 101

Section 8.1

Kids and Their Bone Health

This section includes text excerpted from "Kids and Their Bones: A Guide for Parents," National Institutes of Health (NIH), March 2015.

Typically, when parents think about their children's health, they don't think about their bones. But building healthy bones by adopting healthy nutritional and lifestyle habits in childhood is important to help prevent osteoporosis and fractures later in life.

Osteoporosis, the disease that causes bones to become less dense and more prone to fractures, has been called "a pediatric disease with geriatric consequences," because the bone mass attained in childhood and adolescence is an important determinant of lifelong skeletal health. The health habits your kids are forming now can make, or literally break, their bones as they age.

Why Is Childhood Such an Important Time for Bone Development?

Bones are the framework for your child's growing body. Bone is living tissue that changes constantly, with bits of old bone being removed and replaced by new bone. You can think of bone as a bank account, where (with your help) your kids make "deposits" and "withdrawals" of bone tissue. During childhood and adolescence, much more bone is deposited than withdrawn as the skeleton grows in both size and density.

For most people, the amount of bone tissue in the skeleton (known as bone mass) peaks by their late twenties. At that point, bones have reached their maximum strength and density. Up to 90 percent of peak bone mass is acquired by age 18 in girls and age 20 in boys, which makes youth the best time for your kids to "invest" in their bone health.

How Can I Help Keep My Kids' Bones Healthy?

The same healthy habits that keep your kids going and growing will also benefit their bones. One of the best ways to encourage healthy habits in your children is to be a good role model yourself. Believe it or not, your kids are watching, and your habits, both good and bad, have a strong influence on theirs.

The two most important lifelong bone health habits to encourage now are proper nutrition and plenty of physical activity.

Eating for healthy bones means getting plenty of foods that are rich in calcium and vitamin D. Most kids do not get enough calcium in their diets to help ensure optimal peak bone mass. Are your kids getting enough calcium?

Table 8.1. Recommended Calcium Intakes

Age	Amount of Calcium (Milligrams)
Infants	
Birth to 6 months	200
6 months to 1 year	260
Children/Young Adults	
1–3 years	700
4–8 years	1,000
9–18 years	1,300
Adult Women and Men	
19–50 years old	1,000
51–70 years males	1,000
51–70 years females	1,200
70+ years	1,200
Pregnant or Lactating Women	
14–18 years	1,300
19–50 years	1,000

Source: Food and Nutrition Board (FNB), Institute of Medicine (IOM), National Academy of Sciences (NAS), 2010.

Calcium is found in many foods, but the most common source is milk and other dairy products. Drinking one 8-ounce (oz) glass of milk provides 300 milligrams (mg) of calcium, which is about one-third of the recommended intake for younger children and about one-fourth of the recommended intake for teens. In addition, milk supplies other minerals and vitamins needed by the body. Table 8.1 lists the calcium content for several high calcium foods and beverages. Your kids need several servings of these foods each day to meet their need for calcium.

How Does Physical Activity Help My Kids' Bones?

Muscles get stronger when we use them. The same idea applies to bones: the more work they do, the stronger they get. Any kind of physical exercise is great for your kids, but the best ones for their bones are weight-bearing activities like walking, running, hiking, dancing, tennis, basketball, gymnastics, and soccer. (Children who tend to play outside will also have higher vitamin D levels.) Swimming and bicycling promote your kids' general health, but are not weight-bearing exercises and will not help build bone density. Organized sports can be fun and build confidence, but they are not the only way to build healthy bones.

The most important thing is for your kids to spend less time sitting and more time on their feet and moving. Alone or with friends, at home or at the park, one of the best gifts you can give your kids is a lifelong love of physical activity.

Bone-building activities includes:

- Walking
- Tennis
- Running
- Volleyball
- Hiking
- Ice hockey/field hockey
- Dancing
- Skiing

- Soccer
- Skateboarding
- Gymnastics
- In-line skating
- Basketball
- Lifting weights
- Jumping rope
- Aerobics

What Else Can My Kids Do Besides Eating Calcium-Rich Foods and Getting Plenty of Weight-Bearing Exercise to Keep Their Bones Healthy?

They should avoid smoking. You probably know that smoking is bad for the heart and lungs, but you may not know that it's harmful to bone tissue. Smoking may harm your bones both directly and indirectly. Several studies have linked smoking to higher risk of fracture. The many dangers associated with smoking make it a habit to be avoided.

You may think it's too early to worry about smoking, but the habit typically starts during childhood or adolescence. In fact, most people who use tobacco products start before they finish high school. The good news? If your kids finish high school as nonsmokers, they will probably stay that way for life.

Section 8.2

What Is Childhood Arthritis?

This section includes text excerpted from "Juvenile Arthritis," National Institute of Arthritis and Musculoskeletal and Skin Diseases (NIAMS), June 30, 2015.

Juvenile arthritis (JA) is a term that describes arthritis in children. "Arthritis" means joint inflammation. Arthritis refers to a group of diseases that cause pain, swelling, stiffness, and loss of motion in the joints. A joint is where two or more bones come together. JA commonly affects the knees and the joints in the hands and feet.

There are more than 100 arthritic or rheumatic diseases that may affect the joints but can also cause pain, swelling, and stiffness in other supporting structures of the body such as muscles, tendons, ligaments, and bones. Some rheumatic diseases can also affect other parts of the body, including various internal organs.

Children can develop almost all types of arthritis that affect adults, but the most common type that affects children is juvenile idiopathic arthritis (JIA).

JIA is an umbrella term, or classification system, for all of the more specific types of chronic, or long-lasting, arthritis in children. These conditions used to fall under the term, juvenile rheumatoid arthritis (JRA), which is no longer used.

Who Gets Childhood Arthritis

In the United States, JA and other rheumatic conditions affect nearly 294,000 children age 0–17.

Types of Childhood Arthritis

There are seven separate subtypes of JIA, each with distinct symptoms. However, with every subtype, a child will have arthritis symptoms of joint pain, swelling, tenderness, warmth, or stiffness that last for more than 6 continuous weeks.

The subtypes are:

- **Systemic JIA (formerly known as systemic JRA).** Systemic means the arthritis can affect the whole body, rather than just a specific organ or joint. A child has arthritis with, or just after, a fever that has lasted for at least 2 weeks. The fever has come and gone, but spiked, or hit its highest temperature, for at least 3 days. The fever occurs with at least one or more of the following:

  - Generalized enlargement of the lymph nodes

  - Enlargement of the liver or spleen

  - Inflammation of the lining of the heart (pericarditis) or the lungs (pleuritis)

  - The characteristic rheumatoid rash, which is flat, pale, pink, and generally not itchy. The individual spots of the rash are usually the size of a quarter or smaller. They are present for a few minutes to a few hours, and then disappear without any changes in the skin. The rash may move from one part of the body to another.

- **Oligoarticular JIA (formerly known as pauciarticular JRA).** A child has arthritis affecting one to four joints during the first 6 months of disease. Two subcategories of this type are:

  - Persistent oligoarthritis, which means the child never has more than four joints involved throughout the disease course

  - Extended oligoarthritis, which means that more than four joints are involved after the first 6 months of the disease

- **Polyarticular JIA–rheumatoid factor negative (formerly known as polyarticular JRA–rheumatoid factor negative).** A child has arthritis in five or more joints during the first 6 months of disease, and all tests for rheumatoid factor (proteins produced by the immune system that can attack healthy tissue, which is commonly found in RA and JA) are negative.

- **Polyarticular JIA–rheumatoid factor positive (formerly known as polyarticular RA–rheumatoid factor positive).** A child has arthritis in five or more joints during the first six months of the disease. Also, at least two tests for rheumatoid factor, at least three months apart, are positive.

- **Psoriatic JIA.** A child has both arthritis and psoriasis (a skin disease), or has arthritis and at least two of the following:

  - Inflammation and swelling of an entire finger or toe (this is called dactylitis)

  - Nail pitting or splitting

  - A first-degree relative with psoriasis

- **Enthesitis-related JIA.** The enthesis is the point at which a ligament, tendon, or joint capsule attaches to the bone. If this point becomes inflamed, it can be tender, swollen, and painful with use. The most common locations are around the knee and at the Achilles tendon on the back of the ankle. A child is diagnosed with this condition if he or she has both arthritis and inflammation of an enthesitis site, or has either arthritis or enthesitis with at least two of the following:

  - Inflammation of the sacroiliac joints (at the bottom of the back) or pain and stiffness in the lumbosacral area (in the lower back)

  - A positive blood test for the human leukocyte antigen (HLA) B27 gene

  - Onset of arthritis in males after age six years

  - A first-degree relative diagnosed with ankylosing spondylitis, enthesitis-related arthritis, or inflammation of the sacroiliac joint in association with inflammatory bowel disease (IBD) or acute inflammation of the eye

- **Undifferentiated arthritis.** A child is said to have this condition if the signs and symptoms of arthritis do not fulfill the criteria for one of the other six categories or if they fulfill the criteria for more than one category.

Symptoms of Childhood Arthritis

The most common symptom of all types of JA is persistent joint swelling, pain, and stiffness that is typically worse in the morning or after a nap. The pain may limit movement of the affected joint, although many children, especially younger ones, will not complain of pain.

One of the earliest signs of JA may be limping in the morning because of an affected knee.

Besides joint symptoms, children with systemic JA may have:

- A high fever that may appear and disappear very quickly
- A skin rash that may appear and disappear very quickly
- Swollen lymph nodes located in the neck and other parts of the body
- Inflammation of internal organs, including the heart (fewer than half of the cases) and the lungs (very rarely)

Causes of Childhood Arthritis

Most forms of JA are autoimmune disorders in which the body's immune system—which normally helps to fight off bacteria or viruses—mistakenly attacks some of its own healthy cells and tissues. The result is inflammation, marked by redness, heat, pain, and swelling. Inflammation can cause joint damage.

Doctors do not know why the immune system attacks healthy tissues in children who develop JA. Scientists suspect that it is a two-step process. First, something in a child's genetic makeup gives him or her a tendency to develop JA; then an environmental factor, such as a virus, triggers the development of the disease.

Not all cases of JA are autoimmune; however, research has shown that some people, such as many with systemic arthritis, have what is called an autoinflammatory condition. Although the two terms sound similar, the disease processes behind autoimmune and autoinflammatory disorders are different.

Autoimmune Disorders

When the immune system is working properly, foreign invaders such as bacteria and viruses provoke the body to produce proteins called antibodies. Antibodies attach to these invaders so the immune system can recognize and destroy them. In an autoimmune reaction, the antibodies attach to the body's own healthy tissues by mistake, signaling the body to attack them. Because they target the self, these proteins are called autoantibodies.

Autoinflammatory Disorders

Like autoimmune disorders, autoinflammatory conditions also cause inflammation. And like autoimmune disorders, they also involve an overactive immune system. However, autoinflammation is not caused by autoantibodies. Instead, autoinflammation involves a more primitive part of the immune system that, in healthy people, causes white blood cells to destroy harmful substances. When this system goes awry, it causes inflammation for unknown reasons. Besides inflammation, autoinflammatory diseases often cause fever and rashes.

Diagnosis of Childhood Arthritis

For a doctor to diagnose your child with JA, symptoms must have started before age 16. Doctors usually suspect JA, along with several other possible conditions, when they see children with persistent joint pain or swelling, unexplained skin rashes, and fever associated with swelling of lymph nodes or inflammation of internal organs. A doctor also considers a diagnosis of JA in children with an unexplained limp or excessive clumsiness.

There is no single test that a doctor can use to diagnose JA. A doctor will carefully examine your child and consider his or her medical history and the results of several tests that help confirm JA or rule out other conditions. Specific findings or problems that relate to the joints are the main factors that go into making a JA diagnosis.

Symptoms of Childhood Arthritis

When diagnosing JA, a doctor must consider not only the symptoms your child has, but also the length of time these symptoms have been present. Joint swelling or other joint changes that the doctor can see must be present continuously for at least 6 weeks.

You can help your child's doctor correctly diagnose JA by keeping a record of your child's symptoms and changes in the joints, noting when they first appeared and when they are worse or better.

Family History

It is very rare for more than one member of a family to have JA. But children with a family member who has JA are at a slightly increased risk of developing it as well.

Research shows that JA is also more likely in families with a history of any autoimmune disease. One study showed that families of children with JA are more likely to have a member with an autoimmune disease such as rheumatoid arthritis (RA), multiple sclerosis (MS), or thyroid inflammation (Hashimoto thyroiditis) than are families of children without JA. For that reason, having an autoimmune disease in your family may raise the doctor's suspicions that your child's joint symptoms are caused by JA or some other autoimmune disease.

Lab Tests

Lab tests, usually blood tests, cannot alone provide the doctor with a clear diagnosis. But a doctor can use these tests to help rule out other conditions and classify the type of JA that your child has. A doctor may order blood tests for:

- **Anti-cyclic citrullinated peptide (anti-CCP) antibodies.** Anti-CCP antibodies may be detected in healthy people years before onset of clinical RA. They may predict the eventual development of undifferentiated arthritis into RA.

- **Rheumatoid factor (RF).** RF, an autoantibody that is produced in large amounts in adults with RA, also may be detected in children with JA, although it is rare. The RF test helps the doctor differentiate among the different types of JA.

- **Antinuclear antibody (ANA).** An autoantibody directed against substances in the cells' nuclei, ANA is found in some JA patients. However, the presence of ANA in children generally points to some type of connective tissue disease, helping the doctor to narrow down the diagnosis. A positive test in a child with oligoarthritis markedly raises his or her risk of developing eye disease in the future.

- **Erythrocyte sedimentation rate (ESR or sed rate).** This blood test, which measures how fast red blood cells fall to the bottom of a test tube, can tell the doctor if inflammation is present. Inflammation is the key sign of JA and a number of other conditions.

X-Rays

Your child's doctor will order X-rays if he or she suspects injury to the bone or unusual bone development. Early in the disease, some X-rays can show changes in soft tissue. In general, X-rays are more useful later in the disease, when bones may be affected.

Other Tests

Because there are many causes of joint pain and swelling, the doctor may use other lab tests to help rule out other conditions before diagnosing JA. Some of these conditions include:

- Physical injury
- Bacterial or viral infection
- Lyme disease
- Inflammatory bowel disease (IBD)
- Lupus
- Dermatomyositis
- Some forms of cancer

Treatment

The main goals of treatment are to:

- Preserve a high level of physical and social functioning
- Maintain a good quality of life

To achieve these goals, doctors recommend treatments that:

- Reduce swelling
- Maintain full movement in the affected joints
- Relieve pain
- Prevent, identify, and treat complications

Most children with JA need a combination of medication and other treatments to reach these goals.

Medications

- **Nonsteroidal anti-inflammatory drugs (NSAIDs).** Aspirin, ibuprofen, naproxen, and naproxen sodium are examples of NSAIDs. They are often the first type of medication doctors prescribe for JA. All NSAIDs work similarly by blocking substances called prostaglandins that add to inflammation and pain. However, each NSAID is a different chemical, and each has a slightly different effect on the body. For unknown reasons, some children seem to respond better to one NSAID than another. NSAIDs should only be used at the lowest dose possible for the shortest time needed.

You can buy some NSAIDs over the counter, while several others, including a subclass called cyclooxygenase-2 (COX-2) inhibitors, need a prescription.

91

All NSAIDs can have significant side effects, so consult your child's doctor before giving any of them. Your child's doctor should monitor your child if he or she takes NSAIDs regularly to control JA.

Side effects of NSAIDs include stomach problems; skin rashes; high blood pressure; fluid retention; and liver, kidney, and heart problems. The longer a person uses NSAIDs, the more likely he or she is to have side effects, ranging from mild to serious. Many other medicines cannot be taken when a person is taking NSAIDs because NSAIDs alter the way the body uses or eliminates these other medicines.

- **Disease-modifying antirheumatic drugs (DMARDs).** If NSAIDs do not relieve symptoms of your child's JA, the doctor may prescribe this type of medication. DMARDs slow the progression of JA, but because they may take weeks or months to relieve symptoms, they often are taken with an NSAID. Although there are many different types of DMARDs, many doctors prescribe one called methotrexate.

   Researchers have learned that methotrexate is safe and effective for some children with JA whose symptoms are not relieved by other medications. Because children only need small doses of methotrexate for the relief of arthritis symptoms, potentially dangerous side effects rarely occur. The most serious complication can be liver damage, which a doctor can help prevent with regular blood tests and check-ups. Careful monitoring for side effects is important for people taking methotrexate. When side effects are noticed early, the doctor can reduce the dose and eliminate the side effects.

- **Corticosteroids.** If your child has very severe JA, stronger medicines may be needed to stop serious symptoms, such as inflammation of the sac around the heart (pericarditis). Corticosteroids, such as prednisone, may be added to the treatment plan to control severe symptoms. This medication can be given by IV (intravenous), mouth, or injection directly into a joint. Corticosteroids are powerful anti-inflammatory medicines. Corticosteroids can interfere with your child's normal growth and can cause other side effects, such as a round face, weakened bones, and an increased chance of having infections. Once the medication controls severe symptoms, the doctor will reduce the dose gradually and, in time, stop it completely. It can be dangerous to stop taking corticosteroids suddenly. Carefully follow the doctor's instructions about how to take or reduce the dose. For inflammation in one or just a few joints, injecting a corticosteroid compound into the affected joint or joints can often bring quick relief without the systemic side effects of oral or IV medication.

- **Biologic agents.** If your child has received little relief from other medications, he or she may be given one of a newer class of medications called biologic response modifiers, or biologic agents. These are based on compounds made by living cells. Tumor necrosis factor (TNF) inhibitors are biologic agents that work by blocking the actions of TNF, a naturally occurring protein in the body that helps cause inflammation. Other biologic agents block other inflammatory proteins, such as interleukin-1 or immune cells called T cells. Different biologics tend to work better for the different subtypes of the disease.

All medicines can have side effects. Some medicines and side effects are mentioned in this publication. Some side effects may be more severe than others. You should review the package insert that comes with your medicine and asks your child's healthcare provider or pharmacist if you have any questions about the possible side effects.

Other Treatments

- **Physical therapy.** A regular, general exercise program is an important part of a child's treatment plan. Exercise can help to maintain muscle tone and preserve and recover the range of motion of the joints. A physiatrist (rehabilitation specialist) or a physical therapist can design an appropriate exercise program for your child. The specialist also may recommend using splints and other devices to help maintain normal bone and joint growth.

- **Complementary and alternative therapies.** Many adults seek alternative ways of treating arthritis, such as special diets, supplements, acupuncture, massage, or even magnetic jewelry or mattress pads. Research shows that increasing numbers of children are using alternative and complementary therapies as well.

Although there is little research to support many alternative treatments, some people seem to benefit from them. If your child's doctor feels the approach has value and is not harmful, you can incorporate it into the treatment plan. However, do not neglect regular healthcare or treatment of serious symptoms.

Section 8.3

Juvenile Rheumatoid Arthritis and Vision Loss

"Juvenile Rheumatoid Arthritis and Vision Loss,"
© 2018 Omnigraphics. Reviewed April 2018.

Juvenile rheumatoid arthritis (JRA), otherwise known as juvenile idiopathic arthritis (JIA), is the most common cause of arthritis in children. JRA occurs in children under the age of 16 and is characterized by inflammation of the eyes. Problems with vision are common as a result of treating juvenile rheumatoid arthritis.

Uveitis

Uveitis is a type of inflammation that reduces vision, occurring mostly in children and teens with oligoarticular arthritis. Uveitis, or iridocyclitis, affects the anterior part of the eye—the iris and the ciliary body. It occurs regardless of how severe JIA is and may even start before JIA is diagnosed. However, uveitis is not always related to how active JIA is. The eyes may be unaffected despite inflammation of the joints or there may be inflammation of the eyes even when the joints are healthy.

Uveitis may affect one eye without spreading to the other or may affect both eyes simultaneously. It can only be diagnosed by an ophthalmologist or optometrist. An optometrist can usually check the colored part around the pupil for signs of uveitis since it occurs without any signs of redness in the eyes. Corticosteroid eye drops, pills, injections, or intravenous medications are used to treat uveitis and protect the eyes. Therefore, it is important to have the child's eyes checked periodically to detect signs of uveitis in its early stages.

Cataracts

Cataracts affect the lens of the eye and blur regular vision. Although cataracts rarely affect young people, they may affect those with JIA. With cataracts, the lens of the eye becomes cloudy and blocks light from the retina, resulting in a loss of vision. The child's vision may be affected based on how much of the lens has become cloudy. Cataracts can affect both eyes and can also be a side effect of treating JIA with corticosteroids. Though rare—and largely dependent on how much corticosteroid is used—some young people are more sensitive to the treatment than others for reasons that remain unknown. While mild cataracts do not affect vision, surgical intervention is necessary to treat cataracts and usually does not require an overnight stay in the hospital.

Glaucoma

Glaucoma is an eye disorder caused by damage to the optic nerve that carries information from the eye to the brain. Glaucoma is the second leading cause of blindness in the United States. Glaucoma occurs when there is high pressure inside the eye—a condition called ocular hypertension. Glaucoma is dangerous because there are usually no symptoms until the disease has progressed to a point where loss of vision has already begun and treatment may not be possible. Glaucoma causes peripheral vision loss, which leads to blindness. Glaucoma may also be caused by an increased use of the corticosteroids that are administered to treat JIA. Meeting with an ophthalmologist regularly is mandatory to check for glaucoma since there are no obvious symptoms. Prevention is foremost in the case of glaucoma; however, if the child has contracted glaucoma, primary treatment can be administered by eye drops or oral medication. Depending on the severity of the disease, surgery may be necessary if glaucoma has progressed.

Symptoms

It is important to go to an eye doctor if your eyes become red or if you feel pain in your eyes. Redness or pain may develop over time or may occur suddenly, but these signs require immediate action:

- Medical history
- Blurred vision
- Hypersensitivity to light

- Red eyes
- Floaters (dark spots that appear in the line of sight)
- Eye pain

The likelihood of contracting uveitis is higher in the case of trauma or following previous eye surgeries. The risk is also higher if you have:

- AIDS
- Ankylosing spondylitis, a type of arthritis
- Lupus
- Multiple sclerosis
- Psoriasis
- Rheumatoid arthritis
- Shingles
- Tuberculosis
- Ulcerative colitis

Diagnosis

Your doctor may perform the following tests to diagnose if you have an eye disorder.

Eye Examination

The usual eye examination will have the following procedures:

- Apply eye drops to see the inside of your eyes.
- Ask you to read an eye chart.
- Check your peripheral vision.
- Advise you to follow an object with your eyes as it moves up and down and left and right while keeping your head in one position.

Tonometry Test

Using special tools, your doctor will check the pressure in your eyes to see if they are healthy and if fluids are able to drain out of your eyes easily.

Slit Lamp Examination

The doctor will use a slit lamp (microscope) to shine some light into each eye, checking for any signs of swelling or inflammation.

Blood Tests

A blood test will help your doctor determine if you have uveitis. This test will also help the doctor rule out any other eye disorders. Depending on the results of these tests, your doctor may refer you to particular specialist.

Other Tests

There are other tests a doctor may ask to take in order to test for uveitis. X-ray, a magnetic resonance imaging (MRI) or computed tomography (CT) scan, or a skin test may help your doctor test for uveitis.

Prevention

Medical research has yielded no proven method for stopping uveitis. However, effective measures can be taken to reduce the risk of developing or contracting uveitis.

Diagnose Symptoms Early

Tenderness of the eyes, sensitivity to light, and floaters are reminders to get your eyes checked as soon as possible. Addressing these possible symptoms of uveitis early will leave you better prepared to recognize if you are having an attack and help you address it quickly if you are.

Change Lifestyle Habits

Maintaining a healthy diet with plenty of fruits and vegetables will reduce trans-fatty acids and provide antioxidants that will benefit your eyes. Taking time to relax your mind and body is also essential. Going out for a walk and immersing yourself in activities that will take your mind off your worries will reduce stress and the recurrence of uveitis.

Reduce Exposure to Infections

Tuberculosis, malaria, Lyme disease, toxoplasmosis, syphilis, and herpes are some of the infections that can lead to uveitis. Awareness on these infections can largely reduce the risk of being exposed to these infections.

Medical research has yielded no proven method for stopping uveitis. However, effective measures can be taken to reduce the risk of developing or contracting uveitis.

Treatment

It is essential that children take all the medicines that are prescribed by their doctors. Regular checkups with the rheumatologist and ophthalmologist are also necessary. Schedule an appointment with the rheumatologist, depending on the nature of juvenile arthritis and the medical history of the child.

- A child with oligoarticular arthritis must have an eye examination every 3 months.

- A child with polyarthritis must have an eye examination every 6 months.

- A child with systemic juvenile arthritis must have an eye exam every 12 months.

- Eye examinations do not end after juvenile arthritis has been treated. Regular visits are required. If problems persist, the eye doctor will prescribe eye drops that your child will have to take regularly. These eye drops dilate the pupils and prevent scarring.

Sometimes, the doctor might prescribe steroid eye drops. Long-term use of cortisone and other steroid eye drops may result in glaucoma and cataracts, though. In the case of recurring inflammation, your doctor might prescribe anti-inflammatory drugs. For prolonged side effects of steroid eye drops, your doctor will administer methotrexate either as a shot or orally. However, each case of uveitis can differ largely based on the severity of the eye disorder and your doctor may prescribe a different kind of drug.

References

1. "Eye Problems and Juvenile Idiopathic Arthritis," AboutKidsHealth, January 31, 2017.

2. "How Juvenile Arthritis Affects the Eyes," WebMD LLC. April 22, 2017.

3. "Eye Problems," The Cleveland Clinic Foundation, 2017.

Section 8.4

Juvenile Idiopathic Arthritis

This section includes text excerpted from "Juvenile
Idiopathic Arthritis," Genetics Home Reference (GHR),
National Institutes of Health (NIH), February 2015.

Juvenile idiopathic arthritis (JIA) refers to a group of conditions
involving joint inflammation (arthritis) that first appears before the
age of 16. This condition is an autoimmune disorder, which means
that the immune system malfunctions and attacks the body's organs
and tissues, in this case the joints.

Researchers have described seven types of JIA. The types are distinguished by their signs and symptoms, the number of joints affected,
the results of laboratory tests, and the family history.

Systemic JIA causes inflammation in one or more joints. A high
daily fever that lasts at least 2 weeks either precedes or accompanies
the arthritis. Individuals with systemic arthritis may also have a skin
rash or enlargement of the lymph nodes (lymphadenopathy), liver
(hepatomegaly), or spleen (splenomegaly).

Oligoarticular JIA (also known as oligoarthritis) has no features
other than joint inflammation. Oligoarthritis is marked by the occurrence of arthritis in four or fewer joints in the first 6 months of the
disease. It is divided into two subtypes depending on the course of disease. If the arthritis is confined to four or fewer joints after 6 months,
then the condition is classified as persistent oligoarthritis. If more than
four joints are affected after 6 months, this condition is classified as
extended oligoarthritis.

Rheumatoid factor-positive polyarticular JIA (also known as polyarthritis, rheumatoid factor positive) causes inflammation in five or
more joints within the first 6 months of the disease. Individuals with
this condition also have a positive blood test for proteins called rheumatoid factors. This type of arthritis closely resembles rheumatoid
arthritis (RA) as seen in adults.

Rheumatoid factor negative polyarticular JIA (also known as polyarthritis, rheumatoid factor negative) is also characterized by arthritis in five or more joints within the first 6 months of the disease.

Individuals with this type, however, test negative for rheumatoid factor in the blood.

Psoriatic JIA involves arthritis that usually occurs in combination with a skin disorder called psoriasis. Psoriasis is a condition characterized by patches of red, irritated skin that are often covered by flaky white scales. Some affected individuals develop psoriasis before arthritis while others first develop arthritis. Other features of psoriatic arthritis include abnormalities of the fingers and nails or eye problems.

Enthesitis-related JIA is characterized by tenderness where the bone meets a tendon, ligament or other connective tissue. This tenderness, known as enthesitis, accompanies the joint inflammation of arthritis. Enthesitis-related arthritis may also involve inflammation in parts of the body other than the joints.

The last type of JIA is called undifferentiated arthritis. This classification is given to affected individuals who do not fit into any of the above types or who fulfill the criteria for more than one type of JIA.

Frequency

The incidence of JIA in North America and Europe is estimated to be 4–16 in 10,000 children. One in 1,000 or approximately 294,000 children in the United States are affected. The most common type of JIA in the United States is oligoarticular JIA, which accounts for about half of all cases. For reasons that are unclear, females seem to be affected with JIA somewhat more frequently than males. However, in enthesitis-related JIA males are affected more often than females. The incidence of JIA varies across different populations and ethnic groups.

Genetic Changes

JIA is thought to arise from a combination of genetic and environmental factors. The term "idiopathic" indicates that the specific cause of the disorder is unknown. Its signs and symptoms result from excessive inflammation in and around the joints. Inflammation occurs when the immune system sends signaling molecules and white blood cells to a site of injury or disease to fight microbial invaders and facilitate tissue repair. Normally, the body stops the inflammatory response after healing is complete to prevent damage to its own cells and tissues. In people with JIA, the inflammatory response is prolonged, particularly during movement of the joints. The reasons for this excessive inflammatory response are unclear.

Researchers have identified changes in several genes that may influence the risk of developing JIA. Many of these genes belong to a family of genes that provide instructions for making a group of related proteins called the human leukocyte antigen (HLA) complex. The HLA complex helps the immune system distinguish the body's own proteins from proteins made by foreign invaders (such as viruses and bacteria). Each *HLA* gene has many different normal variations, allowing each person's immune system to react to a wide range of foreign proteins. Certain normal variations of several *HLA* genes seem to affect the risk of developing JIA, and the specific type of the condition that a person may have.

Normal variations in several other genes have also been associated with JIA. Many of these genes are thought to play roles in immune system function. Additional unknown genetic influences and environmental factors, such as infection and other issues that affect immune health, are also likely to influence a person's chances of developing this complex disorder.

Inheritance Pattern

Most cases of JIA are sporadic, which means they occur in people with no history of the disorder in their family. A small percentage of cases of JIA have been reported to run in families, although the inheritance pattern of the condition is unclear. A sibling of a person with JIA has an estimated risk of developing the condition that is about 12 times that of the general population.

Section 8.5

Biologics: New Treatments for Juvenile Arthritis

This section includes text excerpted from "Juvenile Arthritis: Discoveries Lead to Newer Treatments," U.S. Food and Drug Administration (FDA), July 14, 2016.

Arthritis is a disease that mostly affects older people, right? Not necessarily.

Juvenile arthritis is one of the most common chronic illnesses affecting children. In fact, nearly 300,000 youngsters nationwide have been diagnosed with the disease. The most common symptoms include joint pain, inflammation (swelling), tenderness and stiffness. One early sign may be limping in the morning.

Nikolay Nikolov, a rheumatologist and clinical team leader at the Food and Drug Administration (FDA), says that children with juvenile arthritis and their parents have reason to be optimistic. In the last several years, new therapies have been developed by drug companies and approved by the FDA that moderate the effects and control the disease, likely preventing significant disability in later years.

While no one knows exactly what causes juvenile arthritis, scientists do know it is an autoimmune disorder. The immune system, which normally helps the body fight infection, attacks the body's own tissue.

There are several subgroups of juvenile arthritis. Known collectively as Juvenile Idiopathic Arthritis (JIA), these diseases start before age 16 and cause swelling in one or more joints lasting at least six weeks.

JIA affects large joints such as knees, wrists, and ankles as well as small joints. Polyarticular JIA, the largest JIA subgroup, affects many joints. Another subgroup is Systemic JIA, which affects the whole body, and usually causes fever and skin rashes.

In the past, the first line of treatment for children with juvenile arthritis has been to relieve pain and inflammation with nonsteroidal anti-inflammatory drugs (NSAIDs) such as aspirin and ibuprofen. Children with severe juvenile arthritis have been treated also with drugs that suppress the body's immune response such as corticosteroids and methotrexate.

But polyarticular and systemic JIA are now also treated with newer medicines called biologics, which are manufactured in or extracted from biological sources.

Biologics: New Treatments for Juvenile Arthritis

"As science at the molecular level has advanced, we've learned more about what drives arthritis—the mechanism of the disease—and we are able to identify important targets," Nikolov says.

These targets include cytokines (molecules that control and drive inflammation in the body) such as tumor necrosis factor (TNF), interleukins (IL), and other naturally occurring proteins involved in stimulating the body's immune response. Biologics used in the treatment of juvenile arthritis are generally given intravenously or subcutaneously (under the skin), and usually are taken for years. Different biologics tend to work better for different subgroups of the disease. In recent years, FDA has approved several of these treatments. Here are their names, the type of JIA they treat and approval dates:

- Humira (adalimumab) for polyarticular JIA, February 2008

- Orencia (abatacept) for polyarticular JIA, April 2008

- Enbrel (etanercept) for polyarticular JIA, May 1999

- Actemra (tocilizumab) for systemic JIA, April 2011 and polyarticular JIA, April 2013

- Ilaris (canakinumab) for systemic JIA, May 2013.

"In addition to improving the signs, symptoms and physical functioning of patients, many of these biologics have been shown to reduce joint destruction in adults with rheumatoid arthritis (RA), a disease that is related to juvenile arthritis, and thus to change the natural history of the disease," Nikolov says.

While researchers don't yet have a lot of long-term safety information on use of these drugs in children, there is significant experience with their use in adults with RA. Biologics used for the treatment of patients with juvenile arthritis are potent drugs that suppress the immune system and can increase the risk of serious infections, including opportunistic (unusual) infections and tuberculosis.

Expanding Use of New Treatments to Children

When a drug is found to benefit adults with RA in large clinical trials, drug manufacturers may study it in children with juvenile arthritis to find out if the drug works for them too. In addition, FDA considers the known and potential risks of the drug to determine whether its benefits in treating juvenile arthritis outweigh these risks.

"It's possible that safety issues might come up in kids that we have not found in adults. For example, these drugs may affect the developing body and immune system in children, and that may warrant changes in the labels to let both healthcare providers and patients know what are the risks involved, and how to recognize and respond to potential problems," Nikolov says.

Meantime, scientists continue to work on improving existing treatments for children and search for new treatments that will work better with fewer side effects.

Chapter 9

Ankylosing Spondylitis

Ankylosing spondylitis (AS) is a type of arthritis that affects the spine. AS often involves redness, heat, swelling, and pain in the spine or in the joint where the bottom of the spine (sacrum) joins the pelvic bone (ilium).

In some people, AS can also affect the shoulders, ribs, hips, knees, and feet. It can also affect areas where the tendons and ligaments attach to the bones. Sometimes it can affect the eyes, bowel, and very rarely, the heart and lungs.

Many people with AS have mild back pain that comes and goes. Others have severe pain that doesn't go away. Sometimes the spine becomes stiff. In the worst cases, the swelling can cause two or more bones of the spine to fuse. This may stiffen the rib cage, making it hard to take a deep breath.

Who Gets Ankylosing Spondylitis (AS)

A combination of genes may make it more likely you will get AS. The environment also probably plays a role. Men are about twice more likely than women to get AS.

This chapter includes text excerpted from "Ankylosing Spondylitis," National Institute of Arthritis and Musculoskeletal and Skin Diseases (NIAMS), June 30, 2016.

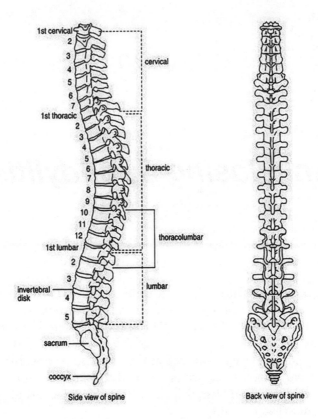

Figure 9.1. *Side and Back Views of the Spine*

Causes of AS

The cause of AS is unknown. It's likely that genes (passed from parents to children) and the environment both play a role. The main gene associated with the risk for AS is called *HLA-B27*. Having the gene doesn't mean you will get AS. Fewer than 1 of 20 people with *HLA-B27* gets AS. Scientists have discovered two more genes (*IL23R* and *ERAP1*) that, along with *HLA-B27*, make it more likely you will get AS.

Diagnosis of AS

To test for AS, your doctor will need:

• A medical history

- A physical exam
- Images of your bones and joints
- Blood tests

Treatment of AS

There is no cure for AS. Some treatments help symptoms and may keep the disease from getting worse. In most cases, your treatment will include medicine, exercise, and a healthy diet. In some cases, surgery can repair some joint damage.

- **Medicines:** Several types of medicines are used to treat AS. It is important to work with your doctor to find the safest and most effective medicine for you. Medicines for AS include:

- **Nonsteroidal anti-inflammatory drugs (NSAIDs).** These drugs relieve pain and swelling. Aspirin, ibuprofen, and naproxen are examples of NSAIDs.

- **Corticosteroids.** These strong drugs are similar to the cortisone made by your body. They fight pain and swelling.

- **Disease-modifying antirheumatic drugs (DMARDs).** These drugs work in different ways to reduce pain and swelling in AS.

- **Biologic agents.** These are newer types of medicine. They block proteins involved with pain and swelling.

- **Exercise:** Exercise and stretching may help painful, stiff joints. It should be done carefully and increased gradually. Before beginning an exercise program, it's important to speak with a doctor to decide on an exercise program. Many people with AS find it helpful to exercise in water. Two types of exercises may help:

  - Exercises to make you stronger

  - Exercises where you gently straighten and bend your joints as far as they will comfortably go

- **Diet:** A healthy diet is good for everyone and may be very helpful if you have AS. Keeping a healthy weight reduces stress on painful joints. Omega-3 fatty acids, found in coldwater fish (such as tuna and salmon), flax seeds, and walnuts, might help. This is still being studied.

- **Surgery:** If AS causes joint damage that makes daily activities difficult, joint replacement may be an option. The knee and hip are the joints most often replaced. In very rare cases, your doctor may suggest surgery to straighten the spine. This can only be done by a surgeon with a lot of experience in the procedure.

Healthcare Team

A rheumatologist usually diagnoses you with AS. This is a doctor trained to treat arthritis and related conditions. Because AS can affect different parts of your body, you may need to see more than one doctor. Some other doctors who treat AS symptoms are:

- An ophthalmologist, who treats eye disease
- A gastroenterologist, who treats bowel disease
- A physiatrist, who specializes in physical medicine and rehabilitation
- A physical therapist, who provides stretching and exercise programs

Living with It

These are important things you can do:

- See your doctor often
- Follow the treatment plan that your doctor gave you
- Stay active with regular exercise
- Maintain a healthy diet
- Practice good posture
- Don't smoke

Chapter 10

Behçet Disease

What Is Behçet Disease?

Behçet disease can affect different parts of your body. If you have the disease, you probably have sores in the mouth or on the genitals (sex organs). More serious symptoms can include swelling, heat, redness, and pain in the eyes and other parts of the body. The disease is named after the doctor who first described it, Dr. Hulusi Behçet.

Who Gets It

Behçet disease is common in some parts of the world, but it is rare in the United States. Behçet disease tends to develop in people in their twenties or thirties, but people of all ages can develop this disease.

What Are the Symptoms?

The symptoms of Behçet disease differ for each person. Some people have only mild symptoms, such as sores in the mouth. Others have more severe problems, such as vision loss. Symptoms may appear,

This chapter contains text excerpted from the following sources: Text beginning with the heading "What Is Behçet Disease?" is excerpted from "Behçet's Disease," National Institute of Arthritis and Musculoskeletal and Skin Diseases (NIAMS), August 30, 2015; Text under the heading "How Is It Treated?" is excerpted from "Behçet disease," Genetic and Rare Diseases Information Center (GARD), National Center for Advancing Translational Sciences (NCATS), November 2, 2016.

disappear, and then reappear. If you are having symptoms, then you are going through a "flare."

The five most common symptoms of Behçet disease are:

- Mouth sores

- Genital sores

- Other skin sores

- Swelling of parts of the eye

- Arthritis (pain, swelling, and stiffness in the joints)

   Less common symptoms include:

- Swelling in the brain and spinal cord

- Blood clots

- Swelling in the digestive system (the parts of the body that digest food)

- Blindness

What Causes It

Most symptoms of Behçet disease are due to swelling of the blood vessels. Doctors aren't sure what causes this. You may have a gene that causes a problem in your immune system, making it more likely you will get the disease. Something in the environment, such as bacteria or viruses, may then cause the immune system to attack its blood vessels. You can't give Behçet disease to someone else.

Is There a Test?

Behçet disease is hard to diagnose because:

- The symptoms do not usually appear all at once.

- There are other illnesses that have similar symptoms.

- There is no single test to diagnose Behçet disease.

   Symptoms used to determine if you have the disease include:

- Mouth sores at least three times in 12 months

- Two of the following:

   - Genital sores that go away and come back

- Swelling of parts of the eye (with vision loss)

- Skin sores

- Small red bumps that appear after your doctor pricks your skin with a needle

Because it may take months or even years for all symptoms to appear, it may take a long time before you will know if you have Behçet disease. You can help your doctor diagnose the disease by keeping a record of your symptoms and when they occur.

How Is It Treated?

Although there is no cure for Behçet disease, people can usually control symptoms with proper medication, rest, exercise, and a healthy lifestyle. The goal of treatment is to reduce discomfort and prevent serious complications such as disability from arthritis or blindness. The type of medicine and the length of treatment depend on the person's symptoms and their severity. It is likely that a combination of treatments will be needed to relieve specific symptoms. Patients should tell each of their doctors about all of the medicines they are taking so that the doctors can coordinate treatment.

Topical medicine is applied directly on the sores to relieve pain and discomfort. For example, doctors prescribe rinses, gels, or ointments. Creams are used to treat skin and genital sores. The medicine usually contains corticosteroids (which reduce inflammation), other anti-inflammatory drugs, or an anesthetic, which relieves pain.

Doctors also prescribe medicines taken by mouth to reduce inflammation throughout the body, suppress the overactive immune system, and relieve symptoms. Doctors may prescribe one or more of the medicines listed below to treat the various symptoms of Behçet disease.

- Corticosteroids

- Immunosuppressive drugs (Azathioprine, Chlorambucil or Cyclophosphamide, Cyclosporine, Colchicine, or a combination of these treatments)

- Methotrexate

Interferon-alfa, azathioprine, and TNF-α blockers may be tried in rare cases of patients with resistant, prolonged, and disabling attacks.

The European League Against Rheumatism (EULAR) has recommendations for the management of Behçet disease.

For ocular disease, azathioprine is the first medication that should be used. For severe eye disease (such as drop-in visual acuity, retinal vasculitis, or macular involvement), either cyclosporine A or infliximab may be used in combination with azathioprine and corticosteroids. Interferon-alfa, alone or in combination with corticosteroids, appears to be the second choice in this eye disease.

Chapter 11

Bone Spurs, Bursitis, and Tendonitis

Chapter Contents

Section 11.1—Bone Spurs.. 114

Section 11.2—Bursitis 118

Section 11.3—Tendonitis.. 121

Section 11.1

Bone Spurs

A bone spur, formally known as an osteophyte, is an abnormal growth or projection that develops along the edge of a bone. Although osteoarthritis is one of the main causes of bone spurs, they can form as a result of any type of joint damage or degeneration. When the protective cartilage layer in a joint wears away, the body often responds by trying to repair or regenerate the bone in that area. This natural process creates small, bony outgrowths around the joint. As these bony projections put pressure on the surrounding nerves and soft tissues, patients may experience pain in the affected area.

Common Sites of Bone Spurs

Bone spurs can form anywhere in the body. Some of the most common sites include:

- **Hips:** When a bone spur develops in the hip area, pain often extends down the legs and into the knees. Depending on their growth, bone spurs in this area can restrict movement of the hip joint and cause patients to have difficulty walking.

- **Heels:** Bone spurs usually begin in the front of the heel bone and spread toward the back of the heel. Bone spurs in this area are often painless.

- **Fingers:** When they develop in the joints of the fingers, bone spurs appear as a hard lump beneath the skin, making the knuckles appear knobby

- **Shoulders:** Bone spurs in the shoulder joint can rub on the rotator cuff—a group of muscles and tendons that secure the upper arm within the shoulder socket—resulting in swelling and restriction of shoulder movement

- **Neck:** Bone spurs in the neck vertebrae (cervical osteophytes) can cause cervical spondylosis or neck arthritis. When the bone spurs put pressure on a nerve, they produce pain and stiffness that may radiate to the shoulders and arms. In some cases the osteophytes may impinge on the spinal cord, creating a condition called cervical myelopathy.

- **Spine:** Bone spurs often appear in the spine as it slowly degenerates as part of the aging process. Although they may not cause pain directly, they may compress nerves that pass through the spinal cord, creating a condition called spinal stenosis. People who develop this condition may experience back pain as well as tingling, numbness, or pain that radiates to the shoulders, arms, buttocks, or legs.

Common Causes of Bone Spurs

Some of the main causes of bone spurs include:

- osteoarthritis and other arthritic conditions
- bone or joint degeneration due to normal "wear and tear"
- the aging process (people over age sixty often show signs of bone spurs)
- poor posture while sitting or standing
- traumatic injury to a bone or joint
- inherited genetic traits
- poor nutrition

Symptoms of Bone Spurs

Bone spurs tend to form slowly over a number of years, and in many cases these small, calcified outgrowths do not cause obvious symptoms. As a result, many people develop bone spurs without even realizing it. Patients usually notice osteophytes when they begin to put pressure on surrounding soft tissues, such as ligaments, tendons, muscles, and nerves. Over time, the impingement of bone spurs can damage the tissues, causing swelling, tenderness, and pain in the affected area.

The most common symptom indicating the presence of a bone spur is a persistent pain felt in and around a joint during normal activities like sitting, standing, or walking. If the pain is severe, or movement in the joint is restricted, patients should seek medical attention. In extreme cases, a bone spur can cause a complete loss of motion in a joint.

Diagnosis of Bone Spurs

A complete physical examination is the first step in diagnosing bone spurs. The doctor will evaluate the range of motion in the joint and take note of any pain the patient experiences. The only definitive way to diagnose a bone spur, however, is through imaging tests. The doctor will order an X-ray of the affected joint, which will usually indicate whether a bone spur has formed. Further tests, such as a computerized tomography (CT) scan or magnetic resonance imaging (MRI) scan, may be used to determine whether the bone spur has caused damage to surrounding nerves or soft tissues.

Treatment of Bone Spurs

There are many different approaches to treating bone spurs. Depending on the severity of pain and other symptoms, treatment options range from conservative nonsurgical modalities to total joint replacement surgery. Some of the most commonly used forms of treatment include:

- **Medications:** Nonsteroidal anti-inflammatory drugs (NSAIDs) like ibuprofen, acetaminophen, or naproxen sodium are often prescribed to alleviate the pain and inflammation caused by minor-to-moderate bone spurs. To help relieve severe pain or stiffness in the affected joints, the doctor may prescribe a corticosteroid injection.

- **Rest:** In cases where pain and inflammation tend to flare up following physical activity, the doctor may advise a short period of complete rest to help heal the soft tissues.

- **Cold or heat therapy:** Applying ice packs helps reduce inflammation and relieve pain, while applying moist heat helps improve circulation and reduce stiffness. Doctors often recommend alternating hot and cold treatments for optimum effect.

- **Physical therapy:** Simple stretching exercises can improve the flexibility of the affected joints. Massaging the area may help break up scar tissue that restricts movement, thus increasing flexibility and relieving pain. Taping can provide support to the joint and relieve strain during activity.

- **Orthotic devices:** Bone spurs of the foot and heel can often be managed by changing to more comfortable footwear or using padding, a heel cup, or an orthotic insert to take the pressure off the affected joints.

- **Complementary and alternative medicines (CAM):** A variety of alternative treatments can help alleviate the symptoms of bone spurs, whether they are used in place of or in conjunction with more traditional therapies. Many patients find that acupuncture and acupressure treatments provide relief from back and foot pain associated with bone spurs. Chiropractic adjustments to the spine can also help reduce pain and improve function of the neck and back. Yoga may help people with bone spurs by strengthening muscles, improving flexibility, and reducing stress on the joints. Other natural remedies that have shown some effectiveness in treating bone spurs include ginger and turmeric supplements and apple cider vinegar tonics.

- **Surgery.** Surgery becomes an option when conservative treatment modalities fail to relieve symptoms. Bone spurs that impinge on surrounding tissues or restrict joint movement can often be removed through minimally invasive arthroscopic surgery. In cases where osteoarthritis has caused extensive damage and deformity, the joint may be surgically replaced with a prosthetic component.

References

1. "Bone Spurs (Osteophytes) and Back Pain," Spine-health, 2015.

2. Driver, Catherine Burt. "Bone Spurs," eMedicineHealth, 2015.

3. Weil, Andrew. "Heel Spurs," Dr.Weil.com, 2015.

Section 11.2

Bursitis

This section includes text excerpted from "Bursitis,"
National Institute of Arthritis and Musculoskeletal and
Skin Diseases (NIAMS), February 28, 2017.

Bursitis is a common condition that causes swelling and pain
around muscles and bones. Bursitis is the swelling of the bursa, a
small, fluid-filled sac that acts as a cushion between a bone and other
moving parts, such as muscles, tendons, or skin.

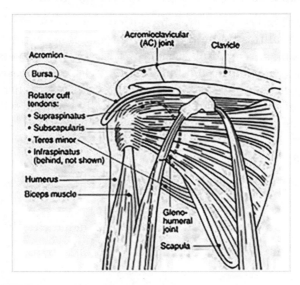

Figure 11.1. *Bursa*

Who Gets Bursitis

You are more likely to get bursitis if you do the same kinds of
movements every day or put stress on your joints. People like carpenters, gardeners, musicians, and athletes often get bursitis. Infection,
arthritis, gout, thyroid disease, and diabetes can also cause bursitis.
Bursitis is more likely the older you get.

Symptoms of Bursitis

Bursitis causes swelling and pain around muscles and bones, especially around joints. Bursae are found throughout the body, but bursitis is most common in shoulders, elbows, wrists, hips, knees, and ankles.

Causes of Bursitis

Bursitis is usually caused by overusing a joint, but it can also be caused by direct trauma. Kneeling or leaning your elbows on a hard surface for a long time can make you more likely to get bursitis.

Diagnosis of Bursitis

To diagnose bursitis, your doctor will probably ask questions about your medical history and conduct a physical examination. Your doctor will probably ask you to describe your pain and will ask when and where you hurt and whether anything makes the pain better or worse.

Your doctor may also do other tests, such as:

- Touching the joint to see whether the tendons, which are another part of your joints, are swollen

- X-rays, which do not show the bursae, but can help rule out other problems

- A magnetic resonance imaging (MRI) test, which can show whether the bursae is swollen

- Taking fluid from the swollen area to test for an infection

Treatment of Bursitis

Treating bursitis can reduce pain and swelling. Some common treatments include:

- Resting and elevating the injured area

- Limiting your activity, in order to reduce further injury

- Taking medicines that will reduce swelling, such as aspirin, naproxen, or ibuprofen

- Gentle stretching and strengthening exercises

- Applying compression to the injured area

- Putting a brace, splint, or band on the injured joint

If an infection is causing your bursitis, your doctor will probably prescribe antibiotics. Your doctor may also recommend ice for sudden, severe injuries, but most cases of bursitis are long term, and ice does not help.

If your bursitis does not improve, your doctor may inject a corticosteroid medicine into the area surrounding the inflamed bursa. Although these injections are common, they must be used with caution because they can lead to weakening or rupture of tendons. If your bursitis does not improve after 6 months to a year, your doctor may recommend surgery to repair damage and relieve pressure on your bursae.

Healthcare Team

Several types of healthcare professionals may treat you, including:

- A primary care physician
- Physical therapists, who help to improve joint function
- Orthopaedists, who treat and perform surgery for bone and joint diseases
- Rheumatologists, who treat arthritis and other diseases of the bones, joints, and muscles

Prevention Strategies

Bursitis typically happens when a person overuses their joints. Here are some tips to protect your joints:

- Exercise regularly
- Start new activities or exercise regimens slowly, so you can see if an exercise is putting too much stress on your joints
- Take breaks from repetitive tasks often
- Use two hands to hold heavy tools, and use a two-handed backhand in tennis
- Don't sit still for long periods
- Practice good posture throughout the day

Section 11.3

Tendonitis

This section includes text excerpted from "Tendonitis,"
National Institute of Arthritis and Musculoskeletal and Skin
Diseases (NIAMS), February 28, 2017.

Tendonitis is swelling and pain in a joint. It is a common condition, usually caused by repeated injuries to a tendon, which is the part of the joint that connects muscles to bones.

Who Gets Tendonitis

You are more likely to get tendonitis if you do the same kinds of movements every day or put stress on your joints. People like carpenters, gardeners, musicians, and athletes often get tendonitis. You are more likely to get tendonitis the older you get.

Types of Tendonitis

Some types of tendonitis are named after the activities that often cause them. Here are some common types:

- **Tennis elbow,** which is an injury to the outer elbow tendon, often caused by repetitive wrist turning or hand gripping.

- **Golfer's elbow,** which is an injury to the inner elbow tendon, often caused by repetitive wrist turning or hand gripping.

- **Biceps tendonitis,** which causes pain in the front or side of the shoulder that may travel down the arm, and sometimes pain when the arm is raised overhead.

- **Rotator cuff tendonitis,** which causes pain at the tip of the shoulder and the upper, outer arm; pain may become worse when reaching, pushing, pulling, lifting, raising the arm, or lying on the shoulder.

- **Jumper's knee,** more common among people who play sports that require jumping, such as basketball, which causes the knee tendon to become inflamed or tear from overuse.

- **Achilles tendonitis,** which is tendonitis in the tendon on the back of the heel.

Symptoms of Tendonitis

Tendonitis causes pain just outside a joint, especially when you move it, and swelling.

Causes of Tendonitis

Tendonitis is usually caused by repeated injuries to a tendon. Infection, arthritis, gout, thyroid disease, and diabetes can also cause tendonitis.

Diagnosis of Tendonitis

To diagnose tendonitis, your doctor will probably ask questions about your medical history and conduct a physical examination. Your doctor will probably ask you to describe your pain and will ask when and where you hurt and whether anything makes the pain better or worse.

Your doctor may also do other tests, such as:

- Touching the joint to see where your joint is swollen

- X-rays, which do not show tendons, but can help rule out other problems

- A magnetic resonance imaging test (MRI), which can show whether the tendon is swollen

- Taking fluid from the swollen area to test for an infection

- Injecting an anesthetic to see if the pain goes away

Treatment of Tendonitis

Treating tendonitis can reduce pain and swelling. Some common treatments include:

- Resting and elevating the injured area

- Limiting your activity to reduce further injury

- Taking medicines that will reduce swelling, such as aspirin, naproxen, or ibuprofen

- Gentle stretching and strengthening exercises

- Applying compression to the injured area

- Soft tissue massage

- Putting a brace, splint, or band on the injured joint

Your doctor may also recommend ice for sudden, severe injuries, but most cases of tendonitis are long term, and ice does not help.

If your tendonitis does not improve, your doctor may inject a medicine into the area surrounding the swollen tendon.

If your tendon is completely torn, you may need surgery. If your tendon is partially or completely torn, you may also need several months of physical therapy and exercises to restore your strength and prevent further injury.

Healthcare Team

Diagnosing and treating tendonitis is a team effort involving you and several types of healthcare professionals. Depending on the severity of the condition, these may include:

- A primary care physician

- Physical therapists, who help to improve joint function

- Orthopaedists, who specialize in the treatment of, and surgery for, bone and joint diseases or injuries

- Rheumatologists, who specialize in arthritis and other diseases of the bones, joints, and muscles

Prevention of Tendonitis

Here are some tips to help reduce the risk and severity of tendonitis:

- Warm up and stretch before exercising

- Strengthen the muscles around your joints

- Take breaks from repetitive tasks

- Increase the gripping surface on tools by using gloves, grip tape, or another padding. Use an oversized grip on golf clubs

- Use two hands to hold heavy tools or hit a backhand in tennis

- Don't sit still for long periods, and have good posture

- Begin new activities and exercises slowly

- Strengthen muscles around the joint

- Stop activities that cause pain

- Cushion the affected joint. Use foam for kneeling, or elbow pads. Increase the gripping surface of tools with gloves or padding. Apply grip tape or an oversized grip to golf clubs

- Consider talking with your doctor or physical therapist before starting new exercises and activities

Chapter 12

Carpal Tunnel Syndrome (CTS)

Carpal tunnel syndrome (CTS) occurs when the median nerve, which runs from the forearm into the palm of the hand, becomes pressed or squeezed at the wrist. The carpal tunnel—a narrow, rigid passageway of ligament and bones at the base of the hand—houses the median nerve and the tendons that bend the fingers. The median nerve provides feeling to the palm side of the thumb and to the index, middle, and part of the ring fingers (although not the little finger). It also controls some small muscles at the base of the thumb.

Sometimes, thickening from the lining of irritated tendons or other swelling narrows the tunnel and causes the median nerve to be compressed. The result may be numbness, weakness, or sometimes pain in the hand and wrist, or occasionally in the forearm and arm. CTS is the most common and widely known of the entrapment neuropathies, in which one of the body's peripheral nerves is pressed upon.

Symptoms of CTS

Symptoms usually start gradually, with frequent burning, tingling, or itching numbness in the palm of the hand and the fingers, especially the thumb and the index and middle fingers. Some carpal tunnel sufferers say their fingers feel useless and swollen, even though little or no swelling is apparent. The symptoms often first appear in one or both

This chapter includes text excerpted from "Carpal Tunnel Syndrome Fact Sheet," National Institute of Neurological Disorders and Stroke (NINDS), January 2017.

125

hands during the night, since many people sleep with flexed wrists. A person with CTS may wake up feeling the need to "shake out" the hand or wrist. As symptoms worsen, people might feel tingling during the day. Decreased grip strength may make it difficult to form a fist, grasp small objects, or perform other manual tasks. In chronic and/ or untreated cases, the muscles at the base of the thumb may waste away. Some people are unable to tell between hot and cold by touch.

Causes of CTS

CTS is often the result of a combination of factors that reduce the available space for the median nerve within the carpal tunnel, rather than a problem with the nerve itself. Contributing factors include trauma or injury to the wrist that causes swelling, such as sprain or fracture; an overactive pituitary gland; an underactive thyroid gland; and rheumatoid arthritis (RA). Mechanical problems in the wrist joint, work stress, repeated use of vibrating hand tools, fluid retention during pregnancy or menopause, or the development of a cyst or tumor in the canal also may contribute to the compression. Often, no single cause can be identified.

Risk Factors for Developing CTS

Women are three times more likely than men to develop CTS, perhaps because the carpal tunnel itself may be smaller in women than in men. The dominant hand is usually affected first and produces the most severe pain. Persons with diabetes or other metabolic disorders that directly affect the body's nerves and make them more susceptible to compression are also at high risk. CTS usually occurs only in adults.

The risk of developing CTS is not confined to people in a single industry or job, but is especially common in those performing assembly line work manufacturing, sewing, finishing, cleaning, and meat, poultry, or fish packing. In fact, CTS is three times more common among assemblers than among data-entry personnel.

Diagnosis of CTS

Early diagnosis and treatment are important to avoid permanent damage to the median nerve.

- A medical history and physical examination of the hands, arms, shoulders, and neck can help determine if the person's discomfort is related to daily activities or to an underlying disorder, and can rule out other conditions that cause similar symptoms. The wrist is examined for tenderness, swelling, warmth, and discoloration. Each finger should be tested for sensation and the muscles at the base of the hand should be examined for strength and signs of atrophy.

- Routine laboratory tests and X-rays can reveal fractures, arthritis, and detect diseases that can damage the nerves, such as diabetes.

- Specific tests may reproduce the symptoms of CTS. In the Tinel test, the doctor taps on or presses over the median nerve in the person's wrist. The test is positive when tingling occurs in the affected fingers. Phalen maneuver (or wrist-flexion test) involves the person pressing the backs of the hands and fingers together with their wrists flexed as far as possible. This test is positive if tingling or numbness occurs in the affected fingers within 1–2 minutes. Doctors may also ask individuals to try to make a movement that brings on symptoms.

- Electrodiagnostic tests may help confirm the diagnosis of CTS. A nerve conduction study measures the electrical activity of the nerves and muscles by assessing the nerve's ability to send a signal along the nerve or to the muscle. Electromyography (EMG) is a special recording technique that detects electrical activity of muscle fibers and can determine the severity of damage to the median nerve.

- Ultrasound imaging can show the abnormal size of the median nerve. Magnetic resonance imaging (MRI) can show the anatomy of the wrist but to date has not been especially useful in diagnosing CTS.

Treatment of CTS

Treatments for CTS should begin as early as possible, under a doctor's direction. Underlying causes such as diabetes or arthritis should be treated first.

Nonsurgical Treatments

- **Splinting.** Initial treatment is usually a splint worn at night.

- **Avoiding daytime activities that may provoke symptoms.** Some people with slight discomfort may wish to take frequent breaks from tasks, to rest the hand. If the wrist is red, warm and swollen, applying cool packs can help.

- **Over-the-counter (OTC) drugs.** In special circumstances, drugs can ease the pain and swelling associated with CTC. Nonsteroidal anti-inflammatory drugs, such as aspirin, ibuprofen, and other nonprescription pain relievers, may provide some short-term relief from discomfort but haven't been shown to treat CTS itself.

- **Prescription medicines.** Corticosteroids (such as prednisone) or the drug lidocaine can be injected directly into the wrist or taken by mouth (in the case of prednisone) to relieve pressure on the median nerve in people with mild or intermittent symptoms. (Caution: Individuals with diabetes and those who may be predisposed to diabetes should note that prolonged use of corticosteroids can make it difficult to regulate insulin levels.)

- **Alternative therapies.** Yoga has been shown to reduce pain and improve grip strength among those with CTS. Some people report relief using acupuncture and chiropractic care but the effectiveness of these therapies remains unproven.

Surgery

Carpal tunnel release is one of the most common surgical procedures in the United States. Generally, surgery involves severing a ligament around the wrist to reduce pressure on the median nerve. Surgery is usually done under local or regional anesthesia (involving some sedation) and does not require an overnight hospital stay. Many people require surgery on both hands. While all carpal tunnel surgery involves cutting the ligament to relieve the pressure on the nerve, there are two different methods used by surgeons to accomplish this.

- **Open release surgery,** the traditional procedure used to correct CTS, consists of making an incision up to 2 inches in the wrist and then cutting the carpal ligament to enlarge the carpal tunnel. The procedure is generally done under local anesthesia on an outpatient basis, unless there are unusual medical conditions.

- **Endoscopic surgery** may allow somewhat faster functional recovery and less postoperative discomfort than traditional open release surgery, but it may also have a higher risk of complications and the need for additional surgery. The surgeon makes one or two incisions (about ½ inch each) in the wrist and palm, inserts a camera attached to a tube, observes the nerve, ligament, and tendons on a monitor, and cuts the carpal ligament (the tissue that holds joints together) with a small knife that is inserted through the tube.

Following surgery, the ligaments usually grow back together and allow more space than before. Although symptoms may be relieved immediately after surgery, full recovery from carpal tunnel surgery can take months. Almost always there is a decrease in grip strength, which improves over time. Some individuals may develop infections, nerve damage, stiffness, and pain at the scar. Most people need to modify work activity for several weeks following surgery, and some people may need to adjust job duties or even change jobs after recovery from surgery.

Although recurrence of CTS following treatment is rare, fewer than half of individuals report their hand(s) feeling completely normal following surgery. Some residual numbness or weakness is common.

Prevention of CTS

At the workplace, workers can do on-the-job conditioning, perform stretching exercises, take frequent rest breaks, and ensure correct posture and wrist position. Wearing fingerless gloves can help keep hands warm and flexible. Workstations, tools, tool handles, and tasks can be redesigned to enable the worker's wrist to maintain a natural position during work. Jobs can be rotated among workers. Employers can develop programs in ergonomics, the process of adapting workplace conditions and job demands to the capabilities of workers. However, research has not conclusively shown that these workplace changes prevent the occurrence of CTS.

Chapter 13

Fibromyalgia

Chapter Contents

Section 13.1—Understanding Fibromyalgia 132

Section 13.2—Drugs Approved to Manage Pain 137

Section 13.3—Mind and Body Therapy for
Fibromyalgia 141

Section 13.1

Understanding Fibromyalgia

This section contains text excerpted from the following sources:
Text beginning with the heading "What Is Fibromyalgia?"
is excerpted from "Fibromyalgia," Office on Women's Health
(OWH), U.S. Department of Health and Human Services (HHS),
September 25, 2017; Text under the heading "Feeling Better with
Fibromyalgia" is excerpted from "Focusing on Fibromyalgia—A
Puzzling and Painful Condition," *NIH News in Health*, National
Institutes of Health (NIH), February 2016.

What Is Fibromyalgia?

Fibromyalgia, or fibromyalgia syndrome, is a condition that causes aches and pain all over the body. People with fibromyalgia often experience other symptoms, such as extreme tiredness or sleeping, mood, or memory problems. Fibromyalgia affects more women than men. The pain, extreme tiredness, and lack of sleep that fibromyalgia causes can affect your ability to work or do daily activities. Fibromyalgia may be caused by a problem in the brain with nerves and pain signals. In other words, in people with fibromyalgia, the brain misunderstands everyday pain and other sensory experiences, making the person more sensitive to pressure, temperature (hot or cold), bright lights, and noise compared to people who do not have fibromyalgia. Treatment can help relieve pain and help prevent flare-ups of symptoms.

Fibromyalgia has been compared to arthritis. Like arthritis, fibromyalgia causes pain and fatigue. But, unlike arthritis, fibromyalgia does not cause redness and swelling, or damage to your joints.

Who Gets Fibromyalgia

Fibromyalgia affects as many as 4 million Americans 18 and older. The average age range at which fibromyalgia is diagnosed is 35–45 years old, but most people have had symptoms, including chronic pain, that started much earlier in life. Fibromyalgia is more common in women than in men.

Are Some Women More at Risk for Fibromyalgia?

Maybe. Fibromyalgia is more common in people who:

- Are obese

- Smoke

- Have another rheumatic (related to the joints) condition, such as rheumatoid arthritis or lupus

- Have a close relative with fibromyalgia. Researchers think a gene or genes may cause pain when the pain would not normally happen.

- Have or had trauma to the brain or spinal cord. Physical trauma may come from an injury or repeated injuries, illness, or an accident. Emotional stress or trauma, such as posttraumatic stress disorder, may also lead to fibromyalgia.

What Are the Symptoms of Fibromyalgia?

Chronic (long-term), widespread pain is the most common symptom of fibromyalgia. You may feel the pain all over your body. Or, you may feel it more in the muscles you use most often, like in your back or legs. The pain may feel like a deep muscle ache, or it may throb or burn. Your pain may also be worse in the morning.

Other symptoms of fibromyalgia include:

- Extreme tiredness, called fatigue, that does not get better with sleep or rest

- Cognitive and memory problems (sometimes called "fibro fog")

- Trouble sleeping

- Mood problems

- Morning fatigue

- Muscle fatigue, causing them to twitch or cramp

- Headaches

- Irritable bowel syndrome (IBS)

- Painful menstrual periods

- Numbness or tingling of hands and feet

- Restless legs syndrome

- Temperature sensitivity

- Sensitivity to loud noises or bright lights

- Depression or anxiety

Women with fibromyalgia often have more morning fatigue, pain all over the body, and IBS symptoms than men with fibromyalgia have.

What Causes Fibromyalgia Symptoms to Flare

Fibromyalgia symptoms can happen without warning. But certain events may trigger flare-ups, including:

- **Hormonal changes during the menstrual cycle or pregnancy.** You may have more trouble sleeping, more widespread pain, or headaches just before your period when your hormone levels drop. Your periods may also be more painful.

- **Stress.** Chronic (long-term) stress may raise your risk for getting fibromyalgia. Also, short-term stress, such as work stress, or stressful events, such as a death of a loved one, can trigger flare-ups in people who have fibromyalgia.

- **Changes in weather.** Some women report pain with changes in barometric pressure (such as when the temperature drops from warm to cold) or on hot, humid days.

What Causes Fibromyalgia

Researchers are not sure exactly what causes fibromyalgia. Genetics may play a role.

Studies also show that the brains of people with fibromyalgia may not process pain in the same way as people who do not have fibromyalgia. Lower levels of certain brain neurotransmitters, such as serotonin or norepinephrine, may cause you to be more sensitive to pain and have a more severe reaction to pain. Imaging studies of the brain show that people with fibromyalgia feel pain when people without fibromyalgia do not. Some medicines prescribed to treat fibromyalgia try to bring the levels of those neurotransmitters back into balance.

How Is Fibromyalgia Diagnosed?

Your doctor or nurse will ask about your symptoms and your medical history. There is no lab test for fibromyalgia. Instead, your doctor will make a diagnosis based upon two criteria:

- You have experienced widespread (in many places on the body) pain for longer than three months

- You have other symptoms, such as fatigue, or memory or sleep problems

You may have to see several doctors before getting a diagnosis. One reason for this may be that pain and fatigue, the main symptoms of fibromyalgia, also are symptoms of many other conditions, such as myalgic encephalomyelitis (ME)/chronic fatigue syndrome (CFS), rheumatoid arthritis (RA), and lupus. Doctors try to figure out if fibromyalgia or another health problem is causing your symptoms.

How Is Fibromyalgia Treated?

Treatment for fibromyalgia may include:

- **Medicine to treat your pain.** The U.S. Food and Drug Administration (FDA) has approved three medicines to treat fibromyalgia: pregabalin, duloxetine, and milnacipran. Your doctor may also suggest pain relievers or antidepressants to treat certain symptoms or to prevent flare-ups.

- **Talk therapy.** Counseling sessions with a trained counselor can teach you different skills and techniques you can use to better control your pain. This type of therapy can be either one on one or in groups with a therapist. Living with a chronic condition like fibromyalgia can be difficult. Support groups may also give you emotional support and help you cope.

Your doctor or nurse may also suggest taking steps at home to relieve your symptoms.

What Steps Can I Take at Home to Relieve Fibromyalgia Symptoms?

You can take the following steps at home to help relieve your symptoms:

- **Getting enough sleep.** Most adults should try to get 7–8 hours of sleep every night. But fibromyalgia can make it hard to fall asleep and stay asleep. Talk to your doctor about any sleep problems you have and ways to treat them. Your doctor may recommend:

  - Going to bed at the same time and getting up at the same time every day

- Not drinking caffeine, alcohol, or eating spicy meals before bedtime

- Not taking daytime naps

- Doing relaxing activities, such as listening to soft music or taking a warm bath, that prepare your body for sleep

- **Reducing stress.** Stress can trigger a flare-up of fibromyalgia symptoms. Strategies such as meditation, massage, and talk therapy may help. Get tips on relieving stress.

- **Getting regular physical activity.** Pain and fatigue may make exercise and daily activities harder to do. But studies show that for many women with fibromyalgia, the regular physical activity can reduce pain. Any activity, even walking around your home or neighborhood, can help relieve your symptoms. Start at a very low level, and slowly increase the amount of activity you get.

- **Trying complementary or alternative therapies.** Some women say their symptoms got better from trying complementary or alternative therapies, such as:

  - Physical therapy
  - Massage
  - Myofascial release therapy
  - Acupuncture
  - Relaxation exercises
  - Tai chi
  - Yoga

Will Fibromyalgia Get Better with Time?

Maybe. Fibromyalgia is a chronic disease that is often a lifelong condition. But fibromyalgia is not a progressive disease, meaning it will not get worse over time. It also does not cause damage to your joints, muscles, or organs.

Taking steps to treat fibromyalgia can help relieve your symptoms.

Will I Still Be Able to Work with Fibromyalgia?

Usually. Most people with fibromyalgia continue to work, but you may have to make changes to do so. You can cut down the number of hours you work, switch to a less demanding job, or adapt a current job. If you face challenges at work, an occupational therapist can help you design a more comfortable workstation or find more efficient and less painful ways to do your job. A number of federal laws protect your rights.

However, if you cannot work because of your fibromyalgia, you may qualify for disability benefits through your employer or the Social Security Administration (SSA).

Feeling Better with Fibromyalgia

- **Get enough sleep.** Getting the right kind of sleep can help ease pain and fatigue. Discuss any sleep problems with your doctor.

- **Exercise.** Research has shown that regular exercise is one of the most effective treatments for fibromyalgia.

- **Try a complementary health approach.** Practices such as tai chi, qi gong, yoga, massage therapy, and acupuncture may help relieve some symptoms.

- **Consider medicines.** Talk to your healthcare provider about an approved medication for treating fibromyalgia.

Section 13.2

Drugs Approved to Manage Pain

This section includes text excerpted from "Living with Fibromyalgia, Drugs Approved to Manage Pain," U.S. Food and Drug Administration (FDA), June 11, 2017.

Approved Drugs

People with fibromyalgia are typically treated with pain medicines, antidepressants, muscle relaxants, and sleep medicines. In June 2007, Lyrica (pregabalin) became the first FDA approved drug for specifically treating fibromyalgia; a year later, in June 2008, Cymbalta (duloxetine hydrochloride) became the second; and in January 2009, Savella (milnacipran hydrochloride (HCI)) became the third.

Lyrica, Cymbalta, and Savella reduce pain and improve function in some people with fibromyalgia. While those with fibromyalgia have been shown to experience pain differently from other people, the mechanism by which these drugs produce their effects is unknown. There is data suggesting that these drugs affect the release of neurotransmitters in the brain. Neurotransmitters are chemicals that transmit signals from one neuron to another. Treatment with Lyrica, Cymbalta, and Savella may reduce the level of pain experienced by some people with fibromyalgia.

Lyrica, marketed by Pfizer Inc., was previously approved to treat seizures, as well as pain from damaged nerves that can happen in people with diabetes (diabetic peripheral neuropathy) and in those who develop pain following the rash of shingles. Side effects of Lyrica including sleepiness, dizziness, blurry vision, weight gain, trouble concentrating, swelling of the hands and feet, and dry mouth. Allergic reactions, although rare, can occur.

Cymbalta, marketed by Eli Lilly and Co., was previously approved to treat depression, anxiety, and diabetic peripheral neuropathy. Cymbalta's side effects include nausea, dry mouth, sleepiness, constipation, decreased appetite, and increased sweating. Like some other antidepressants, Cymbalta may increase the risk of suicidal thinking and behavior in people who take the drug for depression. Some people with fibromyalgia also experience depression.

Savella, marketed by Forest Pharmaceuticals, Inc., is the first drug introduced primarily for treating fibromyalgia. Savella is not used to treat depression in the United States, but acts like medicines that are used to treat depression (antidepressants) and other mental disorders. Antidepressants may increase suicidal thoughts or actions in some people. Side effects include nausea, constipation, dizziness, insomnia, excessive sweating, vomiting, palpitations or increased heart rate, dry mouth and high blood pressure.

Studies of both drugs showed that a substantial number of people with fibromyalgia received good pain relief, but there were others who didn't benefit.

Lyrica and Cymbalta are approved for use in adults 18 years and older. The drug manufacturers have agreed to study their drugs in children with fibromyalgia and in breastfeeding women.

Debilitating Effects

Matallana, who is now president of NFA, says she was a partner in an advertising firm when her life turned completely upside down because of her symptoms. "I finally had to stop working in 1995 and spent most of the next two years in bed," she says. Her husband quit his job and became a consultant working from home so that he could care for her.

"I had a yoga instructor coming to my house three times a week to help me get out of bed. The pain and exhaustion were so bad that there were days that the only activity I was able to do was walk from my bed to the mailbox and back to bed. Each day seemed like an eternity and so I had to focus on just getting through one day at a time."

People with fibromyalgia can experience pain anywhere, but common sites of pain include the neck, shoulders, back, hips, arms, and legs. In addition to pain and fatigue, other symptoms include difficulty sleeping, morning stiffness, headaches, painful menstrual periods, tingling or numbness of hands or feet, and difficulty thinking and remembering. Some people with the condition may also experience irritable bowel syndrome (IBS), pelvic pain, restless leg syndrome, and depression.

What Causes Fibromyalgia

Scientists believe that the condition may be due to injury, emotional distress, or viruses that change the way the brain perceives pain, but the exact cause is unclear. People with rheumatoid arthritis, lupus, and spinal arthritis may be more likely to have the illness.

According to ACR, people with fibromyalgia can have abnormal levels of Substance P in their spinal fluid. This chemical helps transmit and amplify pain signals to and from the brain.

Researchers are looking at the role of Substance P and other neurotransmitters, and studying why people with fibromyalgia have increased sensitivity to pain and whether there is a gene or genes that make a person more likely to have it.

Getting a Diagnosis

Matallana says she felt her suffering was being dismissed as she went from doctor to doctor looking for answers.

"Many doctors suggested that it was just stress," she says. "Some of them even made references that it was all in my head. I was eventually misdiagnosed as having lupus."

When Matallana was 39, a rheumatologist who was just starting his practice finally diagnosed her with fibromyalgia. "With my doctor's help, I started to feel better," she says. "It made all the difference that I had a healthcare provider who could give me insights as to what fibromyalgia research was showing, and that there were other people feeling what I was feeling."

Family physicians, general internists, and rheumatologists are the doctors who typically treat fibromyalgia. There is no diagnostic test for it. Doctors make a diagnosis by conducting physical examinations, evaluating symptoms, and ruling out other conditions. For example, fibromyalgia can be distinguished from arthritis because arthritis causes inflammation of tissues and joints and fibromyalgia does not. Another condition with similar symptoms, hypothyroidism, can be confirmed with a blood test.

Diagnostic criteria set forth by ACR include a history of widespread pain for at least three months and pain in at least 11 of 18 tender point sites.

More than Medicine

People with fibromyalgia may find relief of symptoms with pain relievers, sleep medicines, antidepressants, muscle relaxants, and anti-seizure medications. But medication is just one part of the treatment approach.

What helped Matallana was a combination of medicines for pain and sleep, treatment for some of the overlapping conditions like migraines and irritable bowel syndrome, and a combination of water therapy, massage, and yoga. Walking, jogging, biking, gently stretching muscles, and other exercises also can be helpful.

Emotional support also is essential, Matallana says. "My husband always believed me, and when you have that kind of support it makes a difference. It's really about facing chronic pain for the rest of your life. So dealing with the emotional impact and not just the physical side is very important."

Section 13.3

Mind and Body Therapy for Fibromyalgia

This section contains text excerpted from the following sources:
Text in this section begins with text excerpted from "Mind and
Body Therapy for Fibromyalgia," *NIH News in Health*, National
Institutes of Health (NIH), August 2014. Reviewed April 2018; Text
under the heading "Mind and Body Practices for Fibromyalgia:
What the Science Says" is excerpted from "Mind and Body Practices
for Fibromyalgia: What the Science Says," National Center for
Complementary and Integrative Health (NCCIH), September 2017.

Fibromyalgia is a long-lasting disorder marked by widespread pain,
tenderness, fatigue, and other symptoms that can interfere with daily
life. An estimated 5 million American adults have the condition. It
most often affects women, although men and children also can have the
disorder. Unfortunately, despite ongoing research, its causes remain
unknown.

Fibromyalgia can be difficult to diagnose and treat. Individualized
therapy may include conventional medications as well as mind and
body approaches, such as exercise, strength training, massage, and
acupuncture. But what does the science say about mind and body
practices for fibromyalgia?

The research is still preliminary, but encouraging results suggest that tai chi, qi gong, yoga, massage therapy, acupuncture, and
balneotherapy (hydrotherapy) may help relieve some fibromyalgia
symptoms.

Be sure to speak with your healthcare provider before starting to
use any mind and body practice

Mind and Body Practices for Fibromyalgia: What the Science Says

Recent systematic reviews and randomized clinical trials provide
encouraging evidence that practices such as tai chi, qi gong, yoga,
acupuncture, mindfulness, and biofeedback may help relieve some
fibromyalgia symptoms. There is insufficient evidence that any natural

products can relieve fibromyalgia pain, with the possible exception of vitamin D supplementation, which may reduce pain in people with fibromyalgia who have vitamin D deficiencies.

Current diagnostic criteria are available from the American College of Rheumatology. Treatment often involves an individualized approach that may include both pharmacologic therapies (prescription drugs, analgesics, and NSAIDs) and nonpharmacologic interventions such as exercise, muscle strength training, cognitive-behavioral therapy, movement/body awareness practices, massage, acupuncture, and balneotherapy.

Tai Chi, Qi Gong, Yoga

Findings from some randomized controlled trials suggest that meditative movement therapies such as tai chi, qi gong, and yoga may provide modest relief of some fibromyalgia symptoms.

Massage

Results of a recent systematic review and meta-analysis concluded that massage therapy with a duration of 5 weeks or longer had beneficial immediate effects on improving pain, anxiety, and depression.

Acupuncture

Limited evidence suggests that when compared to a control, acupuncture may help improve symptoms of fibromyalgia such as pain and stiffness.

Balneotherapy (Hydrotherapy)

There is some qualitative evidence that suggests that balneotherapy (hydrotherapy) may provide a small improvement in pain and health-related quality of life for patients with fibromyalgia syndrome.

Mindfulness Meditation

Mindfulness meditation may provide short-term improvements in pain and quality of life in patients with fibromyalgia; however, the evidence is limited by a small number of studies with low methodological quality.

Biofeedback

There is some low-quality evidence that biofeedback, compared to usual care, has an effect on physical functioning, pain, and mood in patients with fibromyalgia; however, due to the lack of quality evidence, it is unknown if biofeedback has any therapeutic effect on these outcomes.

Guided Imagery

Studies on the effects of guided imagery for fibromyalgia symptoms have had inconsistent results.

Chapter 14

Gout and Chondrocalcinosis 2

Chapter Contents

Section 14.1—Understanding Gout 146
Section 14.2—Chondrocalcinosis 2.. 149

Section 14.1

Understanding Gout

This section contains text excerpted from the following sources:
Text beginning with the heading "What Is Gout?" is excerpted from
"Gout," National Institute of Arthritis and Musculoskeletal and Skin
Diseases (NIAMS), April 30, 2016; Text under the heading "If You
Have Gout" is excerpted from "Gripped by Gout—Avoiding the Ache
and Agony," *NIH News in Health*, National Institutes of
Health (NIH), February 2014. Reviewed April 2018.

What Is Gout?

Gout is a kind of arthritis that causes painful and stiff joints. Gout
is caused by the buildup of crystals made of a substance called uric acid
in your joints. It often starts in the big toe and can also cause lumps
under the skin and kidney stones.

Who Gets It

Millions of people have gout at some time in their lives. Usually,
people who get gout get it when they are middle-aged or older, but
children and young adults occasionally get it. Men, especially those
between ages 40–50, are more likely to develop gout than women.
Women rarely develop gout before menopause.

You are more likely to get gout if you:

• Have a family history of gout

• Have had an organ transplant

• Are a man

• Are an adult

• Are overweight

• Drink alcohol

• Eat a lot of foods rich in purines

• Have been exposed to lead

Some other health problems can make it more likely for you to have too much uric acid in the blood. These include:

- Renal insufficiency, a condition in which your kidneys don't get rid of enough waste

- High blood pressure

- Hypothyroidism, or an underactive thyroid gland

- Conditions that make your cells reproduce and shed more quickly than usual, such as psoriasis, hemolytic anemia, and some cancers

- Kelley-Seegmiller syndrome (KSS) or Lesch-Nyhan syndrome (LNS), two rare conditions in which your body doesn't have enough of the enzyme that helps control uric acid levels.

Some medications make you more likely to develop gout, including:

- Diuretics, which are taken to rid the body of excess fluid in condition like hypertension, edema, and heart disease. Diuretics reduce the amount of uric acid passed in the urine.

- Drugs with salicylate, such as aspirin

- Niacin, a vitamin also known as nicotinic acid

- Cyclosporine, a medication that blocks the body's immune system to treat some autoimmune diseases and to prevent the body from rejecting transplanted organs

- Levodopa, a medicine used to treat Parkinson disease (PD)

What Are the Symptoms?

Gout causes pain in your joints, often in the big toe. Many people get their first attack of gout in one of their big toes, but it can also affect other joints in your feet, arms, and legs. In addition to pain, your joint may feel swollen, red, warm, and stiff.

In the early stages of gout, you may have attacks that start at night and come on suddenly. Intense pain and swelling may be bad enough to wake you up. Gout attacks are often triggered by stressful events, alcohol, drugs, or another illness.

Usually, a gout attack will get better in 3–10 days, even without treatment. After that, you may not have another attack for months or even years. Over time, however, your attacks may last longer and happen more often.

After a long period of time, such as 10 years or so, gout can sometimes advance and cause permanent damage to your joints and kidneys. With proper treatment, however, most people with gout do not have permanent damage.

What Causes It

Your body has substances called purines in its tissues. Purines are also found in many foods, including liver, dried beans and peas, and anchovies. When purines break down, they become uric acid.

Normally, uric acid dissolves in your blood and passes out of your body when you pee. When you have too much uric acid in your blood, it can start to form crystals in your joints and under your skin, causing gout.

Things that can cause uric acid to build up in the blood include:

- Your body increasing the amount of uric acid it makes

- Your kidneys not getting rid of enough uric acid

- Eating too many foods high in purines

Is There a Test?

Your doctor can test your blood to see if you have high levels of uric acid. They may also draw a sample of fluid from one of your painful joints to look for crystals of uric acid.

How Is It Treated?

Proper treatment can reduce the pain from gout attacks, help prevent future attacks, and prevent damage to your joints.

Your doctor may recommend medications to treat your pain. These may include:

- Nonsteroidal anti-inflammatory drugs (NSAIDs), which can reduce pain and swelling

- Corticosteroids, such as prednisone, which are strong anti-inflammatory hormones

- Colchicine, which works best when taken within the first 12 hours of a gout attack

- Other medications to reduce symptoms or reduce the buildup of uric acid in your blood

Your doctor may also recommend diet and lifestyle changes, such as losing weight, if you are overweight, and eating fewer foods that are high in purines.

If You Have Gout

To ease or prevent gout attacks:

- Eat a heart-healthy diet. Avoid foods that are high in purines (such as liver, dried beans and peas, gravy, and anchovies)

- Avoid high-fructose, corn syrup-sweetened beverages and foods

- Drink plenty of water, and limit alcohol

- Exercise regularly and maintain a healthy weight

- If you're overweight, ask your doctor how to lose weight safely. Fast or extreme weight loss can raise uric acid levels.

- Tell your healthcare provider about all the medicines and vitamins you take

- Take prescribed medicines as directed

Section 14.2

Chondrocalcinosis 2

This section includes text excerpted from
"Chondrocalcinosis 2," Genetic and Rare Diseases
Information Center (GARD), National Center for Advancing
Translational Sciences (NCATS), January 12, 2018.

Chondrocalcinosis 2 is a rare disease characterized by the accumulation of calcium pyrophosphate dihydrate (CPP) crystals in and around the joints. A buildup of these crystals can lead to joint pain and damage that is progressive (worsens over time). Signs and symptoms of the disease include chronic joint pain or sudden, recurrent episodes of pain, as well as stiffness or swelling of the joints.

Chondrocalcinosis 2 is actually a familial form of chondrocalcinosis (also known as calcium pyrophosphate deposition disease or CPPD), which is caused by a similar buildup of CPP crystals but is associated with the aging process. The age-related chondrocalcinosis is quite common, whereas chondrocalcinosis 2 is not. In addition, people with chondrocalcinosis 2 are more likely to have symptoms that develop earlier in adulthood than the age-related form.

Chondrocalcinosis 2 is caused by changes in the *ANKH* gene. The disease is inherited in an autosomal dominant manner. Chondrocalcinosis 2 is diagnosed based on imaging such as X-rays. The diagnosis can be confirmed with genetic testing of the *ANKH* gene. Treatment may include the use of corticosteroids, pain relievers, and physical therapy.

Symptoms of Chondrocalcinosis 2

Some people with chondrocalcinosis 2 may not have any symptoms of the disease other than showing calcium deposits in and around joints on X-rays. Others may experience symptoms such as joint pain and swelling and difficulty moving the joints. These symptoms can be similar to the symptoms of arthritis or gout, and they may be described as "pseudoarthritis" or "pseudogout."

The symptoms can be chronic (occurring all the time) or may occur in sudden episodes. If the pain occurs in episodes, it can last anywhere from several hours to several weeks. In some cases, episodes of pain may cause fevers. The attack may affect only one joint or multiple joints. Joints that are most commonly affected include the knees, wrists, hips, or shoulders. Some people with chondrocalcinosis 2 may experience pain in the back if calcium deposits develop around the bones of the spine.

Cause of Chondrocalcinosis 2

Chondrocalcinosis 2 is caused by changes in the *ANKH* gene. When a genetic change causes a disease, it is also known as a pathogenic variation. The *ANKH* gene provides instructions to make a protein that may interact with or regulate other proteins involved in the controlling the formation of CPP mineralization. Mineralization is the process by which calcium and phosphorus form crystals to become part of the bone structure. Although the exact function of the *ANKH* protein is not known, it is known that the pathogenic variation in the *ANKH* gene allows too many CPP crystals to build up in the cartilage of joints. The buildup of crystals weakens the cartilage and causes it to break down more easily, leading to the joint pain and other symptoms associated with chondrocalcinosis 2.

Inheritance of Chondrocalcinosis 2

Chondrocalcinosis 2 is inherited in an autosomal dominant manner. This means that people with chondrocalcinosis 2 have a disease-causing change (pathogenic variation) in only one copy of the ANKH gene in each cell of the body. Most genes, including the ANKH gene, come in pairs, and a person inherits one copy of each gene from their mother and the other from their father.

When a person with chondrocalcinosis 2 has children, each child has a:

- 50 percent chance to inherit the changed copy of ANKH, meaning they may develop chondrocalcinosis 2

- 50 percent chance to inherit the working copy of ANKH, meaning they will not develop chondrocalcinosis 2

In some cases, a person with chondrocalcinosis 2 inherits the disease from an affected parent. In other cases, the pathogenic variation that causes the disease is new (de novo) in the affected person, and there is no history of the disease in the family. However, a person with a new pathogenic variation in the ANKH gene has a 50 percent chance of passing this disease-causing change on to each of his or her children.

Diagnosis of Chondrocalcinosis 2

A diagnosis of chondrocalcinosis 2 is often suspected based on signs and symptoms of the disease, as well as the age the symptoms begin. Doctors may wish to take a thorough personal and family history to evaluate for other possible causes of chondrocalcinosis and to determine if there are other family members who may be affected. Specialized testing, such as analysis of the fluid in the joints (synovial fluid), can confirm the diagnosis. X-rays or other imaging techniques may also be used to identify calcium deposits in the cartilage of joints.

If a doctor suspects that a person has chondrocalcinosis caused by a change (pathogenic variation) in the ANKH gene, genetic testing may be ordered to confirm the diagnosis and identify other family members who may have the same pathogenic variation.

Treatment of Chondrocalcinosis 2

There is currently no cure for chondrocalcinosis 2. However, therapies are available to manage the signs and symptoms of the disease. During episodes of joint pain, stiffness, or swelling, the following treatments may be recommended to relieve symptoms:

- Joint aspiration (draining of fluid from the affected joint)

- Corticosteroid injections

- Nonsteroidal anti-inflammatory drugs (NSAIDs), including aspirin or ibuprofen

For people who have frequent episodes of pain or for whom other medications are not effective, small doses of a medication called colchicine may be recommended. However, this medication has side effects and may not help everyone with chondrocalcinosis 2.

In some cases, people with chondrocalcinosis 2 may be required to wear a splint or brace to prevent too much movement. In other cases, physical therapy may be recommended for safe movement of the affected joint.

Prognosis of Chondrocalcinosis 2

For some people with chondrocalcinosis 2, medications and other therapies work well to treat signs and symptoms of the disease. For others, the buildup of CPP crystals is severe and can cause pain that is not relieved with treatment. At this time, there is, unfortunately, no way to prevent or remove the buildup of CPP crystals in the joints. In some cases, the pain associated with chondrocalcinosis 2 can be severe and very disabling.

Chapter 15

Infectious Forms of Arthritis

Chapter Contents

Section 15.1—Arthritis Associated with Lyme
    Disease.. 154

Section 15.2—Reactive Arthritis... 159

Section 15.3—Septic Arthritis (Infectious Arthritis)............... 161

Section 15.1

Arthritis Associated with Lyme Disease

This section includes text excerpted from "A History of Lyme Disease, Symptoms, Diagnosis, Treatment and Prevention," National Institute of Allergy and Infectious Disease (NIAID), April 30, 2015.

A History of Lyme Disease

In the early 1970s, a mysterious group of rheumatoid arthritis (RA) cases occurred among children in Lyme, Connecticut, and two neighboring towns. Puzzled, researchers looked at several possible causes, such as contact with germs (microbes) in water or air. Realizing that most of the children with arthritis lived and played near wooded areas, they then focused their attention on deer ticks.

Researchers knew that the children's first symptoms typically started during the summer, the height of tick season. Several children reported having a skin rash just before developing arthritis, and many of them recalled being bitten by a tick where the rash appeared. By the mid-1970s, researchers began describing the signs and symptoms of this new disease, now termed Lyme disease, to help physicians diagnose patients.

However, it was not until 1981 that National Institute of Allergy and Infectious Disease (NIAID) researchers at Rocky Mountain Laboratories (RML) in Hamilton, Montana, identified the cause of Lyme disease and discovered the connection between the deer tick and the disease. European researchers had described a skin rash similar to that of Lyme disease in early 20th century medical literature.

Willy Burgdorfer, Ph.D., an NIAID scientist studying Rocky Mountain spotted fever, also caused by a tick bite, wondered whether the European rash, called erythema migrans (EM), and Lyme disease might have the same cause. Along with his RML colleague Alan Barbour, M.D., Dr. Burgdorfer continued to study spiral-shaped bacteria, or spirochetes, from infected deer ticks. In November 1981, the two scientists found that a spirochete caused both Lyme disease and EM. The *spirochete* was later named Borrelia burgdorferi in honor of Dr. Burgdorfer's role in its discovery.

Symptoms of Lyme Disease

Typically, the first symptom of Lyme disease is a rash known as EM, which starts as a small red spot at the site of the tick bite and gets larger over a period of days or weeks, forming a circular or oval-shaped red rash. The rash may look like a bull's eye, appearing as a red ring around a clear area with a red center. It appears within a few weeks of a tick bite and usually occurs at the place of the bite. The rash can range in size from that of a small coin to the width of a person's back. As infection spreads, rashes can appear at different sites on the body. The rash is often accompanied by other symptoms, such as fever, headache, stiff neck, body aches, and fatigue.

Although these symptoms may be like those of common viral infections, such as the flu, Lyme disease symptoms tend to last longer or may come and go over time.

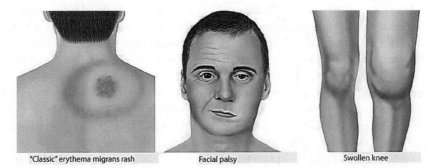

"Classic" erythema migrans rash Facial palsy Swollen knee

Figure 15.1. *Symptoms of Lyme Disease* (Source: "Signs and Symptoms of Untreated Lyme Disease," Centers for Disease Control and Prevention (CDC).)

Some people who have Lyme disease may develop arthritis or nervous system problems and more rarely, heart problems.

Lyme disease may also cause eye inflammation, hepatitis (liver disease), and severe fatigue. However, these problems usually only appear in conjunction with other symptoms of the disease.

Diagnosis of Lyme Disease

Healthcare providers may have difficulty diagnosing Lyme disease because many of its symptoms are similar to those of other illnesses, such as the flu. The bull's eye rash is the only symptom that is unique to Lyme disease, but not everyone infected with Lyme bacteria develops the rash.

Research supported by the National Institutes of Health (NIH) and Centers for Disease Control and Prevention (CDC) suggest that a tick must be attached to the body for at least 36 hours to transmit Lyme disease. Although transmission cannot occur without the tick bite, many people may not remember being bitten because the deer tick is tiny and its bite is usually painless.

If a person has symptoms of Lyme disease but does not have the distinctive rash, healthcare providers will rely on a detailed medical history. The medical history includes whether symptoms first appeared during the summer months, if the person had been outdoors in an area where Lyme disease is common, and whether the person was bitten by a tick, along with a careful physical exam and laboratory tests to check for the presence of antibodies to B. burgdorferi to help provide a diagnosis. It takes a few weeks for someone infected with B. burgdorferi to produce antibodies against the bacteria.

Healthcare providers frequently use one of two antibody tests as a first-level screening. The screening tests are designed to be very "sensitive," meaning that almost everyone who has Lyme disease and some people who do not, will test positive. If the screening test is negative, it is highly unlikely that the person has Lyme disease and no further testing is needed. If the screening test is positive or indeterminate, a second, different test known as a Western blot test should be performed. Used appropriately, this test is designed to be "specific," meaning that it will usually be positive only if a person is truly infected. If the Western blot is negative, it suggests that the first test was a false positive.

The CDC does not recommend a Western blot test without conducting the first-level blood screening. Using the Western blot alone increases the potential for false positive results, which may cause individuals to be treated for Lyme disease when they do not have it and, subsequently, not receive treatment for the true cause of their illness. It is also noteworthy that some laboratories offer Lyme disease testing using assays whose accuracy and clinical usefulness have not been adequately established. Tests that use urine or other bodily fluids (other than blood) to diagnose Lyme disease have not been approved by the U.S. Food and Drug Administration (FDA).

Treatment of Lyme Disease

Antibiotics are prescribed to effectively treat Lyme disease. These medicines can help speed healing of the EM rash and keep symptoms, such as arthritis and nervous system problems, from developing. In general, the sooner treatment begins after infection, the quicker and more complete the recovery. Treatment for pregnant women is similar to treatment for others, but certain antibiotics are not used because they may affect the fetus.

After receiving treatment for Lyme disease, patients may still experience muscle or joint aches and nervous system symptoms, such as trouble with memory and concentration. To help combat these problems, researchers are trying to find out how long a person should take antibiotics for the various symptoms that may follow about with Lyme disease.

Individuals who have previously had Lyme disease can be infected again if bitten by an infected tick.

Prevention of Lyme Disease

The best way to prevent Lyme disease is to avoid contact with deer ticks, especially during the summer months when infections are most common. Other useful tips:

- Wear long pants, long sleeves, and long socks to keep ticks off the skin. Tuck shirts into pants, and pant legs into socks or shoes, to keep ticks on the surface of your clothing. If outside for a long period of time, tape the area where pants and socks meet to prevent ticks from crawling under clothing.

- Wear light-colored clothing to make it easier to spot ticks

- Spray clothing with the repellent permethrin, found in lawn and garden stores. Do not apply permethrin directly to the skin.

- Spray exposed clothing and skin with the repellent containing 20–30 percent N,N-Diethyl-meta-toluamide (DEET) to prevent tick bites. Carefully read and understand manufacturer instructions when using repellant, especially when using the products on infants and children.

- Pregnant women, in particular, should avoid ticks in Lyme disease areas as infection may be transmitted to the fetus

- Avoid wooded areas and nearby shady grasslands. Deer ticks are common in these areas, and particularly common where the two areas merge.

- Maintain a clear backyard by removing yard litter and excess brush that could attract deer and rodents

- Once indoors after being outside, check for ticks, especially in the hairy areas of the body, and wash all clothing

- Before letting pets indoors, check them for ticks. Ticks may fall off and then attach to humans. Pets can also develop Lyme disease.

Research supported by the NIH and CDC suggest that a tick must be attached to the body for at least 36 hours to transmit Lyme disease. Risk of infection can be decreased by promptly removing ticks.

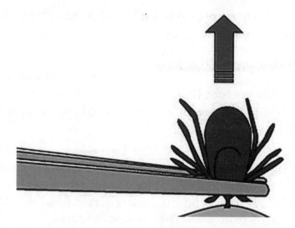

Figure 15.2. *Tick Removal* (Source: "Lyme Disease: What You Need to Know," Centers for Disease Control and Prevention (CDC).)

After finding a tick, remove it using fine-tipped tweezers; do not use petroleum jelly, a hot match, nail polish, or other products. Grab the tick close to the skin and pull up gently so that all parts of the tick are removed. Wash hands afterward with soap and water or waterless alcohol-based hand rub, and clean the area with an antiseptic, such as rubbing alcohol, or soap and water.

Section 15.2

Reactive Arthritis

This section includes text excerpted from "Reactive Arthritis," National Institute of Arthritis and Musculoskeletal Diseases (NIAMS), October 30, 2016.

Reactive arthritis is pain or swelling in a joint that is caused by an infection in your body. You may also have red, swollen eyes and a swollen urinary tract. These symptoms may occur alone, together, or not at all.

Most people with reactive arthritis recover fully from the first flare of symptoms and can return to regular activities 2–6 months later. Some people will have long-term, mild arthritis. A few patients will have long-term, severe arthritis that is difficult to control with treatment and may cause joint damage.

Who Gets Reactive Arthritis

Men between ages 20–40 are most likely to get reactive arthritis. Men are also more likely than women to get the form that is caused by a bacteria passed along during sex. Women and men are at equal risk of getting the disease because of bacteria in food. Women with reactive arthritis often have milder symptoms than men.

Symptoms of Reactive Arthritis

Symptoms of reactive arthritis may be so mild that you do not notice them. They can come and go over a period of weeks or months. In a few people, symptoms can turn into a long-term disease.

Symptoms of reactive arthritis can include:

- Joint swelling and pain
- Inflammation of the urinary and genital tract
- Redness and swelling of the eyes
- Mouth sores and skin rashes

Causes of Reactive Arthritis

Reactive arthritis may be set off by an infection in the bladder or the urethra, which carries urine out of the body. In women, an infection in the vagina can spark the reaction. For both men and women, it can start with bacteria passed on during sex. Another form of reactive arthritis starts with eating food or handling something that has bacteria on it.

You can't pass your reactive arthritis on to someone else. However, you can pass along the bacteria that can trigger the disease.

Doctors do not know why some people develop reactive arthritis and others do not.

Diagnosis of Reactive Arthritis

There is no specific lab test to confirm that you have reactive arthritis. Doctors sometimes find it difficult to diagnose. Tests the doctor may order include:

- Complete medical history
- Blood tests
- Tests for infections
- X-rays

Treatment of Reactive Arthritis

There is no cure for reactive arthritis, but some treatments ease the symptoms. Your doctor might use one or more of the following:

- Nonsteroidal anti-inflammatory drugs (NSAIDs) to treat pain and inflammation
- Corticosteroids injected into painful joints or applied to skin sores
- Antibiotics to fight the bacterial infection that triggered the disease
- Medicines to stop the immune system from attacking its own tissues

Healthcare Team

Diagnosing and treating reactive arthritis requires a team effort involving you and several types of healthcare professionals. These may include:

- Rheumatologists, who specialize in arthritis and other diseases of the bones, joints, and muscles. Your rheumatologist will also coordinate care between your different doctors.

- Ophthalmologists, who treat eye disease

- Urologists or gynecologists, who treat genital symptoms

- Dermatologists, who treat skin symptoms

- Orthopaedists, who perform surgery on severely damaged joints

- Physiatrists, who help with exercise programs

Living with It

Exercise can reduce joint pain and stiffness. It can also help you lose weight to reduce stress on joints. You should speak to your doctor about a safe, well-rounded exercise program.

Section 15.3

Septic Arthritis (Infectious Arthritis)

This section includes text excerpted from "Infectious Arthritis," MedlinePlus, National Institutes of Health (NIH), August 25, 2016.

What Are Joints?

Most kinds of arthritis cause pain and swelling in your joints. Joints are places where two bones meet, such as your elbow or knee.

What Is Infectious Arthritis?

Infectious arthritis is an infection in the joint. The infection comes from a bacterial, viral, or fungal infection that spreads from another part of the body.

What Are the Symptoms of Infectious Arthritis?

Symptoms of infectious arthritis include:

- Intense pain in the joint
- Joint redness and swelling
- Chills and fever
- Inability to move the area with the infected joint

What Is Reactive Arthritis?

One type of infectious arthritis is reactive arthritis. The reaction is to an infection somewhere else in your body. The joint is usually the knee, ankle, or toe. Sometimes, reactive arthritis is set off by an infection in the bladder, or in the urethra, which carries urine out of the body. In women, an infection in the vagina can cause the reaction. For both men and women, it can start with bacteria passed on during sex. Another form of reactive arthritis starts with eating food or handling something that has bacteria on it.

How Is Infectious Arthritis Diagnosed?

To diagnose infectious arthritis, your healthcare provider may do tests of your blood, urine, and joint fluid.

What Is the Treatment for Infectious Arthritis?

Treatment includes medicines and sometimes surgery.

Chapter 16

Lupus

Chapter Contents

Section 16.1—Systemic Lupus Erythematosus........................ 164

Section 16.2—Lupus and Osteoporosis............................... 168

Section 16.3—Lupus and Women 171

Section 16.1

Systemic Lupus Erythematosus

This section includes text excerpted from "Systemic Lupus Erythematosus (Lupus)," National Institute of Arthritis and Musculoskeletal and Skin Diseases (NIAMS), June 30, 2016.

Systemic lupus erythematosus (SLE), also known as lupus, is a disease that can damage many parts of the body, such as the joints, skin, kidneys, heart, lungs, blood vessels, and brain. You can't catch lupus from another person. If you have lupus you will have periods of illness (flares) and periods of wellness (remission).

Lupus occurs when the immune system, which normally helps protect the body from infection and disease, attacks different parts of the body.

Who Gets Systemic Lupus Erythematosus

We know that many more women than men have SLE. Lupus is more common in African American women than in Caucasian women and is also more common in women of Hispanic, Asian, and Native American descent. African American and Hispanic women are also more likely to have active disease and serious organ system involvement. In addition, lupus can run in families, but the risk that a child or a brother or sister of a patient will also have lupus is still quite low.

Although SLE usually first affects people between the ages of 15–45 years, it can occur in childhood or later in life as well.

Symptoms of Systemic Lupus Erythematosus

Each person with SLE has slightly different symptoms that can range from mild to severe. You may have symptoms in only one or in many parts of your body. Symptoms may also come and go over time. Some of the most common symptoms of lupus include:

- Painful or swollen joints (arthritis)
- Unexplained fever

- Extreme fatigue
- Red rashes, most often on the face
- Chest pain upon deep breathing
- Hair loss
- Sensitivity to the sun
- Mouth sores
- Pale or purple fingers and toes from cold and stress
- Swollen glands
- Swelling in the legs or around the eyes

Other symptoms could include:

- Anemia (a decrease in red blood cells)
- Kidney inflammation, which typically requires drug treatment to prevent permanent damage
- Headaches, dizziness, depression, confusion, or seizures if the disease affects the central nervous system
- Inflammation of the blood vessels
- Decreased number of white blood cells or platelets
- Increased risk of blood clots
- Inflammation of the heart or the lining that surrounds it
- Heart valve damage

Causes of Systemic Lupus Erythematosus

No one completely understands what causes SLE. Studies suggest that a number of different genes may determine your risk for developing the disease.

Some environmental factors also appear to play a role in lupus. In particular, scientists are studying the effects of sunlight, stress, hormones, cigarette smoke, certain drugs, and viruses.

Diagnosis of Systemic Lupus Erythematosus

Diagnosing SLE can be difficult and may take months or even years. Although there is no single test for lupus, your doctor may do the following to diagnosis you with the condition:

- Ask you about your medical history

- Give you a physical exam

- Take samples of blood, skin, kidney, or urine for laboratory tests. The most useful tests look for certain antibodies in the blood

Treatment of Systemic Lupus Erythematosus

Treatments for SLE have improved dramatically in recent decades, giving doctors more choices in how to manage the disease. Because some treatments may cause harmful side effects, you should immediately report any new symptoms to your doctor. You should also talk to your doctor before stopping or changing treatments.

Treatments for lupus include:

- **Medications:**

  - **Nonsteroidal anti-inflammatory drugs (NSAIDs)** are used to treat joint or chest pain or fever. Ibuprofen and naproxen sodium are available over the counter, whereas other NSAIDs are available by prescription only.

  - **Antimalarials** prevent and treat malaria, but doctors have found that they also are useful for treating fatigue, joint pain, skin rashes, and inflammation of the lungs caused by lupus. These drugs may also prevent flares from recurring.

  - **Corticosteroids,** strong inflammation-fighting drugs, may be taken by mouth, in creams applied to the skin, by injection, or by intravenous (IV) infusion (dripping the drug into the vein through a small tube). Because they are potent drugs, your doctor will seek the lowest dose required to achieve the desired benefit.

  - **Immunosuppressives** restrain an overactive immune system and may be prescribed if your kidneys or central nervous systems (CNS) are affected by lupus. These drugs may be given by mouth or by IV infusion. The risk for side effects increases with the length of treatment.

  - **B-lymphocyte stimulator (BlyS)-specific inhibitors** reduce the number of abnormal B cells thought to be a problem in lupus.

- Alternative and complementary therapies may improve symptoms, although research has not shown whether they help treat the disease. Examples include:

- Special diets

- Nutritional supplements

- Fish oils

- Ointments and creams

- Chiropractic treatment

- Homeopathy

In many cases, you may need to take medications to treat problems related to lupus, such as high cholesterol, high blood pressure, or infection.

Who Treats Systemic Lupus Erythematosus

Most people will see a rheumatologist for their SLE treatment. A rheumatologist is a doctor who specializes in rheumatic diseases (arthritis and other inflammatory disorders, often involving the immune system). Clinical immunologists (doctors specializing in immune system disorders) may also treat people with lupus. As treatment progresses, other professionals often help, including:

- Primary care doctors, such as a family physician or internal medicine specialist, who coordinates care between the different health providers and treats other problems as they arise.

- Mental health professionals, who help people cope with difficulties in the home and workplace that may result from their medical conditions.

- Nephrologists, who treat kidney disease

- Cardiologists, who specialize in the heart and blood vessels

- Hematologists, who specialize in blood disorders

- Endocrinologists, who treat problems related to the glands and hormones

- Dermatologists, who treat skin problems

Section 16.2

Lupus and Osteoporosis

This section includes text excerpted from "What
People with Lupus Need to Know about Osteoporosis,"
NIH Osteoporosis and Related Bone Diseases~National
Resource Center (NIH ORBD~NRC), April 2016.

What Is Lupus?

Lupus is an autoimmune disease, a disorder in which the body
attacks its own healthy cells and tissues. As a result, various parts
of the body—such as the joints, skin, kidneys, heart, and lungs—can
become inflamed and damaged. There are many different kinds of
lupus. Systemic lupus erythematosus (SLE) is the form of the disease
that is commonly referred to as lupus.

People with lupus can have a wide range of symptoms. Some of
the most commonly reported symptoms are fatigue, painful or swollen joints, fever, skin rashes, and kidney problems. Typically, these
symptoms come and go. When symptoms are present in a person with
the disease, it is known as a flare. When symptoms are not present,
the disease is said to be in remission.

We know that many more women than men have lupus. Lupus is
more common in African American women than in Caucasian women
and is also more common in women of Hispanic, Asian, and Native
American descent. African American and Hispanic women are also
more likely to have active disease and serious organ system involvement. In addition, lupus can run in families, but the risk that a child
or a brother or sister of a patient will also have lupus is still quite low.
It is difficult to estimate how many people in the United States have
the disease, because its symptoms vary widely and its onset is often
hard to pinpoint. Unfortunately, there is no cure for the disease.

What Is Osteoporosis?

Osteoporosis is a condition in which the bones become less dense
and more likely to fracture. Fractures from osteoporosis can result

in significant pain and disability. In the United States, more than 53 million people either already have osteoporosis or are at high risk due to low bone mass.

Risk factors for developing osteoporosis include:

- thinness or small frame

- family history of the disease

- being postmenopausal and particularly having had early menopause

- normal absence of menstrual periods (amenorrhea)

- prolonged use of certain medications, such as those used to treat lupus, asthma, thyroid deficiencies, and seizures

- low calcium intake

- lack of physical activity

- smoking

- excessive alcohol intake

Osteoporosis often can be prevented. It is known as a "silent disease" because, if undetected, bone loss can progress for many years without symptoms until a fracture occurs. Osteoporosis has been called a childhood disease with old age consequences because building healthy bones in youth helps prevent osteoporosis and fractures later in life. However, it is never too late to adopt new habits for healthy bones.

The Link between Lupus and Osteoporosis

Studies have found an increase in bone loss and fracture in individuals with SLE. Individuals with lupus are at increased risk for osteoporosis for many reasons. To begin with, the glucocorticoid medications often prescribed to treat SLE can trigger significant bone loss. In addition, pain and fatigue caused by the disease can result in inactivity, further increasing osteoporosis risk. Studies also show that bone loss in lupus may occur as a direct result of the disease. Of concern is the fact that 90 percent of the people affected with lupus are women, a group already at increased risk for osteoporosis.

Osteoporosis Management Strategies

Strategies for the prevention and treatment of osteoporosis in people with lupus are not significantly different from the strategies for those who do not have the disease.

- **Nutrition.** A well-balanced diet rich in calcium and vitamin D is important for healthy bones. Good sources of calcium include low-fat dairy products; dark green, leafy vegetables; and calcium-fortified foods and beverages. Supplements can help ensure that you get adequate amounts of calcium each day, especially in people with a proven milk allergy. The Institute of Medicine (IOM) recommends a daily calcium intake of 1,000 mg (milligrams) for men and women up to age 50. Women over age 50 and men over age 70 should increase their intake to 1,200 mg daily.

  Vitamin D plays an important role in calcium absorption and bone health. Food sources of vitamin D include egg yolks, saltwater fish, and liver. Many people obtain enough vitamin D naturally, but some individuals may need vitamin D supplements to achieve the recommended intake of 600–800 IU (International Units) each day.

- **Exercise.** Like muscle, bone is living tissue that responds to exercise by becoming stronger. The best activity for your bones is a weight-bearing exercise that forces you to work against gravity. Some examples include walking, climbing stairs, weight training, and dancing.

  Exercising can be challenging for people with lupus who are affected by joint pain and inflammation, muscle pain, and fatigue. However, regular exercise, such as walking, may help prevent bone loss and provide many other health benefits.

- **Healthy lifestyle.** Smoking is bad for bones as well as the heart and lungs. Women who smoke tend to go through menopause earlier, resulting in earlier reduction in levels of the bone-preserving hormone estrogen and triggering earlier bone loss. In addition, smokers may absorb less calcium from their diets. Alcohol also can have a negative effect on bone health. Those who drink heavily are more prone to bone loss and fracture, both because of poor nutrition and an increased risk of falling.

- **Bone density test.** A bone mineral density (BMD) test measures bone density at various parts of the body. This safe and painless test can detect osteoporosis before a fracture occurs and predict one's chances of fracturing in the future. Lupus patients, particularly those receiving glucocorticoid therapy for 2 months or more, should talk to their doctors about whether they might be candidates for a bone density test. The BMD test can help determine whether medication should be considered.

* **Medication.** Like lupus, osteoporosis is a disease with no cure. However, several medications are available for the prevention and/or treatment of osteoporosis, including: bisphosphonates; estrogen agonists/antagonists (also called selective estrogen receptor modulators or SERMS); calcitonin; parathyroid hormone; estrogen therapy; hormone therapy; and a receptor activator of nuclear factor-κB ligand (RANKL) inhibitor.

Section 16.3

Lupus and Women

This section contains text excerpted from the following sources:
Text beginning with the heading "What Is Lupus?" is excerpted from "Lupus and Women," Office on Women's Health (OWH), U.S. Department of Health and Human Services (HHS), May 25, 2017; Text under the heading "Lupus Symptoms" is excerpted from "Lupus Symptoms," Office on Women's Health (OWH), U.S. Department of Health and Human Services (HHS), May 25, 2017; Text under the heading "Lupus Diagnosis and Treatment" is excerpted from "Lupus Diagnosis and Treatment," Office on Women's Health (OWH), U.S. Department of Health and Human Services (HHS), May 25, 2017.

What Is Lupus?

Lupus is a chronic (lifelong) autoimmune disease that can damage any part of the body. With autoimmune diseases, the body's immune (defense) system cannot tell the difference between viruses, bacteria, and other germs and the body's healthy cells, tissues, or organs. Because of this, the immune system attacks and destroys these healthy cells, tissues, or organs.

What Are the Different Types of Lupus?

There are several different types of lupus:

- **Systemic lupus erythematosus (SLE)** is the most common and most serious type of lupus. SLE affects all parts of the body.

- **Cutaneous lupus erythematosus (CLE)**, which affects only the skin

- **Drug-induced lupus,** a short-term type of lupus caused by certain medicines

- **Neonatal lupus,** a rare type of lupus that affect newborn babies

What Is Systemic Lupus Erythematosus (SLE)?

SLE is the most common type of lupus. SLE can be mild or severe and can affect different parts of the body. Common symptoms include fatigue, hair loss, sun sensitivity, painful and swollen joints, unexplained fever, skin rashes, and kidney problems.

There is no one test for SLE. Usually your doctor will ask you about your family and personal medical history and your symptoms. Your doctor will also do some laboratory tests.

What Is Cutaneous Lupus Erythematosus (CLE)?

This type of lupus is a skin disease that can affect people with or without SLE. "Cutaneous" means "skin." Symptoms may include rashes, hair loss, swelling of the blood vessels, ulcers, and sun sensitivity. To find out if you have cutaneous lupus and what kind it is, your doctor will remove a small piece of the rash or sore and look at it under a microscope.

There are two major kinds of cutaneous lupus:

- **Discoid lupus erythematosus (DLE).** A discoid rash usually begins as a red raised rash that becomes scaly or changes color to a dark brown. These rashes often appear on the face and scalp, but they may affect other areas. Many people with DLE have scarring. Sometimes DLE causes sores in the mouth or nose. If you have DLE, there is a small chance that you will later get SLE.

- **Subacute cutaneous lupus erythematosus** causes skin lesions that appear on parts of the body exposed to sun. These lesions do not cause scars.

What Is Drug-Induced Lupus?

Drug-induced lupus is caused by certain medicines. The symptoms of drug-induced lupus are like those of SLE, such as joint pain, muscle pain, and fever. But symptoms are usually not as serious. Also, drug-induced lupus rarely affects major organs. Most often, the disease goes away when the medicine is stopped.

The medicines that most commonly cause drug-induced lupus are used to treat other chronic health problems. These include seizures, high blood pressure, or rheumatoid arthritis. But not everyone who takes these medicines will get drug-induced lupus.

What Is Neonatal Lupus?

Neonatal lupus is a rare condition in infants that is caused by certain antibodies from the mother. These antibodies can be found in mothers who have lupus. But, if you have lupus, this does not mean you will definitely pass it to your baby. Most infants of mothers with lupus are healthy.

It is also possible for an infant to have neonatal lupus even though the mother does not have lupus currently. But, if a baby is born with lupus, often the mother will develop lupus later in life.

At birth, an infant with neonatal lupus may have a skin rash, liver problems, or low blood cell counts. These symptoms often go away completely after several months and have no lasting effects. Infants with neonatal lupus also can have a rare but serious heart defect.

Who Gets Lupus

Anyone can get lupus. It is difficult to know how many people in the United States have lupus, because the symptoms are different for every person. It is estimated that 1.5 million Americans have lupus. Other estimates range from 161,000 to 322,000 Americans with systemic lupus erythematosus (SLE).

About 9 out of 10 diagnoses of lupus are in women ages 15–44.

How Does Lupus Affect Women?

Lupus is most common in women ages 15–44, or during the years they can have children. Having lupus raises your risk of other health problems. Lupus can also make these problems happen earlier in life compared to women who do not have lupus.

These health problems include:

- **Heart disease.** Lupus raises the risk of the most common type of heart disease, called coronary artery disease (CAD). This is partly because people with lupus have more CAD risk factors, which include high blood pressure, high cholesterol, and type 2 diabetes. Lupus causes inflammation (swelling), which also increases the risk for CAD. Women with lupus may be less active because of fatigue, joint problems, and muscle pain, and this also puts them at risk for heart disease. In one study, women with lupus were 50 times more likely to have chest pain or a heart attack than other women of the same age.

- **Osteoporosis.** Medicines that treat lupus may cause bone loss. Bone loss can lead to osteoporosis, a condition that causes weak and broken bones. Also, pain and fatigue can keep women with lupus from getting physical activity. Staying active can help prevent bone loss.

- **Kidney disease.** More than half of all people with lupus have kidney problems, called lupus nephritis. Kidney problems often begin within the first five years after lupus symptoms start to appear. This is one of the more serious complications of lupus. Also, kidney inflammation is not usually painful so you don't know when it's happening. That is why it's important for people with lupus to get regular urine and blood tests for kidney disease. Treatment for lupus nephritis works best if caught early.

How Does Lupus Affect Women of Color?

African-American women are three times more likely to get lupus than white women. Lupus is also more common in Hispanic, Asian, and Native American and Alaskan Native women.

African-American and Hispanic women usually get lupus at a younger age and have more severe symptoms, including kidney problems, than women of other groups. African American with lupus also have more problems with seizures, strokes, and dangerous swelling of the heart. Hispanic women with lupus also have more heart problems than women of other groups. Researchers think that genes play a role in how lupus affects minority women.

What Causes Lupus

Researchers are still studying possible causes of lupus. We do know that lupus is not a disease you can catch from someone else. Genes play an important role but are not the only reason a person will get lupus. Even someone with one or more of the genes associated with lupus has only a small chance of actually getting the disease. Researchers are studying possible causes such as:

- The environment. Sunlight, stress, smoking, certain medicines, and viruses may trigger symptoms in people who are most likely to get lupus due to their genes.

- Hormones such as estrogen. Lupus is more common in women during their childbearing years when estrogen levels are highest.

- Problems with the immune system.

Lupus Symptoms

Lupus symptoms also usually come and go, meaning that you don't have them all of the time. Lupus is a disease of flares (the symptoms worsen and you feel ill) and remissions (the symptoms improve and you feel better).

Lupus symptoms include:

- **Muscle and joint pain.** You may experience pain and stiffness, with or without swelling. This affects most people with lupus. Common areas for muscle pain and swelling include the neck, thighs, shoulders, and upper arms.

- **Fever.** A fever higher than 100 degrees Fahrenheit affects many people with lupus. The fever is often caused by inflammation or infection. Lupus medicine can help manage and prevent fever.

- **Rashes.** You may get rashes on any part of your body that is exposed to the sun, such as your face, arms, and hands. One common sign of lupus is a red, butterfly-shaped rash across the nose and cheeks.

- **Chest pain.** Lupus can trigger inflammation in the lining of the lungs. This causes chest pain when breathing deeply.

- **Hair loss.** Patchy or bald spots are common. Hair loss could also be caused by some medicines or infection.

- **Sun or light sensitivity.** Most people with lupus are sensitive to light, a condition called photosensitivity. Exposure to light can cause rashes, fever, fatigue, or joint pain in some people with lupus.

- **Kidney problems.** Half of people with lupus also have kidney problems, called lupus nephritis. Symptoms include weight gain, swollen ankles, high blood pressure, and decreased kidney function.

- **Mouth sores.** Also called ulcers, these sores usually appear on the roof of the mouth, but can also appear in the gums, inside the cheeks, and on the lips. They may be painless, or you may have soreness or dry mouth.

- **Prolonged or extreme fatigue.** You may feel tired or exhausted even when you get enough sleep. Fatigue can also be a warning sign of a lupus flare.

- **Anemia.** Fatigue could be a sign of anemia, a condition that happens when your body does not have red blood cells to carry oxygen throughout your body.

- **Memory problems.** Some people with lupus report problems with forgetfulness or confusion.

- **Blood clotting.** You may have a higher risk of blood clotting. This can cause blood clots in the legs or lungs, stroke, heart attack, or repeated miscarriages.

- **Eye disease.** You may get dry eyes, eye inflammation, and eye-lid rashes.

Lupus Diagnosis and Treatment

How Is Lupus Diagnosed?

Lupus can be hard to diagnose because it has many symptoms that are often mistaken for symptoms of other diseases. Many people have lupus for a while before they find out they have it. If you have symptoms of lupus, tell your doctor right away.

No single test can tell if a person has lupus. But your doctor can find out if you have lupus in other ways, including:

- **Medical history.** Tell your doctor about your symptoms and other problems. Keep track of your symptoms by writing them down when they happen. Also, track how long they last.

- **Family history of lupus or other autoimmune diseases.** Tell your doctor if lupus or other autoimmune diseases run in your family.

- **Complete physical exam.** Your doctor will look for rashes and other signs that something is wrong.

- **Blood and urine tests.** The antinuclear antibody (ANA) test can show if your immune system is more likely to make the autoantibodies of lupus. Most people with lupus test positive for ANA. But, a positive ANA does not always mean you have lupus. If you test positive for ANA, your doctor will likely order more tests for antibodies that are specific to systemic lupus erythematosus (SLE).

- **Skin or kidney biopsy.** A biopsy is a minor surgery to remove a sample of tissue. The tissue is then viewed under a microscope. Skin and kidney tissue looked at in this way can show signs of an autoimmune disease.

Your doctor may use any or all of these tests to make your diagnosis. They also can help your doctor rule out other diseases that can be confused with lupus.

How Is Lupus Treated?

There is no cure for lupus but treatments can help you feel better and improve your symptoms. Your treatment will depend on your symptoms and needs. The goals of treatment are to:

- Prevent flares

- Treat symptoms when they happen

- Reduce organ damage and other problems

Your treatment might include medicines to:

- Reduce swelling and pain

- Calm your immune system to prevent it from attacking the organs and tissues in your body

- Reduce or prevent damage to the joints

- Reduce or prevent organ damage

What Types of Medicines Treat Lupus?

Several different types of medicines treat lupus. Your doctors and nurses may change the medicine they prescribe for your lupus as your symptoms and needs change.

Types of medicines commonly used to treat lupus include:

- **Nonsteroidal anti-inflammatory drugs (NSAIDs).** Over-the-counter NSAIDs, such as ibuprofen and naproxen, help reduce mild pain and swelling in joints and muscles.

- **Corticosteroids.** Corticosteroids (prednisone) may help reduce swelling, tenderness, and pain. In high doses, they can calm the immune system. Corticosteroids, sometimes just called "steroids," come in different forms: pills, a shot, or a cream to apply to the skin. Lupus symptoms usually respond very quickly to these powerful drugs. Once this has happened, your doctor will lower your dose slowly until you no longer need it. The longer a person uses these drugs, the harder it becomes to lower the dose. Stopping this medicine suddenly can harm your body.

- **Antimalarial drugs.** Medicines that prevent or treat malaria also treat joint pain, skin rashes, fatigue, and lung inflammation. Two common antimalarial medicines are hydroxychloroquine (Plaquenil) and chloroquine phosphate (Aralen). Studies found that taking antimalarial medicine can stop lupus flares and may help people with lupus live longer.

- **BLyS-specific inhibitors.** These drugs limit the amount of abnormal B cells (cells in the immune system that create antibodies) found in people with lupus. A common type of BLyS-specific inhibitor that treats lupus symptoms, belimumab, blocks the action of a specific protein in the body that is important in immune response.

- **Immunosuppressive agents/chemotherapy.** These medicines may be used in severe cases of lupus, when lupus affects major organs and other treatments do not work. These medicines can cause serious side effects because they lower the body's ability to fight off infections.

- **Other medicines.** You may need other medicines to treat illnesses or diseases that are linked to your lupus — such as high blood pressure or osteoporosis. Many people with lupus are also at risk for blood clots, which can cause a stroke or heart attack. Your doctor may prescribe anticoagulants ("blood thinners"), such as warfarin or heparin, to prevent your blood from clotting too easily. You cannot take warfarin during pregnancy.

Talk to your doctor:

- About any side effects you may have
- If your medicines no longer help your symptoms
- If you have new symptoms
- If you want to become pregnant
- About any vitamins or herbal supplements you take — they might not mix well with medicines you use to treat lupus

Can I Treat My Lupus with Alternative Medicine?

Some people with lupus try creams, ointments, fish oil, or supplements they can buy without a prescription. Some people try homeopathy or see a chiropractor to care for their lupus. Some people with lupus who try these types of treatments say that they help.

Research studies have not shown any benefits to these types of treatments. And research studies have not been done to see if these treatments hurt people with lupus.

Talk to your doctor or nurse before trying any alternative medicine. Also, don't stop or change your prescribed treatment without first talking to your doctor or nurse.

Will I Need to See a Special Doctor for My Lupus?

Maybe. Start by seeing your family doctor and a rheumatologist, a doctor who specializes in the diseases of joints and muscles such as lupus. Depending on your symptoms or whether your organs have been hurt by your lupus, you may need to see other types of doctors. These may include nephrologists, who treat kidney problems, and clinical immunologists, who treat immune system disorders.

Can I Die from Lupus?

Yes, lupus can cause death. But, thanks to new and better treatments, most people with lupus can expect to live long, healthy lives. The leading causes of death in people with lupus are health problems that are related to lupus, such as kidney disease, infections, and heart disease.

Work with your doctor to manage lupus. Take your medicine as your doctor tells you to and make healthy choices, such as not smoking, eating healthy foods, getting regular physical activity, and managing your weight.

What Research Is Being Done on Lupus?

Research on lupus focuses on:

- The genes that play a role in lupus and in the immune system
- Ways to change the immune system in people with lupus
- Different symptoms and effects of lupus in different racial and ethnic groups
- Things in the environment that may cause lupus
- The role of hormones in lupus
- Birth control pills and hormone therapy use in women with lupus
- Heart disease in people with lupus
- The causes of nervous system damage in people with lupus
- Treatments for lupus
- Treatments for organ damage caused by lupus, including stem cell transplantation
- Getting a better idea of how many Americans have lupus

Chapter 17

Myositis

Myositis means inflammation of the muscles that you use to move your body. An injury, infection, or autoimmune disease can cause it. Two specific kinds are polymyositis and dermatomyositis. Polymyositis causes muscle weakness, usually in the muscles closest to the trunk of your body. Dermatomyositis causes muscle weakness, plus a skin rash.

Other symptoms of myositis may include

- Fatigue after walking or standing

- Tripping or falling

- Trouble swallowing or breathing

Doctors may use a physical exam, lab tests, imaging tests and a muscle biopsy to diagnose myositis. There is no cure for these diseases, but you can treat the symptoms. Polymyositis and dermatomyositis are first treated with high doses of a corticosteroid. Other options include medications, physical therapy, exercise, heat therapy, assistive devices, and rest.

This chapter contains text excerpted from the following sources: Text in this chapter begins with excerpts from "Myositis," MedlinePlus, National Institutes of Health (NIH), April 17, 2016; Text under the heading "Dermatomyositis" is excerpted from "Dermatomyositis Information Page," National Institute of Neurological Disorders and Stroke (NINDS), May 25, 2017; Text under the heading "Polymyositis" is excerpted from "Polymyositis Information Page," National Institute of Neurological Disorders and Stroke (NINDS), December 4, 2017.

Dermatomyositis

Dermatomyositis is one of a group of muscle diseases known as the inflammatory myopathies, which are characterized by chronic muscle inflammation accompanied by muscle weakness. Dermatomyositis' cardinal symptom is a skin rash that precedes, accompanies, or follows progressive muscle weakness. The rash looks patchy, with purple or red discolorations, and characteristically develops on the eyelids and on muscles used to extend or straighten joints, including knuckles, elbows, knees, and toes. Red rashes may also occur on the face, neck, shoulders, upper chest, back, and other locations, and there may be swelling in the affected areas. The rash sometimes occurs without obvious muscle involvement. Adults with dermatomyositis may experience weight loss, a low-grade fever, inflamed lungs, and be sensitive to light such that the rash or muscle disease gets worse. Children and adults with dermatomyositis may develop calcium deposits, which appear as hard bumps under the skin or in the muscle (called calcinosis). Calcinosis most often occurs 1–3 years after the disease begins. These deposits are seen more often in children with dermatomyositis than in adults. In some cases of dermatomyositis, distal muscles (muscles located away from the trunk of the body, such as those in the forearms and around the ankles and wrists) may be affected as the disease progresses. Dermatomyositis may be associated with collagen-vascular or autoimmune diseases, such as lupus.

Treatment

There is no cure for dermatomyositis, but the symptoms can be treated. Options include medication, physical therapy, exercise, heat therapy (including microwave and ultrasound), orthotics and assistive devices, and rest. The standard treatment for dermatomyositis is a corticosteroid drug, given either in pill form or intravenously. Immunosuppressant drugs, such as azathioprine and methotrexate, may reduce inflammation in people who do not respond well to prednisone. Periodic treatment using intravenous immunoglobulin can also improve recovery. Other immunosuppressive agents used to treat the inflammation associated with dermatomyositis include cyclosporine A, cyclophosphamide, and tacrolimus. Physical therapy is usually recommended to prevent muscle atrophy and to regain muscle strength and range of motion. Many individuals with dermatomyositis may need a topical ointment, such as topical corticosteroids, for their skin disorder. They should wear a high-protection sunscreen and protective clothing. Surgery may be required to remove calcium deposits that cause nerve pain and recurrent infections.

Prognosis

Most cases of dermatomyositis respond to therapy. The disease is usually more severe and resistant to therapy in individuals with cardiac or pulmonary problems.

Polymyositis

Polymyositis is one of a group of muscle diseases known as the inflammatory myopathies, which are characterized by chronic muscle inflammation accompanied by muscle weakness. Polymyositis affects skeletal muscles (those involved with making movement) on both sides of the body. It is rarely seen in persons under age 18; most cases are in adults between the ages of 31–60. Progressive muscle weakness starts in the proximal muscles (muscles closest to the trunk of the body) which eventually leads to difficulties climbing stairs, rising from a seated position, lifting objects, or reaching overhead. People with polymyositis may also experience arthritis, shortness of breath, difficulty swallowing and speaking, and heart arrhythmias. In some cases of polymyositis, distal muscles (muscles further away from the trunk of the body, such as those in the forearms and around the ankles and wrists) may be affected as the disease progresses. Polymyositis may be associated with collagen-vascular or autoimmune diseases, such as lupus. It may also be associated with infectious disorders, such as human immunodeficiency virus infection (HIV) and acquired immunodeficiency syndrome (AIDS).

Treatment

There is no cure for polymyositis, but the symptoms can be treated. Options include medication, physical and occupational therapy, exercise, heat therapy (including microwave and ultrasound), orthotics and assistive devices, and rest. The standard treatment for polymyositis is a corticosteroid drug, given either in pill form or intravenously. Immunosuppressant drugs, such as azathioprine and methotrexate, may reduce inflammation in people who do not respond well to prednisone. Periodic treatment using intravenous immunoglobulin can also improve recovery. Other immunosuppressive agents used to treat the inflammation associated with polymyositis include cyclosporine A, cyclophosphamide, and tacrolimus. Physical therapy is usually recommended to prevent muscle atrophy and to regain muscle strength and range of motion. Occupational therapists can prepare an assessment of daily activities to help address issues such as bathing and eating.

Prognosis

The prognosis for polymyositis varies. Most people respond fairly well to therapy, but some have a more severe disease that does not respond adequately to therapies and are left with significant disability. In rare cases, individuals with severe and progressive muscle weakness will develop respiratory failure or pneumonia. Difficulty swallowing may cause weight loss and malnutrition.

Chapter 18

Osteoporosis

Chapter Contents

Section 18.1—Understanding Osteoporosis 186

Section 18.2—Osteoporosis and Arthritis: Two
Common But Different Conditions..................... 204

Section 18.3—What People with RA Need to Know
about Osteoporosis 207

Section 18.4—Osteoporosis in Women....................................... 210

Section 18.5—Osteoporosis in Men.. 220

Section 18.6—Osteoporosis in Aging 227

Section 18.1

Understanding Osteoporosis

This section includes text excerpted from "Handout on
Health: Osteoporosis," NIH Osteoporosis and
Related Bone Diseases~National Resource Center
(NIH ORBD~NRC), February 2016.

Osteoporosis is a disease marked by reduced bone strength leading
to an increased risk of fractures, or broken bones. Bone strength has
two main features: bone mass (amount of bone) and bone quality. Osteoporosis is the major underlying cause of fractures in postmenopausal
women and the elderly. Fractures occur most often in bones of the hip,
spine, and wrist, but any bone can be affected. Some fractures can be
permanently disabling, especially when they occur in the hip.

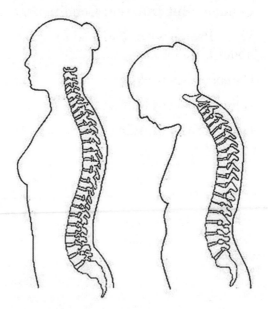

Figure 18.1. *Osteoporosis in the Vertebrae* (Source: "Osteoporosis," Office
on Women's Health (OWH), U.S. Department of Health and Human Services (HHS).)

Osteoporosis is often called a "silent disease," because it usually progresses without any symptoms until a fracture occurs or one or more vertebrae (bones in the spine) collapse. Collapsed vertebrae may first be felt or seen when a person develops severe back pain, loss of height, or spine malformations such as a stooped or hunched posture.

Bones affected by osteoporosis may become so fragile that fractures occur spontaneously or as the result of minor bumps, falls, or normal stresses and strains such as bending, lifting, or even coughing.

Many people think that osteoporosis is a natural and unavoidable part of aging. However, medical experts now believe that osteoporosis is largely preventable. Furthermore, people who already have osteoporosis can take steps to prevent or slow further progress of the disease and reduce their risk of future fractures. Although osteoporosis was once viewed primarily as a disease of old age, it is now recognized as a disease that can stem from less than optimal bone growth during childhood and adolescence, as well as from bone loss later in life.

Who Has Osteoporosis

In the United States, more than 53 million people either already have osteoporosis or are at high risk due to low bone mass. Osteoporosis can occur at any age, although the risk for developing the disease increases as you get older.

Osteoporosis is most common in non-Hispanic white women, but the disease affects many older Americans of any race or sex.

In addition to the financial costs, osteoporosis takes a toll in terms of reduced quality of life for many people who suffer fractures. It can also affect the lives of family members and friends who serve as caregivers.

Of all fractures, hip fractures have the most serious impact. Most hip fractures require hospitalization and surgery; some hip fracture patients require nursing home placement. One in three adults who lived independently before their hip fracture remains in a nursing home for at least a year after their injury. About one in five hip fracture patients over age 50 die in the year following their fracture as a result of associated medical complications. Vertebral fractures also can have serious consequences, including chronic back pain and disability. They have also been linked to increased mortality in older people.

Bone Basics

Bone is a living tissue that supports our muscles, protects vital internal organs, and stores most of the body's calcium. It consists mainly of a framework of tough, elastic fibers of a protein called collagen and crystals of calcium phosphate mineral that harden and strengthen the framework. The combination of collagen and calcium phosphate makes bones strong yet flexible to hold up under stress.

Bone also contains living cells, including some that nourish the tissue and others that control the process known as bone remodeling. Throughout life, our bones are constantly being renewed by means of this remodeling process, in which old bone is removed (bone resorption) and replaced by new bone (bone formation). Bone remodeling is carried out through the coordinated actions of bone-removing cells called osteoclasts and bone-forming cells called osteoblasts.

During childhood and the teenage years, new bone is added to the skeleton faster than old bone is removed or resorbed. As a result, bones grow in both size and strength. After you stop growing taller, bone formation continues at a faster pace than resorption until around the early twenties, when women and men reach their peak bone mass, or maximum amount of bone. Peak bone mass is influenced by various genetic and external, or environmental, factors, including whether you are male or female (your sex), hormones, nutrition, and physical activity. Genetic factors may determine as much as 50–90 percent of bone mass; environmental factors account for the remaining 10–50 percent. This means you have some control over your peak bone mass.

After your early twenties, your bone mass may remain stable or decrease very gradually for a period of years, depending on a variety of lifestyle factors such as diet and physical activity. Starting in midlife, both men and women experience an age-related decline in bone mass. Women lose bone rapidly in the first 4–8 years after menopause (the completion of a full year without a menstrual period), which usually occurs between ages 45–55. By age 65, men and women tend to be losing bone tissue at the same rate, and this more gradual bone loss continues throughout life.

Causes of Osteoporosis

Less than optimal bone growth during childhood and adolescence can result in a failure to reach optimal peak bone mass. Thus, peak bone mass attained early in life is an important factor affecting your risk of osteoporosis in later years. People who start out with greater reserves of bone (higher peak bone mass) are less likely to develop osteoporosis when bone loss occurs as a result of aging, menopause, or other factors. Other causes of osteoporosis are bone loss due to a greater than expected rate of bone resorption, a decreased rate of bone formation, or both.

A major contributor to bone loss in women during later life is the reduction in estrogen production that occurs with menopause. Estrogen is a sex hormone that plays a critical role in building and maintaining bone. Decreased estrogen, whether due to natural menopause, surgical removal of the ovaries, or chemotherapy or radiation treatments for cancer, can lead to bone loss and eventually osteoporosis. After menopause, the rate of bone loss speeds up as the amount of estrogen produced by a woman's ovaries drops dramatically. Bone loss is most rapid in the first few years after menopause but continues into the postmenopausal years.

In men, sex hormone levels also decline after middle age, but the decline is more gradual. These declines probably also contribute to bone loss in men after around age 50.

Osteoporosis can also result from bone loss that may accompany a wide range of disease conditions, eating disorders, and certain medications and medical treatments. For instance, osteoporosis may be caused by long-term use of some antiseizure medications (anticonvulsants) and glucocorticoid medications such as prednisone and cortisone. Glucocorticoids are anti-inflammatory drugs used to treat many diseases, including rheumatoid arthritis (RA), lupus, asthma, and Crohn's disease. Other causes of osteoporosis include alcoholism, anorexia nervosa, abnormally low levels of sex hormones, hyperthyroidism, kidney disease, and certain gastrointestinal (GI) disorders. Sometimes osteoporosis results from a combination of causes.

Risk Factors for Osteoporosis

Factors that are linked to the development of osteoporosis or contribute to an individual's likelihood of developing the disease are called risk factors. Many people with osteoporosis have several risk factors for the disease, but others who develop osteoporosis have no identified risk factors. There are some risk factors that you cannot change, and others that you can or may be able to change.

Risk Factors You Cannot Change

- **Sex:** Your chances of developing osteoporosis are greater if you are a woman. Women have lower peak bone mass and smaller bones than men. They also lose bone more rapidly than men in middle age because of the dramatic reduction in estrogen levels that occurs with menopause.

- **Age:** The older you are, the greater your risk of osteoporosis. Bone loss builds up over time, and your bones become weaker as you age.

- **Body size:** Slender, thin-boned women are at greater risk, as are, surprisingly, taller women.

- **Race:** Caucasian (white) women are at highest risk, but the disease affects many older Americans of any race or sex.

- **Family history:** Susceptibility to osteoporosis and fractures appears to be, in part, hereditary. People whose parents have a history of fractures also tend to have reduced bone mass and an increased risk for fractures.

Risk Factors You Can or May Be Able to Change

- **Sex hormone deficiencies:** The most common manifestation of estrogen deficiency in premenopausal women is amenorrhea, the abnormal absence of menstrual periods. Missed or irregular periods can be caused by various factors, including hormonal disorders as well as extreme levels of physical activity combined with restricted calorie intake—for example, in female marathon runners, ballet dancers, and women who spend a great deal of time and energy working out at the gym. Low estrogen levels in women after menopause and low testosterone levels in men also increase the risk of osteoporosis. Lower than normal estrogen levels in men may also play a role. Low testosterone and estrogen levels are often a cause of osteoporosis in men being treated with certain medications for prostate cancer.

- **Diet:** From childhood into old age, a diet low in calcium and vitamin D can increase your risk of osteoporosis and fractures. Excessive dieting or inadequate caloric intake can also be bad for bone health. People who are very thin and do not have much body fat to cushion falls have an increased risk of fracture.

- **Certain medical conditions:** In addition to sex hormone problems and eating disorders, other medical conditions—including a variety of genetic, endocrine, gastrointestinal, blood, and rheumatic disorders—are associated with an increased risk for osteoporosis. Anorexia nervosa, for example, is an eating disorder that leads to abnormally low body weight, malnutrition, amenorrhea, and other effects on the body that adversely affect bone health. Late onset of puberty and early menopause reduce lifetime estrogen exposure in women and also increase the risk of osteoporosis.

- **Medications:** Long-term use of certain medications, including glucocorticoids and some anticonvulsants, leads to bone loss and increased risk of osteoporosis. Other drugs that may lead to bone loss include anticlotting drugs, such as heparin; drugs that suppress the immune system, such as cyclosporine; and drugs used to treat prostate cancer.

- **An inactive lifestyle or extended bed rest:** Low levels of physical activity and prolonged periods of inactivity can contribute to an increased rate of bone loss. They also leave you in poor physical condition, which can increase your risk of falling and breaking a bone.

- **Excessive use of alcohol:** Chronic heavy drinking is a significant risk factor for osteoporosis.

- **Smoking:** Most studies indicate that smoking is a risk factor for osteoporosis and fracture, although the exact reasons for the harmful effects of tobacco use on bone health are unclear.

Diagnosing Osteoporosis

Diagnosing osteoporosis involves several steps, starting with a physical exam and a careful medical history, blood and urine tests, and possibly a bone mineral density assessment. When recording information about your medical history, your doctor will ask questions to find out whether you have risk factors for osteoporosis and fractures. The doctor may ask about any fractures you have had, your lifestyle (including diet, exercise habits, and whether you smoke), current or past health problems and medications that could contribute to low bone mass and increased fracture risk, your family history of osteoporosis and other diseases, and, for women, your menstrual history. The doctor will also do a physical exam that should include checking for loss of height and changes in posture and may include checking your balance and gait (the way you walk).

If you have back pain or have experienced a loss in height or a change in posture, the doctor may request an X-ray of your spine to look for spinal fractures or malformations due to osteoporosis. However, X-rays cannot necessarily detect osteoporosis. The results of laboratory tests of blood and urine samples can help your doctor identify conditions that may be contributing to bone loss, such as hormonal problems or vitamin D deficiency. If the results of your physical exam, medical history, X-rays, or laboratory tests indicate that you may have osteoporosis or that you have significant risk factors for the disease, your doctor may recommend a bone density test.

Mineral is what gives hardness to bones, and the density of mineral in the bones is an important determinant of bone strength. Bone mineral density (BMD) testing can be used to definitively diagnose osteoporosis, detect low bone mass before osteoporosis develops, and help predict your risk of future fractures. In general, the lower your bone density, the higher your risk for fracture. The results of a bone density test will help guide decisions about starting therapy to prevent or treat osteoporosis. BMD testing may also be used to monitor the effectiveness of ongoing therapy.

The most widely recognized test for measuring bone mineral density is a quick, painless, noninvasive technology known as central dual-energy X-ray absorptiometry (DXA). This technique, which uses low levels of X-rays, involves passing a scanner over your body while you are lying on a cushioned table. DXA can be used to determine BMD of the entire skeleton and at various sites that are prone to fractures, such as the hip, spine, or wrist. Bone density measurement by DXA at the hip and spine is generally considered the most reliable way to diagnose osteoporosis and predict fracture risk.

The doctor will compare your BMD test results to the average bone density of young, healthy people and to the average bone density of other people of your age, sex, and race. For both women and men, the diagnosis of osteoporosis using DXA measurements of BMD is currently based on a number called a T-score. Your T-score represents the extent to which your bone density differs from the average bone density of young, healthy people. If you are diagnosed with osteoporosis or very low bone density, or if your bone density is below a certain level and you have other risk factors for fractures, the doctor will talk with you about options for treatment or prevention of osteoporosis.

The U.S. Preventive Services Task Force (USPSTF), an independent panel of experts in primary care and prevention, recommends that all women age 65 and older be screened for osteoporosis. The task force also recommends screening for women under the age of 65 who are at high risk for fractures. Men over the age 65 who are at high risk for fractures should talk to their doctor about screening. If you are over 50 and have broken a bone, you may have osteoporosis or be at increased risk for the disease. You should also ask your doctor about osteoporosis if you notice that you have lost height or your posture has become stooped or hunched, or if you experience sudden back pain.

You may also want to be evaluated for osteoporosis and fracture risk if you have a chronic disease or eating disorder known to increase the risk of osteoporosis, are taking one or more medications known to cause bone loss, or have multiple risk factors for osteoporosis and osteoporosis-related fractures.

When to Talk to Your Doctor about Osteoporosis

Consider talking to your doctor about being evaluated for osteoporosis if:

- You are a man or woman over age 50 or a postmenopausal woman and you break a bone

- You are a woman age 65 or older

- You are a woman younger than age 65 and at high risk for fractures

- You are a man age 65 or older and at high risk for fractures

- You have lost height, developed a stooped or hunched posture, or experienced sudden back pain with no apparent cause

- You have been taking glucocorticoid medications such as prednisone, cortisone, or dexamethasone for 2 months or longer or are taking other medications known to cause bone loss

- You have a chronic illness or are taking a medication that is known to cause bone loss

- You have anorexia nervosa or a history of this eating disorder

- You are a premenopausal woman, not pregnant, and your menstrual periods have stopped, are irregular, or never started when you reached puberty

Treating Osteoporosis

The primary goal in treating people with osteoporosis is preventing fractures. A comprehensive treatment program includes a focus on proper nutrition, exercise, and prevention of falls that may result in fractures.

Your doctor may also prescribe one of several medications that have been shown to slow or stop bone loss or build new bone, increase bone density, and reduce fracture risk. If you take medication to prevent or treat osteoporosis, it is still essential that you obtain the recommended amounts of calcium and vitamin D. Exercising and maintaining other aspects of a healthy lifestyle are also important.

For people with osteoporosis resulting from another condition, the best approach is to identify and treat the underlying cause. If you are taking a medication that causes bone loss, your doctor may be able to reduce the dose of that medication or switch you to another medication that is effective but not harmful to your bones. If you have a disease that requires long-term glucocorticoid therapy, such as RA or lupus, you can also take certain medications approved for the prevention or treatment of osteoporosis associated with aging or menopause. Staying as active as possible, eating a healthy diet that includes adequate calcium and vitamins, and avoiding smoking and excess alcohol use are also important for people with osteoporosis resulting from other conditions. Children and adolescents with such conditions as juvenile rheumatic diseases and asthma can also be diagnosed with this kind of osteoporosis.

Medical specialists who treat osteoporosis include family physicians, internists, endocrinologists, geriatricians, gynecologists, orthopedic surgeons, rheumatologists, and physiatrists (doctors specializing in physical medicine and rehabilitation). Physical and occupational therapists and nurses may also participate in the care of people with osteoporosis.

Nutrition

A healthy, balanced diet that includes plenty of fruits and vegetables; enough calories; and adequate calcium, vitamin D, and vitamin K is essential for minimizing bone loss and maintaining overall health. Calcium and vitamin D are especially important for bone health. Calcium is the most important nutrient for preventing osteoporosis and for reaching peak bone mass. For healthy postmenopausal women who are not consuming enough calcium (1,200 mg per day) in their diet, calcium and vitamin D supplements help to preserve bone mass and prevent hip fracture. Calcium is also needed for the heart, muscles, and nerves to work properly and for blood to clot normally. We take in calcium from our diet and lose it from the body mainly through urine, feces, and sweat. The body depends on dietary calcium to build healthy new bone and avoid excessive loss of calcium from bone to meet other needs. The Institute of Medicine (IOM) of the National Academy of Sciences (NAS) recommends specific amounts of dietary calcium and vitamin D for various stages of life. Men and women up to age 50 need 1,000 mg of calcium per day, and the recommendation increases to 1,200 mg for women after age 50 and for men after age 70.

Many people in the United States consume much less than the recommended amount of calcium in their diets. Good sources of calcium include low-fat dairy products; dark green leafy vegetables, including broccoli, bok choy, collards, and turnip greens; sardines and salmon with bones; soybeans, tofu, and other soy products; and calcium-fortified foods such as orange juice, cereals, and breads. If you have trouble getting enough calcium in your diet, you may need to take a calcium supplement such as calcium carbonate, calcium phosphate, or calcium citrate. If you are between the ages of 19–50, your daily calcium intake should not exceed 2,500 mg because too much calcium can cause problems such as kidney stones. (After age 50, intakes should not exceed 2,000 mg per day.) Calcium coming from food sources provides better protection from kidney stones. Anyone who has had a kidney stone should increase their dietary calcium and decrease the amount from supplements as well as increase fluid intake.

Vitamin D is required for proper absorption of calcium from the intestine. It is made in the skin after exposure to sunlight. Only a few foods naturally contain significant amounts of vitamin D, including fatty fish and fish oils. Foods fortified with vitamin D, such as milk and cereals, are a major dietary source of vitamin D. Although many people obtain enough vitamin D naturally, studies show that vitamin D production decreases in older adults, in people who are housebound, and during the winter—especially in northern latitudes. If you are at risk for vitamin D deficiency, you can take multivitamins or calcium supplements that contain vitamin D to meet the recommended daily intake of 600 International Units (IU) for men and women up to the age of 70 and 800 IU for people over 70. Doses of more than 2,000 IU per day are not advised unless under the supervision of a doctor. Larger doses can be given initially to people who are deficient as a way to replenish stores of vitamin D.

Lifestyle

In addition to a healthy diet, a healthy lifestyle is important for optimizing bone health. You should avoid smoking and, if you drink alcohol, do so in moderation (no more than one drink per day is a good general guideline). It is also important to recognize that some prescription medications can cause bone loss or increase your risk of falling and breaking a bone. Talk to your doctor if you have concerns about any medications you are taking.

Exercise

Exercise is an important part of an osteoporosis treatment program. Physical activity is needed to build and maintain bone throughout adulthood, and complete bed rest leads to serious bone loss. The evidence suggests that the most beneficial physical activities for bone health include strength training or resistance training. Exercise can help maintain or even modestly increase bone density in adulthood and, together with adequate calcium and vitamin D intake, can help minimize age-related bone loss in older people. Exercise of various sorts has other important benefits for people with osteoporosis. It can reduce your risk of falling by increasing muscle mass and strength and improving coordination and balance. In older people, exercise also improves function and delays loss of independence.

Although exercise is beneficial for people with osteoporosis, it should not put any sudden or excessive strain on your bones. If you have osteoporosis, you should avoid high impact exercise. To help ensure against fractures, a physical therapist or rehabilitation medicine specialist can recommend specific exercises to strengthen and support your back, teach you safe ways of moving and carrying out daily activities, and recommend an exercise program that is tailored to your circumstances. Other trained exercise specialists, such as exercise physiologists, may also be able to help you develop a safe and effective exercise program.

Fall Prevention

Fall prevention is a critical concern for men and women with osteoporosis. Falls increase your likelihood of fracturing a bone in the hip, wrist, spine, or other part of the skeleton. Fractures can affect your quality of life and lead to loss of independence and even premature death. A host of factors can contribute to your risk of falling.

Falls can be caused by impaired vision or balance, loss of muscle mass, and chronic or short-term illnesses that impair your mental or physical functioning. They can also be caused by the effects of certain medications, including sedatives or tranquilizers, sleeping pills, antidepressants, anticonvulsants, muscle relaxants, some heart medicines, blood pressure pills, and diuretics. Use of four or more prescription medications has also been shown to increase the risk for falling. Drinking alcoholic beverages is another risk factor. If you have osteoporosis, it is important to be aware of any physical changes you may be experiencing that affect your balance or gait and to discuss these changes with your doctor or other healthcare provider. It is also important to have regular checkups and tell your doctor if you have had problems with falling.

The force or impact of a fall (how hard you land) plays a major role in determining whether you will break a bone. Catching yourself so that you land on your hands or grabbing onto an object as you fall can prevent a hip fracture. You may break your wrist or arm instead, but the consequences are not as serious as if you break your hip. Studies have shown that wearing a specially designed garment that contains hip padding may reduce hip fractures resulting from falls in frail, elderly people living in nursing homes or residential care facilities, but use of the garments by residents is often low.

Falls can also be caused by factors in your environment that create unsafe conditions. Some tips to help eliminate the environmental factors that lead to falls include:

Outdoors and Away from Home

- Use a cane or walker for added stability

- Wear shoes that give good support and have thin nonslip soles. Avoid wearing slippers and athletic shoes with deep treads.

- Walk on grass when sidewalks are slippery; in winter, sprinkle salt or kitty litter on slippery sidewalks.

- Be careful on highly polished floors that are slick and dangerous, especially when wet, and walk on plastic or carpet runners when possible

- Stop at curbs and check their height before stepping up or down

Indoors

- Keep rooms free of clutter, especially on floors

- Keep floor surfaces smooth but not slippery

- Wear shoes that give good support and have thin nonslip soles. Avoid wearing slippers and athletic shoes with deep treads.

- Be sure carpets and area rugs have skid-proof backing or are tacked to the floor. Use double-stick tape to keep rugs from slipping.

- Be sure stairwells are well lit and that stairs have handrails

- Install grab bars on bathroom walls near tub, shower, and toilet

- Use a rubber bathmat or slip-proof seat in the shower or tub

- Improve the lighting in your home. Use a nightlight or flashlight if you get up at night.

- Use stepladders that are stable and have a handrail

- Install ceiling fixtures or lamps that can be turned on by a switch near the room's entrance

- If you live alone (or spend large amounts of time alone), consider purchasing a cordless phone; you won't have to rush to answer the phone when it rings and you can call for help if you do fall

- Consider having a personal emergency-response system; you can use it to call for help if you fall

Preventing Falls among Seniors

Falls are not just the result of getting older. Many falls can be prevented. Falls are usually caused by a number of things. By changing some of these things, you can lower your chances of falling:

Begin a regular exercise program. Exercise is one of the most important ways to reduce your chances of falling. It makes you stronger and helps you feel better. Exercises that improve balance and coordination (like tai chi) are the most helpful. Lack of exercise leads to weakness and increases your chances of falling. Ask your doctor or healthcare worker about the best type of exercise program for you.

Make your home safer. About half of all falls happen at home. To make your home safer:

- Remove things you can trip over (such as papers, books, clothes, and shoes) from stairs and places where you walk

- Remove small throw rugs or use double-sided tape to keep the rugs from slipping

- Keep items you use often in cabinets you can reach easily without using a step stool

- Have grab bars put in next to your toilet and in the tub or shower

- Use nonslip mats in the bathtub and on shower floors

- Improve the lighting in your home. As you get older, you need brighter lights to see well. Lamp shades or frosted bulbs can reduce glare.

- Have handrails and lights put in on all staircases

- Wear shoes that give good support and have thin nonslip soles. Avoid wearing slippers and athletic shoes with deep treads

Have your healthcare provider review your medicines. Have your doctor or pharmacist look at all the medicines you take (including the ones that don't need prescriptions, such as cold medicines). As you get older, the way some medicines work in your body can change. Some medicines, or combinations of medicines, can make you drowsy or lightheaded, which can lead to a fall.

Have your vision checked. Have your eyes checked by an eye doctor. You may be wearing the wrong glasses or have a condition such as glaucoma or cataracts that limits your vision. Poor vision can increase your chances of falling.

Medications

The U.S. Food and Drug Administration (FDA) has approved several medications for prevention or treatment of osteoporosis, based on their ability to reduce fractures.

*Medications Associated with Osteoporosis**

- Anticoagulants (heparin)

- Anticonvulsants (some)

- Aromatase inhibitors

- Cyclosporine A and tacrolimus

- Cancer chemotherapy drugs

- Glucocorticoids (and adrenocorticotropic hormone [ACTH])

- Gonadotropin-releasing hormone agonists

- Lithium

- Methotrexate

- Proton pump inhibitors

- Selective serotonin reuptake inhibitors (SSRIs)

- Thyroxine

Not an inclusive list

Side Effects of Medicines

All medicines can have side effects. Some medicines and side effects are mentioned in this publication. Some side effects may be more severe than others. You should review the package insert that comes with your medicine and ask your healthcare provider or pharmacist if you have any questions about the possible side effects.

Bisphosphonates. Several bisphosphonates are approved for the prevention or treatment of osteoporosis. These medications reduce the activity of cells that cause bone loss.

Parathyroid hormone. A form of human parathyroid hormone (PTH) is approved for postmenopausal women and men with osteoporosis who are at high risk for having a fracture. Use of the drug for more than 2 years is not recommended.

RANK ligand (RANKL) inhibitor. A RANK ligand (RANKL) inhibitor is approved for postmenopausal women with osteoporosis and men who are at high risk for fracture.

Estrogen agonists/antagonists. An estrogen agonist/antagonist (also called a selective estrogen receptor modulator or SERM) is approved for the prevention and treatment of osteoporosis in postmenopausal women. SERMs are not estrogens, but they have estrogen-like effects on some tissues and estrogen-blocking effects on other tissues.

Calcitonin. Calcitonin is approved for the treatment of osteoporosis in women who are at least 5 years beyond menopause. Calcitonin is a hormone involved in calcium regulation and bone metabolism.

Estrogen and hormone therapy. Estrogen and combined estrogen and progestin (hormone therapy) are approved for the prevention of postmenopausal osteoporosis as well as the treatment of moderate to severe hot flashes and vaginal dryness that may accompany menopause. Estrogen without an added progestin is recommended only for women who have had a hysterectomy (surgery to remove the uterus), because estrogen increases the risk of developing cancer of the uterine lining and progestin reduces that risk.

The FDA has recommended that women use hormone therapy at the lowest dose and for the shortest time, and carefully consider and discuss with their doctor other approved osteoporosis treatments.

Alternative Therapies

Isoflavones are naturally occurring compounds found in soybeans. Because they are structurally similar to estrogen, researchers have thought that they may hold promise as an alternative to estrogen therapy to protect postmenopausal women from osteoporosis. Several studies have explored the effects of soy isoflavones on bone health, but results have been mixed, ranging from a modest impact to no effect. Most of these studies had various limitations, including their short duration and small sample size, making it difficult to fully evaluate the impact of these compounds on bone health. Moreover, reports from National Institutes of Health (NIH)-supported clinical trials have failed to demonstrate a bone-sparing effect of soy isoflavones.

Preventing Osteoporosis

Preventing osteoporosis is a lifelong endeavor. To reach optimal peak bone mass and minimize loss of bone as you get older, there are several factors you should consider. Addressing all of these factors is the best way to optimize bone health throughout life.

An inadequate supply of calcium over a lifetime is thought to play a significant role in the development of osteoporosis.

Calcium

An inadequate supply of calcium over a lifetime is thought to play a significant role in the development of osteoporosis. Many published studies show that low calcium intakes are associated with low bone mass, rapid bone loss, and high fracture rates. National surveys suggest that the average calcium intake of individuals is far below the levels recommended for optimal bone health. Individuals who consume adequate amounts of calcium and vitamin D throughout life are more likely to achieve optimal skeletal mass early in life and are less likely to lose bone later in life.

Calcium needs change during your lifetime. The body's demand for calcium is greater during childhood and adolescence, when the skeleton is growing rapidly, and in women during pregnancy and breastfeeding. Postmenopausal women and older men also need to consume more calcium. Increased calcium requirements in older people may be related to vitamin D deficiencies that reduce intestinal absorption of calcium. Also, as you age, your body becomes less efficient at absorbing calcium and other nutrients. Older adults are also more likely to have chronic medical problems and to use medications that may impair calcium absorption. Calcium and vitamin D supplements may help slow bone loss and prevent hip fracture.

Adolescence is the most critical period for building bone mass that helps protect against osteoporosis later in life. Yet studies show that among children age 9–19 in the United States, few meet the recommended levels. Therefore, it is especially important for parents, other caregivers, and pediatricians to talk to children and young teens about developing bone-healthy habits, including eating calcium-rich foods and getting enough exercise.

Table 18.1. Recommended Calcium and Vitamin D Intakes

Life-Stage Group	Calcium (mg/day)	Vitamin D (IU/day)
Infants 0–6 months	200	400
Infants 6–12 months	260	400
1–3 years old	700	600
4–8 years old	1,000	600
9–13 years old	1,300	600
14–18 years old	1,300	600
19–30 years old	1,000	600
31–50 years old	1,000	600
51- to 70-year-old males	1,000	600
51- to 70-year-old females	1,200	600
>70 years old	1,200	800
14–18 years old, pregnant/lactating	1,300	600
19–50 years old, pregnant/lactating	1,000	600

Vitamin D

Vitamin D plays an important role in calcium absorption and bone health. It is made in the skin after exposure to sunlight and can also be obtained through the diet, as described in the section of this publication on treating osteoporosis. Although many people are able to obtain enough vitamin D naturally, vitamin D production decreases in the elderly, in people who are housebound or do not get enough sun, and in some people with chronic neurological or gastrointestinal diseases. These individuals and others at risk for vitamin D deficiency may require vitamin D supplementation. The recommended daily intake of vitamin D is 400 International Units (IU) for infants, 600 IU for children and adults up to age 70, and 800 IU for people over 70.

Overall Nutrition

A healthy, balanced diet that includes lots of fruits and vegetables and enough calories is also important for lifelong bone health.

Exercise

Like muscle, bone is living tissue that responds to exercise by becoming stronger. There is good evidence that physical activity early in life contributes to higher peak bone mass. (However, remember that excessive exercise can be bad for bone health.) The best exercise for building and maintaining bone mass is weight-bearing exercise: exercise that you do on your feet and that forces you to work against gravity. Weight-bearing exercises include jogging, aerobics, hiking, walking, stair climbing, gardening, weight training, tennis, and dancing. High-impact exercises may provide the most benefit. Bicycling and swimming are not weight-bearing exercises, but they have other health benefits. Exercise machines that provide some degree of weight-bearing exercise include treadmills, stair-climbing machines, ski machines, and exercise bicycles.

Strength training to build and maintain muscle mass and exercises that help with coordination and balance are also important. Later in life, the benefits of exercise for building and maintaining bone mass are not nearly as great, but staying active and doing weight-bearing exercise is still important. A properly designed exercise program that builds muscles and improves balance and coordination provides other benefits for older people, including helping to prevent falls and maintaining overall health and independence. Experts recommend 30 minutes or more of moderate physical activity on most (preferably all) days of the week, including a mix of weight-bearing exercises, strength training (two or three times a week), and balance training.

Smoking

Smoking is bad for your bones and for your heart and lungs. Women who smoke have lower levels of estrogen compared to nonsmokers and frequently go through menopause earlier.

Alcohol

People who drink heavily are more prone to bone loss and fractures because of poor nutrition and harmful effects on calcium balance and hormonal factors. Drinking too much also increases the risk of falling, which is likely to increase fracture risk.

Section 18.2

Osteoporosis and Arthritis: Two Common But Different Conditions

This section includes text excerpted from "Osteoporosis and Arthritis: Two Common but Different Conditions," NIH Osteoporosis and Related Bone Diseases~National Resource Center (NIH ORBD~NRC), May 1, 2016.

About Osteoporosis

Osteoporosis is a condition in which the bones become less dense and more likely to fracture. In the United States, more than 53 million people either already have osteoporosis or are at high risk due to low bone mass. In osteoporosis, there is a loss of bone tissue that leaves bones less dense and more likely to fracture. It can result in a loss of height, severe back pain, and change in one's posture. Osteoporosis can impair a person's ability to walk and can cause prolonged or permanent disability.

Risk factors for developing osteoporosis include:

- thinness or small frame
- family history of the disease
- being postmenopausal and particularly having had early menopause
- abnormal absence of menstrual periods (amenorrhea)
- prolonged use of certain medications, such as those used to treat lupus, asthma, thyroid deficiencies, and seizures
- low calcium intake
- lack of physical activity
- smoking
- excessive alcohol intake

Osteoporosis is known as a silent disease because it can progress undetected for many years without symptoms until a fracture occurs.

Osteoporosis is diagnosed by a bone mineral density test, which is a safe and painless way to detect low bone density.

Although there is no cure for the disease, the U.S. Food and Drug Administration (FDA) has approved several medications to prevent and treat osteoporosis. In addition, a diet rich in calcium and vitamin D, regular weight-bearing exercise, and a healthy lifestyle can prevent or lessen the effects of the disease.

About Arthritis

Arthritis is a general term for conditions that affect the joints and surrounding tissues. Joints are places in the body where bones come together, such as the knees, wrists, fingers, toes, and hips. Two common types of arthritis are osteoarthritis (OA) and rheumatoid arthritis (RA).

- **OA** is a painful, degenerative joint disease that often involves the hips, knees, neck, lower back, or small joints of the hands. OA usually develops in joints that are injured by repeated overuse from performing a particular task or playing a favorite sport or from carrying around excess body weight. Eventually this injury or repeated impact thins or wears away the cartilage that cushions the ends of the bones in the joint. As a result, the bones rub together, causing a grating sensation. Joint flexibility is reduced, bony spurs develop, and the joint swells. Usually, the first symptom of OA is pain that worsens following exercise or immobility. Treatment usually includes analgesics, topical creams, or nonsteroidal anti-inflammatory drugs (NSAID), appropriate exercises or physical therapy; joint splinting; or joint replacement surgery for seriously damaged larger joints, such as the knee or hip.

- **RA** is an autoimmune inflammatory disease that usually involves various joints in the fingers, thumbs, wrists, elbows, shoulders, knees, feet, and ankles. An autoimmune disease is one in which the body releases enzymes that attack its own healthy tissues. In RA, these enzymes destroy the linings of joints. This causes pain, swelling, stiffness, malformation, and reduced movement and function. People with RA also may have systemic symptoms, such as fatigue, fever, weight loss, eye inflammation, anemia, subcutaneous nodules (bumps under the skin), or pleurisy (a lung inflammation).

Two Common but Different Conditions

Although osteoporosis and osteoarthritis are two very different medical conditions with little in common, the similarity of their names causes great confusion. These conditions develop differently, have different symptoms, are diagnosed differently, and are treated differently.

Osteoporosis and arthritis do share many coping strategies. With either or both of these conditions, many people benefit from exercise programs that may include physical therapy and rehabilitation. In general, exercises that emphasize stretching, strengthening, posture, and range of motion are appropriate. Examples include low-impact aerobics, swimming, tai chi, and low-stress yoga. However, people with osteoporosis must take care to avoid activities that include bending forward from the waist, twisting the spine, or lifting heavy weights. People with arthritis must compensate for limited movement in affected joints. Always check with your doctor to determine whether a certain exercise or exercise program is safe for your specific medical situation.

Most people with arthritis will use pain management strategies at some time. This is not always true for people with osteoporosis. Usually, people with osteoporosis need pain relief when they are recovering from a fracture. In cases of severe osteoporosis with multiple spine fractures, pain control also may become part of daily life. Regardless of the cause, pain management strategies are similar for people with osteoporosis, OA, and RA.

Section 18.3

What People with RA Need to Know about Osteoporosis

This section includes text excerpted from "What People With Rheumatoid Arthritis Need to Know About Osteoporosis," National Institute of Arthritis and Musculoskeletal and Skin Diseases (NIAMS), April 1, 2016.

About Rheumatoid Arthritis (RA)

Rheumatoid arthritis (RA) is an autoimmune disease, a disorder in which the body attacks its own healthy cells and tissues. When someone has RA, the membranes around his or her joints become inflamed and release enzymes that cause the surrounding cartilage and bone to wear away. In severe cases, other tissues and body organs also can be affected.

Individuals with RA often experience pain, swelling, and stiffness in their joints, especially those in the hands and feet. Motion can be limited in the affected joints, curtailing one's ability to accomplish even the most basic everyday tasks. About one-quarter of those with RA develop nodules (bumps) that grow under the skin, usually close to the joints. Fatigue, anemia (low red blood cell count), neck pain, and dry eyes and dry mouth also can occur in individuals with the disease.

Scientists estimate that about 1.5 million people in the United States have RA. The disease occurs in all racial and ethnic groups, but affects 2–3 times as many women as men. RA is more commonly found in older individuals, although the disease typically begins in middle age. Children and young adults can also be affected.

About Osteoporosis

Osteoporosis is a condition in which the bones become less dense and more likely to fracture. Fractures from osteoporosis can result in significant pain and disability. In the United States, more than 53 million people either already have osteoporosis or are at high risk due to low bone mass.

Risk factors for developing osteoporosis include:

- thinness or small frame
- family history of the disease
- being postmenopausal and particularly having had early menopause
- abnormal absence of menstrual periods (amenorrhea)
- prolonged use of certain medications, such as those used to treat lupus, asthma, thyroid deficiencies, and seizures
- low calcium intake
- lack of physical activity
- smoking
- excessive alcohol intake

Osteoporosis often can be prevented. It is known as a silent disease because, if undetected, bone loss can progress for many years without symptoms until a fracture occurs. Osteoporosis has been called a childhood disease with old age consequences because building healthy bones in youth helps prevent osteoporosis and fractures later in life. However, it is never too late to adopt new habits for healthy bones.

The Link between RA and Osteoporosis

Studies have found an increased risk of bone loss and fracture in individuals with RA. People with RA are at increased risk for osteoporosis for many reasons. To begin with, the glucocorticoid medications often prescribed for the treatment of RA can trigger significant bone loss. In addition, pain and loss of joint function caused by the disease can result in inactivity, further increasing osteoporosis risk. Studies also show that bone loss in RA may occur as a direct result of the disease. The bone loss is most pronounced in areas immediately surrounding the affected joints. Of concern is the fact that women, a group already at increased risk for osteoporosis, are 2–3 times more likely than men to have RA as well.

Osteoporosis Management Strategies

Strategies for preventing and treating osteoporosis in people with RA are not significantly different from the strategies for those who do not have the disease.

Nutrition. A well-balanced diet rich in calcium and vitamin D is important for healthy bones. Good sources of calcium include low-fat dairy products; dark green, leafy vegetables; and calcium-fortified foods and beverages. Supplements can help ensure that you get adequate amounts of calcium each day, especially in people with a proven milk allergy. The Institute of Medicine (IOM) recommends a daily calcium intake of 1,000 mg (milligrams) for men and women up to age 50. Women over age 50 and men over age 70 should increase their intake to 1,200 mg daily.

Vitamin D plays an important role in calcium absorption and bone health. Food sources of vitamin D include egg yolks, saltwater fish, and liver. Many people, especially those who are older, may need vitamin D supplements to achieve the recommended intake of 600–800 IU (International Units) each day.

Exercise. Like muscle, bone is living tissue that responds to exercise by becoming stronger. The best activity for your bones is the weight-bearing exercise that forces you to work against gravity. Some examples include walking, climbing stairs, weight training, and dancing.

Exercising can be challenging for people with RA, and it needs to be balanced with rest when the disease is active. However, regular exercise, such as walking, can help prevent bone loss and, by enhancing balance and flexibility, can reduce the likelihood of falling and breaking a bone. Exercise is also important for preserving joint mobility.

Healthy lifestyle. Smoking is bad for bones as well as the heart and lungs. Women who smoke tend to go through menopause earlier, resulting in earlier reduction in levels of the bone-preserving hormone estrogen and triggering earlier bone loss. In addition, smokers may absorb less calcium from their diets. Alcohol also can have a negative effect on bone health. Those who drink heavily are more prone to bone loss and fracture, because of both poor nutrition and increased risk of falling.

Bone density test. A bone mineral density (BMD) test measures bone density in various parts of the body. This safe and painless test can detect osteoporosis before a fracture occurs and can predict one's chances of fracturing in the future. The BMD test can help determine whether medication should be considered. People with RA, particularly those who have been receiving glucocorticoid therapy for 2 months or more, should talk to their doctor about whether a BMD test is appropriate.

Medication. Like RA, osteoporosis has no cure. However, medications are available to prevent and treat osteoporosis. Several medications are available for people with RA who have or are at risk for glucocorticoid-induced osteoporosis.

Section 18.4

Osteoporosis in Women

This section includes text excerpted from "Osteoporosis,"
Office on Women's Health (OWH), U.S. Department of
Health and Human Services (HHS), October 2, 2017.

Osteoporosis is a disease of the bones that causes bones to become weak and break easily. Osteoporosis affects mostly older women, but prevention starts when you are younger. No matter your age, you can take steps to build bone mass and prevent bone loss. Broken bones from osteoporosis cause serious health problems and disability in older women.

Osteoporosis is called a "silent" disease. You may have bone loss for many years without any symptoms until you break a bone. A broken bone can cause severe pain and disability. It can make it harder to do daily tasks on your own, such as walking.

What Is Bone Loss?

Bone loss is the amount of minerals, such as calcium, that your body absorbs (takes) from your bones. Bone loss can happen for several reasons. Some of the most common reasons include:

- **You do not get enough calcium from food.** Your body uses calcium to build healthy bones and teeth and stores calcium in your bones. Your body also uses calcium to send messages through your nervous system, help your muscles contract, and regulate your heart's rhythm. But your body does not make calcium. You have to get all the calcium your body needs from the foods you eat and drink (or from supplements). If you don't get enough calcium each day, your body will take the calcium it needs from your bones.

- **You are past menopause.** As you get older, your bones don't make new bone fast enough to keep up with your body's needs. The calcium taken from your bones causes you to lose bone density. Bone loss also speeds up after menopause and can lead to weak, brittle bones.

Who Gets Osteoporosis

Osteoporosis affects more women than men. Of the estimated 10 million Americans with osteoporosis, more than 8 million (or 80%) are women.
Women are more likely to get osteoporosis because:

- Women usually have smaller, thinner, less dense bones than men

- Women often live longer than men. Bone loss happens naturally as we age

- Women also lose more bone mass after menopause with very low levels of the hormone estrogen. Higher estrogen levels before menopause helps protect bone density.

Osteoporosis is most common in older women. In the United States, osteoporosis affects one in four women 65 or older. But younger women can get osteoporosis. And girls and women of all ages need to take steps to protect their bones.

Are Some Women More at Risk for Osteoporosis?

Yes. Your risk for osteoporosis is higher if you:

- **Are past menopause.** After menopause, your ovaries make very little of the hormone estrogen. Estrogen helps protect bone density. Some women lose up to 25 percent of bone mass in the first 10 years after menopause.

- **Have a small, thin body** (weigh less than 127 pounds)

- **Have a family history of osteoporosis**

- **Are Mexican-American or white.** One in four Mexican-American women and about one in six white women over 50 years old have osteoporosis. Asian-American women also have a higher risk for osteoporosis because they are usually smaller and thinner than other women and, therefore, may have less bone density.

- **Do not get enough calcium and vitamin D.** Calcium and vitamin D work together to build and maintain strong bones.

- **Do not get enough physical activity.** Women of all ages need to get regular weight-bearing physical activity, such as walking, dancing, or playing tennis, to help build and maintain bone density.

- **Have not gotten your menstrual period for three months in a row (called amenorrhea).** If you have amenorrhea and you are not pregnant, breastfeeding, or taking a medicine that stops your periods, talk to your doctor or nurse. Not getting your period means your ovaries may have stopped making estrogen.

- **Have an eating disorder.** Eating disorders, especially anorexia nervosa and bulimia nervosa, can weaken your bones. Anorexia can also lead to amenorrhea.

- **Smoke.** Women who smoke have lower bone density and often go through menopause earlier than nonsmokers. Studies also suggest that smoking raises your risk for broken bones, and this risk goes up the longer you smoke and the more cigarettes you smoke.

- **Have a health problem that raises your risk of getting osteoporosis.** These include diabetes, premature ovarian failure, celiac disease and inflammatory bowel disease (IBD), and depression.

- **Take certain medicines to treat long-term health problems,** such as arthritis, asthma, lupus, or thyroid disease.

- **Drink too much alcohol.** For women, experts recommend no more than one alcoholic drink a day if you choose to drink alcohol. Long-term, heavy drinking can cause many health problems, including bone loss, heart disease, and stroke.

What Are the Symptoms of Osteoporosis?

You may not have any symptoms of osteoporosis until you break (fracture) a bone. A fracture can happen in any bone of the body. But fractures are most common in the hip, wrist, and spine (vertebrae). Vertebrae support your body, helping you to stand and sit up. See the picture.

Osteoporosis in the vertebrae can cause serious problems for women. A fracture in this area can happen during day-to-day activities like climbing stairs, lifting objects, or bending forward when you have osteoporosis.

Fractures in the vertebrae can cause it to collapse and bend forward. If this happens, you may get any or all of these symptoms:

- Sloping shoulders
- Curve in the back
- Height loss
- Back pain
- Hunched posture

What Causes Osteoporosis

Osteoporosis is caused by bone loss. Most often, the reason for bone loss is very low levels of the hormone estrogen. Estrogen plays an important role in building and maintaining your bones.

The most common cause of low estrogen levels is menopause. After menopause, your ovaries make very little estrogen.

Also, your risk for developing osteoporosis is higher if you did not develop strong bones when you were young. Girls develop 90 percent of bone mass by age 18. If an eating disorder, poor eating, lack of physical activity, or another health problem prevents you from building bone mass early in life, you will have less bone mass to draw on later in life.

How Is Osteoporosis Diagnosed?

Your doctor will do a bone density test to see how strong or weak your bones are. A common test is a central dual-energy X-ray absorptiometry (DXA). A DXA is a special type of X-ray of your bones. This test uses a very low amount of radiation.

Your doctor may also use other screening tools to predict your risk of having low bone density or breaking a bone

Do I Need to Be Tested for Osteoporosis?

Your doctor may suggest a bone density test for osteoporosis if:

- You are 65 or older
- You are younger than 65 and have risk factors for osteoporosis. Bone density testing is recommended for older women whose risk of breaking a bone is the same or greater than that of a

65-year-old white woman with no risk factors other than age. Ask your doctor or nurse whether you need a bone density test before age 65.

How Can I Get Free or Low-Cost Osteoporosis Screening Tests?

Screening for osteoporosis is covered by most insurance plans, including Medicare Part B. Depending on your insurance plan, you may be able to get screenings at no cost to you.

- If you have insurance, check with your insurance provider to find out what's included in your plan

- If you have Medicare, find out about Medicare coverage for bone density tests

- If you have Medicaid, the benefits covered are different in each state, but certain benefits must be covered. Check with your state's Medicaid program to find out what's covered.

- If you don't have insurance, you may be able to get a no-cost or low-cost bone density test

How Is Osteoporosis Treated?

If you have osteoporosis, your doctor may prescribe medicine to prevent more bone loss or build new bone mass. The most common types of medicine to prevent or treat osteoporosis include:

Bisphosphonates. Bisphosphonates help treat bone loss. They may also help build bone mass.

Selective estrogen receptor modulators (SERMs). SERMs may help slow the rate of bone loss after menopause.

Denosumab. This injectable drug may help reduce bone loss and improve bone strength if you are past menopause and at higher risk for broken bones from osteoporosis.

Calcitonin. Calcitonin is a hormone made by your thyroid gland that helps regulate calcium levels in your body and build bone mass. Taking calcitonin can help slow the rate of bone loss.

Menopausal hormone therapy. Often used to treat menopausal symptoms, menopausal hormone therapy may also help prevent bone loss. The U.S. Food and Drug Administration (FDA) recommends taking menopausal hormone therapy at the lowest dose that works for your menopause symptoms for the shortest time needed.

Parathyroid hormone or teriparatide. Teriparatide is an injectable form of human parathyroid hormone. It helps the body build up new bone faster than the old bone is broken down.

Your doctor may also suggest getting more calcium, vitamin D, and physical activity.

All medicines have risks. For example, menopausal hormone therapy may raise your risk of a blood clot, heart attack, stroke, breast cancer, or gallbladder disease. Talk to your doctor or nurse about the benefits and risks of all medicines.

How Can I Prevent Osteoporosis?

One of the best ways to prevent weak bones is to work on building strong ones. Building strong bones during childhood and the teen years is important to help prevent osteoporosis later.

As you get older, your bones don't make new bone fast enough to keep up with the bone loss. And after menopause, bone loss happens even more quickly. But you can take steps to slow the natural bone loss with aging and to prevent your bones from becoming weak and brittle.

- Get enough calcium and vitamin D each day.

- Get active. Choose weight-bearing physical activities like running or dancing to build and strengthen your bones.

- Don't smoke. Smoking raises your risk for broken bones.

- If you drink alcohol, drink in moderation (for women, this is one drink a day at most). Too much alcohol can harm your bones. Also, too much at one time or mixed with certain medicines can affect your balance and lead to falls.

- Talk to your doctor about whether you need medicine to prevent bone loss.

How Does Calcium Help Prevent Osteoporosis?

Calcium is found in your bones and teeth. It helps build bones and keep them healthy. Your body also uses calcium to help your blood clot and your muscles contract. If you don't get enough calcium each day from the foods you eat, your body will take the calcium it needs from your bones, making your bones weak. You can get calcium through food or calcium supplements.

How Much Calcium Do Women Need Each Day?

How much calcium you need depends on your age:

- **9–18 years:** 1,300 mg per day
- **19–50 years:** 1,000 mg per day
- **51 and older:** 1,200 mg per day

Pregnant or nursing women need the same amount of calcium as other women of the same age.

You can get the calcium you need each day from food and/or calcium supplements.

What Foods Contain Calcium?

Calcium is found naturally in some foods:

- Milk
- Cheese
- Yogurt
- Leafy green vegetables, such as broccoli, kale, and mustard greens

Calcium is sometimes added to certain foods, such as:
Breakfast cereals (some have up to 100% of the recommended daily value—or 1,000 milligrams—of calcium in each ¾ cup serving)

- Orange juice
- Tofu
- Soymilk
- Breads and pastas

What Should I Look for When Buying Food with Calcium?

When buying food with calcium, look at the Nutrition Facts label to see how much calcium is in the food. Food labels show the amount of calcium as a percentage of the Daily Value (written as %DV). Foods providing 20 percent DV or more are high sources of calcium, but foods with lower percentages (5% or more) are still good sources of calcium.

What If Dairy Foods Make Me Sick or I Don't like to Eat Them? How Can I Get Enough Calcium?

If you have problems eating foods with dairy or don't like to eat them, try the following tips to make sure you get enough calcium:

- Try lactose-reduced or lactose-free products, such as milk or yogurt

- Take a lactose supplement (in pill or liquid form) before eating dairy foods to help you digest them

- Choose other food sources of calcium. Other good sources of calcium include tofu or orange juice with calcium added, and vegetables such as bok choy, kale, collard greens, mustard greens, and broccoli.

- Ask your doctor or nurse if you need to take calcium supplements

Should I Take a Calcium Supplement?

The answer depends on how much calcium you need each day and how much calcium you get from the foods you eat.

It's best to get the calcium your body needs from food. But if you don't get enough calcium from the foods you eat, you may want to consider taking a calcium supplement.

You can get calcium supplements at the grocery store or drug store. Talk with your doctor or nurse before taking calcium supplements to see which kind is best for you and how much you need to take.

How Does Vitamin D Help Prevent Osteoporosis?

Vitamin D helps your body absorb calcium from the food you eat. Just eating foods with calcium is not enough. You also need to get enough vitamin D to help your body use the calcium it gets.

Your skin makes vitamin D when it is exposed to sunlight. In general, you need 10–15 minutes of sunlight to the hands, arms, and face, 2–3 times a week to make enough vitamin D. The amount of time depends on how sensitive your skin is to light. It also depends on your use of sunscreen, your skin color, the season, the latitude (how far north or south) where you live, and the amount of pollution in the air.

You can also get vitamin D from foods such as milk or from vitamin supplements. The vitamin D you get from food or supplements is measured in international units (IU).

How Much Vitamin D Do Women Need Each Day?

How much vitamin D you need each day depends on your age:

- **Women up to age 70:** 600 international units (IU)
- **Women 71 and older:** 800 IU each day

Pregnant and breastfeeding women need the same amount of vitamin D (600 IU) as other women of the same age.

What Foods Contain Vitamin D?

Although it's hard to get enough vitamin D through food alone, foods with vitamin D include:

- Salmon
- Tuna fish
- Egg yolks

Vitamin D is often added to certain foods, including:

- Breakfast cereals
- Milk
- Orange juice

What Types of Physical Activity Help Prevent Osteoporosis?

Regular physical activity of any type can help slow bone loss, improve muscle strength, and help your balance. But weight-bearing physical activity is especially important to build bone and help prevent bone loss. Weight-bearing physical activity is any activity in which your body works against gravity.

Weight-bearing activities you can try include:

- Dancing
- Gardening

- Lifting weights
- Tennis
- Tai chi
- Yoga
- Running
- Walking

What Can Happen If Osteoporosis Is Not Treated?

Osteoporosis that is not treated can lead to serious bone breaks (fractures), especially in the hip and spine. One in three women is likely to have a fracture caused by osteoporosis in her lifetime.

Hip fractures can cause serious pain and disability and require surgery.

Spinal fractures can cause you to lose height or get a stooped back. They often cause serious pain and require surgery.

Fractures can happen after minor falls, stumbles, or bumps into furniture. Falls are the leading cause of injuries in older adults over age 65.

Does Pregnancy Affect Bone Density?

Maybe. Your unborn baby needs calcium to help his or her bones grow. While in the womb, babies get calcium from what you eat (or the supplements you take). If you don't get enough calcium from food or supplements, your baby will use the calcium in your bones.

You can lose some bone density during pregnancy, but any bone mass lost is usually restored after childbirth (or after breastfeeding). Also, during pregnancy, you absorb calcium from food and supplements (like prenatal vitamins) better than women who are not pregnant. Your body also makes more of the hormone estrogen, which protects bone.

Does Breastfeeding Affect Bone Density?

Yes, women often lose some bone density during breastfeeding. But this loss is temporary. Several studies have shown that when women lose bone mass during breastfeeding, they recover full bone density within six months after breastfeeding stops.

Section 18.5

Osteoporosis in Men

This section contains text excerpted from the following sources: Text in this section begins with excerpts from "Osteoporosis in Men," NIH Osteoporosis and Related Bone Diseases~National Resource Center (NIH ORBD~NRC), June 2015; Text beginning with the heading "Calcium Supplements" is excerpted from "Calcium and Vitamin D: Important at Every Age," NIH Osteoporosis and Related Bone Diseases~National Resource Center (NIH ORBD~NRC), May 2015.

Osteoporosis is a disease that causes the skeleton to weaken and the bones to break. It poses a significant threat to millions of men in the United States.

Despite these compelling figures, surveys suggest that a majority of American men view osteoporosis solely as a "woman's disease." Moreover, among men whose lifestyle habits put them at increased risk, few recognize the disease as a significant threat to their mobility and independence.

Osteoporosis is called a "silent disease" because it progresses without symptoms until a fracture occurs. It develops less often in men than in women because men have larger skeletons, their bone loss starts later and progresses more slowly, and they have no period of rapid hormonal change and bone loss. However, in the past few years the problem of osteoporosis in men has been recognized as an important public health issue, particularly in light of estimates that the number of men above the age of 70 will continue to increase as life expectancy continues to rise.

What Causes Osteoporosis

Bone is constantly changing—that is, old bone is removed and replaced by new bone. During childhood, more bone is produced than removed, so the skeleton grows in both size and strength. For most people, bone mass peaks during the third decade of life. By this age, men typically have accumulated more bone mass than women. After this point, the amount of bone in the skeleton typically begins to decline slowly as removal of old bone exceeds formation of new bone.

Men in their fifties do not experience the rapid loss of bone mass that women do in the years following menopause. By age 65 or 70, however, men and women are losing bone mass at the same rate, and the absorption of calcium, an essential nutrient for bone health throughout life, decreases in both sexes. Excessive bone loss causes bone to become fragile and more likely to fracture.

Fractures resulting from osteoporosis most commonly occur in the hip, spine, and wrist, and can be permanently disabling. Hip fractures are especially dangerous. Perhaps because such fractures tend to occur at older ages in men than in women, men who sustain hip fractures are more likely than women to die from complications.

Primary and Secondary Osteoporosis

There are two main types of osteoporosis: primary and secondary. In cases of primary osteoporosis, either the condition is caused by age-related bone loss (sometimes called senile osteoporosis) or the cause is unknown (idiopathic osteoporosis). The term idiopathic osteoporosis is typically used only for men younger than 70 years old; in older men, an age-related bone loss is assumed to be the cause.

The majority of men with osteoporosis have at least one (sometimes more than one) secondary cause. In cases of secondary osteoporosis, the loss of bone mass is caused by certain lifestyle behaviors, diseases, or medications. The most common causes of secondary osteoporosis in men include exposure to glucocorticoid medications, hypogonadism (low levels of testosterone), alcohol abuse, smoking, gastrointestinal disease, hypercalciuria, and immobilization.

Causes of Secondary Osteoporosis in Men

- glucocorticoid medications
- other immunosuppressive drugs
- hypogonadism (low testosterone levels)
- excessive alcohol consumption
- smoking
- chronic obstructive pulmonary disease and asthma
- cystic fibrosis
- gastrointestinal disease
- hypercalciuria
- anticonvulsant medications

- thyrotoxicosis

- hyperparathyroidism

- immobilization

- osteogenesis imperfecta

- homocystinuria

- neoplastic disease

- ankylosing spondylitis and rheumatoid arthritis (RA)

- systemic mastocytosis

Glucocorticoid medications. Glucocorticoids are steroid medications used to treat diseases such as asthma and RA. Bone loss is a very common side effect of these medications. The bone loss these medications cause may be due to their direct effect on bone, muscle weakness or immobility, reduced intestinal absorption of calcium, a decrease in testosterone levels, or, most likely, a combination of these factors.

When glucocorticoid medications are used on an ongoing basis, bone mass often decreases quickly and continuously, with most of the bone loss in the ribs and vertebrae. Therefore, people taking these medications should talk to their doctor about having a bone mineral density (BMD) test. Men should also be tested to monitor testosterone levels, as glucocorticoids often reduce testosterone in the blood.

A treatment plan to minimize loss of bone during long-term glucocorticoid therapy may include using the minimal effective dose, and discontinuing the drug or administering it through the skin, if possible. Adequate calcium and vitamin D intake is important, as these nutrients help reduce the impact of glucocorticoids on the bones. Other possible treatments include testosterone replacement and osteoporosis medication.

Hypogonadism. Hypogonadism refers to abnormally low levels of sex hormones. It is well known that loss of estrogen causes osteoporosis in women. In men, reduced levels of sex hormones may also cause osteoporosis.

Although it is natural for testosterone levels to decrease with age, there should not be a sudden drop in this hormone that is comparable to the drop in estrogen experienced by women at menopause. However, medications such as glucocorticoids (discussed above), cancer treatments (especially for prostate cancer), and many other factors can affect testosterone levels. Testosterone replacement therapy (TRT) may be helpful in preventing or slowing bone loss. Its success depends on factors such as age and how long testosterone levels have been reduced. Also, it is not yet clear how long any beneficial effect of testosterone replacement will last. Therefore, doctors usually treat the osteoporosis directly, using medications approved for this purpose.

Research suggests that estrogen deficiency may also be a cause of osteoporosis in men. For example, estrogen levels are low in men with hypogonadism and may play a part in bone loss. Osteoporosis has been found in some men who have rare disorders involving estrogen. Therefore, the role of estrogen in men is under active investigation.

Alcohol abuse. There is a wealth of evidence that alcohol abuse may decrease bone density and lead to an increase in fractures. Low bone mass is common in men who seek medical help for alcohol abuse.

In cases where bone loss is linked to alcohol abuse, the first goal of treatment is to help the patient stop, or at least reduce, his consumption of alcohol. More research is needed to determine whether bone lost to alcohol abuse will rebuild once drinking stops, or even whether further damage will be prevented. It is clear, though, that alcohol abuse causes many other health and social problems, so quitting is ideal. A treatment plan may also include a balanced diet with lots of calcium- and vitamin D-rich foods, a program of physical exercise, and smoking cessation.

Smoking. Bone loss is more rapid, and rates of hip and vertebral fracture are higher, among men who smoke, although more research is needed to determine exactly how smoking damages bone. Tobacco, nicotine, and other chemicals found in cigarettes may be directly toxic to bone, or they may inhibit absorption of calcium and other nutrients needed for bone health. Quitting is the ideal approach, as smoking is harmful in so many ways. As with alcohol, it is not known whether quitting smoking leads to reduced rates of bone loss or to a gain in bone mass.

Gastrointestinal disorders. Several nutrients, including amino acids, calcium, magnesium, phosphorus, and vitamins D and K, are important for bone health. Diseases of the stomach and intestines can lead to bone disease when they impair absorption of these nutrients. In such cases, treatment for bone loss may include taking supplements to replenish these nutrients.

Hypercalciuria. Hypercalciuria is a disorder that causes too much calcium to be lost through the urine, which makes the calcium unavailable for building bone. Patients with hypercalciuria should talk to their doctor about having a BMD test and, if bone density is low, discuss treatment options.

Immobilization. Weight-bearing exercise is essential for maintaining healthy bones. Without it, bone density may decline rapidly. Prolonged bed rest (following fractures, surgery, spinal cord injuries (SCIs), or illness) or immobilization of some part of the body often results in significant bone loss. It is crucial to resume weight-bearing exercise (such as walking, jogging, dancing, and lifting weights) as soon as possible after a period of prolonged bed rest. If this is not possible, you should work with your doctor to minimize other risk factors for osteoporosis.

What Are the Risk Factors for Men?

Several risk factors have been linked to osteoporosis in men:

- **Chronic diseases** that affect the kidneys, lungs, stomach, and intestines or alter hormone levels
- **Regular use of certain medications,** such as glucocorticoids
- **Undiagnosed low levels of the sex hormone testosterone**
- **Unhealthy lifestyle habits.** Smoking, excessive alcohol use, low calcium intake, and inadequate physical exercise
- **Age.** The older you are, the greater your risk
- **Race.** Caucasian men appear to be at particularly high risk, but all men can develop this disease

How Is Osteoporosis Diagnosed in Men?

Osteoporosis can be effectively treated if it is detected before significant bone loss has occurred. A medical workup to diagnose osteoporosis will include a complete medical history, X-rays, and urine and blood tests. The doctor may also order a bone mineral density test. This test can identify osteoporosis, determine your risk for fractures (broken bones), and measure your response to osteoporosis treatment. The most widely recognized BMD test is called a central dual-energy X-ray absorptiometry, or central DXA test. It is painless a bit like having an X-ray, but with much less exposure to radiation. It can measure bone density at your hip and spine.

It is increasingly common for women to be diagnosed with osteoporosis or low bone mass using a BMD test, often at midlife when doctors begin to watch for signs of bone loss. In men, however, the diagnosis is often not made until a fracture occurs or a man complains of back pain and sees his doctor. This makes it especially important for men to inform their doctors about risk factors for developing osteoporosis, loss of height or change in posture, a fracture, or sudden back pain.

What Treatments Are Available?

Once a man has been diagnosed with osteoporosis, his doctor may prescribe one of the medications approved by the U.S. Food and Drug Administration (FDA) for this disease.

If bone loss is due to glucocorticoid use, the doctor may prescribe a medication approved to prevent or treat glucocorticoid-induced osteoporosis, monitor bone density and testosterone levels, and suggest using the minimum effective dose of glucocorticoid.

Other possible prevention or treatment approaches include calcium and/or vitamin D supplements and regular physical activity.

If osteoporosis is the result of another condition (such as testosterone deficiency) or exposure to certain other medications, the doctor may design a treatment plan to address the underlying cause.

How Can Osteoporosis Be Prevented?

There have been fewer research studies on osteoporosis in men than in women. However, experts agree that all people should take the following steps to preserve their bone health:

- Avoid smoking, reduce alcohol intake, and increase your level of physical activity.

- Ensure a daily calcium intake that is adequate for your age.

- Ensure an adequate intake of vitamin D. Dietary vitamin D intake should be 600 IU (International Units) per day up to age 70. Men over age 70 should increase their uptake to 800 IU daily.

- The amount of vitamin D found in 1 quart of fortified milk and most multivitamins is 400 IU.

- Engage in a regular regimen of weight-bearing exercises in which bones and muscles work against gravity. This might include walking, jogging, racquet sports, climbing stairs, team sports, weight training, and using resistance machines. A doctor should evaluate the exercise program of anyone already diagnosed with osteoporosis to determine if twisting motions and impact activities, such as those used in golf, tennis, or basketball, need to be curtailed.

- Discuss with your doctor the use of medications that are known to cause bone loss, such as glucocorticoids.

- Recognize and seek treatment for any underlying medical conditions that affect bone health.

Calcium Supplements

If you have trouble getting enough calcium in your diet, you may need to take a calcium supplement. The amount of calcium you will need from a supplement depends on how much calcium you obtain from food sources. There are several different calcium compounds from which to choose, such as calcium carbonate and calcium citrate, among others. Except in people with gastrointestinal disease, all major forms of calcium supplements are absorbed equally well when taken with food.

Calcium supplements are better absorbed when taken in small doses (500 mg or less) several times throughout the day. In many individuals, calcium supplements are better absorbed when taken with food. It is important to check supplement labels to ensure that the product meets United States Pharmacopeia (USP) standards.

Vitamin D

The body needs vitamin D to absorb calcium. Without enough vitamin D, one can't form enough of the hormone calcitriol (known as the "active vitamin D"). This in turn leads to insufficient calcium absorption from the diet. In this situation, the body must take calcium from its stores in the skeleton, which weakens existing bone and prevents the formation of strong, new bone.

Section 18.6

Osteoporosis in Aging

This section includes text excerpted from "Osteoporosis in Aging," *NIH News in Health*, National Institutes of Health (NIH), January 2015.

Bones feel solid, but the inside of a bone is actually filled with holes like a honeycomb. Bone tissues are broken down and rebuilt all the time. While some cells build new bone tissue, others dissolve bone and release the minerals inside.

As we get older, we begin to lose more bone than we build. The tiny holes within bones get bigger, and the solid outer layer becomes thinner. In other words, our bones get less dense. Hard bones turn spongy, and spongy bones turn spongier. If this loss of bone density goes too far, it's called osteoporosis. Over 10 million people nationwide are estimated to have osteoporosis.

It's normal for bones to break in bad accidents. But if your bones are dense enough, they should be able to stand up to most falls. Bones weakened by osteoporosis, though, are more likely to break.

"It's just like any other engineering material," says Dr. Joan McGowan, an NIH expert on osteoporosis. If you fall and slam your weight onto a fragile bone, "it reaches a point where the structures aren't adequate to support the weight you're putting on them." If the bone breaks, it's a major hint that an older person has osteoporosis.

Broken bones can lead to serious problems for seniors. The hip is a common site for osteoporosis, and hip fractures can lead to a downward spiral of disability and loss of independence. Osteoporosis is also common in the wrist and the spine.

The hormone estrogen helps to make and rebuild bones. A woman's estrogen levels drop after menopause, and bone loss speeds up. That's why osteoporosis is most common among older women. But men get osteoporosis, too.

"A third of all hip fractures occur in men, yet the problem of osteoporosis in men is frequently downplayed or ignored," says Dr. Eric Orwoll, a physician-researcher who studies osteoporosis at Oregon

Health and Science University. Men tend to do worse than women after a hip fracture, Orwoll says.

Experts suggest that women start getting screened for osteoporosis at age 65. Women younger than age 65 who are at high risk for fractures should also be screened. Men should discuss screening recommendations with their healthcare providers.

Screening is done with a bone mineral density test at the hip and spine. The most common test is known as DXA, for dual-energy X-ray absorptiometry. It's painless, like having an X-ray. Your results are often reported as a T-score, which compares your bone density to that of a healthy young woman. A T-score of -2.5 or lower indicates osteoporosis.

There's a lot you can do to lower your risk of osteoporosis. Getting plenty of calcium, vitamin D, and exercise is a good start, Orwoll says.

Calcium is a mineral that helps bones stay strong. It can come from the foods you eat—including milk and milk products, dark green leafy vegetables like kale and collard greens—or from dietary supplements. Women over age 50 need 1,200 mg of calcium a day. Men need 1,000 mg a day from ages 51–70 and 1,200 mg a day after that.

Vitamin D helps your body absorb calcium. As you grow older, your body needs more vitamin D, which is made by your skin when you're in the sun. You can also get vitamin D from dietary supplements and from certain foods, such as milk, eggs, fatty fish, and fortified cereals. Talk with your healthcare provider to make sure you're getting a healthy amount of vitamin D. Problems can arise if you're getting too little or too much.

Exercise, especially weight-bearing exercise, helps bones, too. Weight-bearing exercises include jogging, walking, tennis, and dancing. The pull of muscles is a reminder to the cells in your bones that they need to keep the tissue dense.

Smoking, in contrast, weakens bones. Heavy drinking does too—and makes people more likely to fall. Certain drugs may also increase the risk of osteoporosis. Having family members with osteoporosis can raise your risk for the condition as well.

The good news is, even if you already have osteoporosis, it's not too late to start taking care of your bones. Since your bones are rebuilding themselves all the time, you can help push the balance toward more bone growth by giving them exercise, calcium, and vitamin D.

Several medications can also help fight bone loss. The most widely used are bisphosphonates. These drugs are generally prescribed to people diagnosed with osteoporosis after a DXA test, or to those who've had a fracture that suggests their bones are too weak. Bisphosphonates have been tested more thoroughly in women, but are approved for men too.

Researchers are trying to develop drugs that increase bone growth. For now, there's only one available: parathyroid hormone. It's effective at building bone and is approved for women and men with osteoporosis who are at high risk for having a fracture.

Another important way to avoid broken bones is to prevent falling and occasions for fracture in the first place. Unfortunately, more than 2 million so-called fragility fractures (which wouldn't have happened if the bones had been stronger) occur nationwide each year. "To reduce the societal burden of fracture, it's going to take a combined approach of not only focusing on the skeleton but focusing on fall prevention," says Dr. Kristine Ensrud, a physician-researcher who studies aging-related disorders at the University of Minnesota and Minneapolis VA Health Care System.

Many things can affect the risk for a fall, such as how good a person's balance is and how many trip hazards are in the environment. The kind of fall matters, too. Wrist fractures often occur when a person falls forward or backward. "It's the active older person who trips and puts her hand out," McGowan says. Hip fractures often arise when a person falls to the side. Your hip may be strong enough to handle weight that goes up and down, but not an impact from another direction.

"That's why exercise that builds balance and confidence is very good at preventing fractures," McGowan says. For example, she says, tai chi won't provide the loads needed to build bone mass, but it can increase balance and coordination—and make you more likely to catch yourself before you topple.

NIH-funded researchers are looking for better ways to tell how strong your bones are, and how high your chances are of breaking a bone. For now, though, the DXA test is the best measure, and many seniors, even older women, don't get it, Ensrud says. If you're concerned about your bone health, she adds, "Ask your healthcare provider about the possibility of a bone density test."

Chapter 19

Paget Disease of Bone

Chapter Contents

Section 19.1—What Is Paget Disease of Bone? 232

Section 19.2—Paget Disease of Bone and
Osteoarthritis: Different Yet Related 236

Section 19.3—Pain and Paget Disease of Bone 239

Section 19.4—FAQs on Paget Disease of Bone 241

Section 19.1

What Is Paget Disease of Bone?

This section includes text excerpted from "Information for Patients about Paget's Disease of Bone," NIH Osteoporosis and Related Bone Diseases~National Resource Center (NIH ORBD~NRC), May 2015.

Paget disease is a chronic disorder that can result in enlarged and misshapen bones. The excessive breakdown and formation of bone tissue causes affected bone to weaken—resulting in bone pain, misshapen bones, fractures, and arthritis in the joints near the affected bones. Paget disease typically is localized, affecting just one or a few bones, as opposed to osteoporosis, for example, which affects all the bones in the body.

Scientists do not know for sure what causes Paget disease. In some cases, the disease runs in families, and so far two genes have been identified that predispose affected people to develop Paget disease. In most cases, however, scientists suspect that environmental factors play a role. For example, scientists are studying the possibility that a slow-acting virus may cause Paget disease.

Prevalence of Paget Disease of Bone

The disease is more common in older people and those of northern European heritage. Research suggests that a close relative of someone with Paget disease is seven times more likely to develop the disease than someone without an affected relative.

Symptoms of Paget Disease of Bone

Many patients do not know they have Paget disease because they have no symptoms. Sometimes the symptoms may be confused with those of arthritis or other disorders. In other cases, the diagnosis is made only after the patient has developed complications.

Symptoms can include:

- **Pain**, which can occur in any bone affected by the disease or result from arthritis, is a complication that develops in some patients.

- **Headaches and hearing loss**, which may occur when Paget disease affects the skull

- **Pressure on nerves**, which may occur when Paget disease affects the skull or spine

- **Increased head size, bowing of a limb, or curvature of the spine,** which may occur in advanced cases

- **Hip pain**, which may occur when Paget disease affects the pelvis or thighbone.

- **Damage to cartilage of joints,** which may lead to arthritis.

Any bone or bones can be affected, but Paget disease occurs most frequently in the spine, pelvis, legs, or skull. Generally, symptoms progress slowly, and the disease does not spread to normal bones.

Diagnosis of Paget Disease of Bone

Paget disease is almost always diagnosed using X-rays but may be discovered initially by either of the following tests:

- **Alkaline phosphatase blood test.** An elevated level of alkaline phosphatase in the blood can be suggestive of Paget disease.

- **Bone scans.** Bone scans are useful in determining the extent and activity of the condition.

If a blood test or bone scan suggests Paget disease, the affected bone(s) should be X-rayed to confirm the diagnosis.

Early diagnosis and treatment are important to minimize complications. Siblings and children of people with Paget disease may wish to have an alkaline phosphatase blood test every 2 or 3 years starting around the age of 40. If the alkaline phosphatase level is higher than normal, a bone scan may be used to identify which bone or bones are affected and an X-ray of these bones is used to verify the diagnosis of Paget disease.

Prognosis for Paget Disease of Bone

The outlook for people diagnosed with Paget disease is generally good, particularly if treatment is given before major changes have occurred in the affected bones. Treatment can reduce symptoms but is not a cure. Osteogenic sarcoma, a form of bone cancer, is an extremely rare complication that occurs in less than 1 percent of all patients with Paget disease.

Medical Conditions That May Lead to Paget Disease of Bone

Paget disease may lead to other medical conditions, including:

- **Arthritis.** Long bones in the leg may bow, distorting alignment and increasing pressure on nearby joints. In addition, pagetic bone may enlarge, causing joint surfaces to undergo excessive wear and tear. In these cases, pain may be caused by a combination of Paget disease and osteoarthritis (OA).

- **Hearing loss.** Loss of hearing in one or both ears may occur when Paget disease affects the skull and the bone that surrounds the inner ear. Treating Paget disease may slow or stop hearing loss. Hearing aids also may help.

- **Heart disease.** In severe Paget disease, the heart works harder to pump blood to affected bones. This usually does not result in heart failure except in some people who also have hardening of the arteries.

- **Kidney stones.** Kidney stones are more common in patients with Paget disease.

- **Nervous system problems.** Pagetic bone can cause pressure on the brain, spinal cord, or nerves and reduced blood flow to the brain and spinal cord.

- **Sarcoma.** Rarely, Paget disease is associated with the development of a malignant tumor of the bone. When there is a sudden onset or worsening of pain, sarcoma should be considered.

- **Loose teeth.** When Paget disease affects the facial bones, the teeth may loosen. This may make chewing more difficult.

- **Vision loss.** Rarely, when the skull is involved, the nerves to the eye may be affected, causing some loss of vision.

Paget disease is not associated with osteoporosis. Although Paget disease and osteoporosis can occur in the same patient, they are completely different disorders. Despite their marked differences, several medications for Paget disease also are used to treat osteoporosis.

Treatment of Paget Disease of Bone

Healthcare Team

The following types of medical specialists are generally knowledgeable about treating Paget disease:

- **Endocrinologists.** Doctors who specialize in hormonal and metabolic disorders

- **Rheumatologists.** Doctors who specialize in joint and muscle disorders

- **Others.** Orthopedic surgeons, neurologists, and otolaryngologists (doctors who specialize in ear, nose, and throat disorders) may be called on to evaluate specialized symptoms.

Treatment Options

Drug therapy. The U.S. Food and Drug Administration (FDA) has approved several medications to treat Paget disease. The medications work by controlling the excessive breakdown and formation of bone that occurs in the disease. The goal of treatment is to relieve bone pain and prevent progression of the disease. People with Paget disease should talk to their doctors about which medication is right for them. It is also important to get adequate calcium and vitamin D through diet and supplements as prescribed by your doctor, except for patients who have had kidney stones.

Bisphosphonates are a class of drugs used to treat a variety of bone diseases. Several bisphosphonates are currently available to treat Paget disease. Calcitonin is a naturally occurring hormone made by the thyroid gland. The medication may be appropriate for some patients.

Surgery. Medical therapy before surgery helps decrease bleeding and other complications. Patients who are having surgery should discuss pretreatment with their doctor. Surgery may be advised for three major complications of Paget disease:

- **Fractures.** Surgery may allow fractures to heal in better position.

- **Severe degenerative arthritis.** Hip or knee replacement may be considered if disability is severe and medication and physical therapy are no longer helpful.

- **Bone deformity.** Cutting and realigning pagetic bone (a procedure called an osteotomy) may reduce the pain in weight-bearing joints, especially the knees.

Complications resulting from enlargement of the skull or spine may injure the nervous system. However, most neurological symptoms, even those that are moderately severe, can be treated with medication and do not require neurosurgery.

Diet and exercise. There is no special diet to prevent or help treat Paget disease. However, according to the Institute of Medicine (IOM) of the National Academy of Sciences (NAS), women age 50 and older and men age 70 and older should get 1,200 mg of calcium and at least 600 IU (International Units) of vitamin D every day to maintain a healthy skeleton. People age 70 and older need to increase their vitamin D intake to 800 IU. People with a history of kidney stones should discuss calcium and vitamin D intake with their doctor.

Exercise is important because it helps preserve skeletal health, prevent weight gain, and maintain joint mobility. Patients should discuss any new exercise program with their doctor before beginning, to avoid any undue stress on affected bones.

Section 19.2

Paget Disease of Bone and Osteoarthritis: Different Yet Related

This section includes text excerpted from "Paget's Disease of Bone and Osteoarthritis: Different Yet Related," NIH Osteoporosis and Related Bone Diseases~ National Resource Center (NIH ORBD~NRC), May 2015.

Paget disease and osteoarthritis (OA) are completely different disorders that share some of the same symptoms; namely, joint and bone pain. This section describes the differences between Paget disease of bone and OA, the similarities in their symptoms, how Paget disease can cause OA, and issues related to diagnosis and treatment.

About Paget Disease

Paget disease is a chronic disorder that can result in enlarged and misshapen bones. The excessive breakdown and formation of bone tissue causes affected bone to weaken, resulting in pain, misshapen bones, fractures, and other bone and joint problems, including OA. Paget disease typically is localized, affecting just one or a few bones, as opposed to osteoporosis, for example, which affects all the bones in the body. Scientists do not know for sure what causes Paget disease.

About Osteoarthritis (OA)

OA is a condition that causes changes in cartilage, the elastic tissue that cushions the joints. Healthy cartilage allows bones to glide over one another, while absorbing energy from the shock of physical movement. In OA, the surface layer of cartilage breaks down and wears away. This allows bones under the cartilage to rub together, causing pain, swelling, and loss of motion of the joint.

Distinguishing between Paget Disease and OA

Not everyone with Paget disease will develop OA. Among those who have both, some may have OA caused by the Paget disease while others will simply have two unrelated conditions.

Both Paget disease and OA can cause joint and bone pain. In people with both conditions, joint and bone pain can occur in the same areas of the body. This can sometimes make it difficult for doctors to tell which condition is causing the pain.

No single test can diagnose OA. The diagnosis of OA in a person with Paget disease may involve blood tests, X-ray images, or the examination of fluid drawn from the joint. Blood and urine tests may also be used to help find out if something other than Paget disease is causing the arthritis.

The bone changes revealed by X-ray images help doctors diagnose both OA and Paget disease. However, in people who have both conditions in the same area of the body, it is often difficult to distinguish between the two. For this reason, the judgment of the patient's doctor is critically important for accurate diagnosis and effective treatment.

How Paget Disease Can Cause OA

Although they are different conditions, there is a link between Paget disease and OA. The changes that occur in bones affected by Paget disease can also affect the function of nearby joints. As a result, people with Paget disease frequently have OA. Paget disease can cause OA when it:

- Changes the shape of bones under the cartilage of the joint
- Causes long bones (such as the thigh or leg) to bow and bend, placing excess stress on the joints

- Causes changes in the normal curvature of the spine

- Softens the pelvis, affecting the hip joint

Treatment for Paget disease and OA

The treatment strategies for Paget disease and OA are quite different, so it is important to distinguish between the two when making therapy-related decisions. For example, people with both disorders who get good results from their Paget disease treatment may continue to experience OA-related pain. Correctly identifying OA as the source of pain is critical to the selection of effective treatments.

The goal of OA therapy is to improve joint function and control pain and swelling. Treatment approaches include exercise, weight control, rest, joint care, prescription and over-the-counter (OTC) medicines, pain relief techniques, and alternative therapies such as acupuncture and nutritional supplements. In certain cases, surgery on the affected joint may be needed.

The goal of Paget disease therapy is to relieve pain and control the progress of the disorder. Treatment strategies include the use of prescription medications approved for Paget disease, OTC pain medications, appropriate forms of exercise, and, in some cases, surgery on the affected bone or joint.

Because effective therapies are available for both Paget disease and OA, the results of the combination of the two disorders need not be severe. This is particularly true when treatment for Paget disease begins before major complications have developed.

Section 19.3

Pain and Paget Disease of Bone

This section includes text excerpted from "Pain and Paget's Disease of Bone," NIH Osteoporosis and Related Bone Diseases~National Resource Center (NIH ORBD~NRC), May 2015.

Types of Pain

Paget disease can cause several different kinds of pain, as described below.

- **Bone pain:** Small breaks called microfractures can occur in pagetic bone. These breaks can cause pain, especially in weight-bearing bone such as the spine, pelvis, or leg.

- **Joint pain:** Cartilage (a hard but slippery tissue that cushions the joints) can be damaged when Paget disease reaches the end of a long bone or changes the shape of bones located near joints. This can result in osteoarthritis (OA) and joint pain.

- **Muscle pain:** When bone is changed by Paget disease, the muscles that support the bone may have to work harder and at different angles, causing muscle pain.

- **Nervous system pain:** Bones enlarged by Paget disease can put pressure on the brain, spinal cord, or nerves. This can cause headache; pain in the neck, back, and legs; and sciatica, a "shooting" pain that travels down the sciatic nerve from the lower back to the leg.

Available Treatments

It is important for most people with Paget disease to receive medical treatment as soon as possible. Today's treatments can help reduce pain and possibly prevent the development of further complications.

Several types of medicines are used to address the pain caused by Paget disease. A doctor may recommend drugs designed to control the Paget disease or to relieve pain. The doctor also may recommend drugs to address painful complications of Paget disease, such as arthritis.

When severe pain cannot be controlled with medicine, surgery on the affected bone or joint may be needed.

An appropriate program of regular exercise also can help people with Paget disease reduce or eliminate pain.

Medicines used to treat Paget disease help slow the rate at which affected bone is changed, thereby reducing pain. The U.S. Food and Drug Administration (FDA) has approved several bisphosphonates and calcitonin for the treatment of Paget disease.

Several over-the-counter (OTC) drugs can be used to reduce the pain associated with Paget disease. Each of these medicines is taken orally (by mouth), usually in tablet form. Although there are many brand names for these drugs, they can be purchased on the basis of their key ingredient, which is:

- ibuprofen
- naproxen
- aspirin
- acetaminophen

In some cases physicians will recommend the use of pain-relieving medicine that requires a prescription.

Surgery to Manage Pain

Although surgery is rarely required for Paget disease, it should be considered in certain circumstances. Hip or knee replacement surgery may help people with severe pain from Paget disease-related arthritis. Surgery can also realign affected leg bones to reduce the stress and pain at knee and ankle joints or help broken bones heal in a better position.

The Value of Exercise

Physical exercise is an important tool for persons with Paget disease. Regular exercise can help patients:

- maintain bone strength
- avoid weight gain (and the pressure added weight puts on weakened bone)
- keep weight-bearing joints mobile and free of pain

To make sure that pagetic bone is not harmed, patients should discuss their plans with a doctor before beginning any exercise program.

There Is No Need to Be in Pain

Although there is no cure for Paget disease, people with the disorder do not have to live with constant pain. As this section describes, available therapies—especially when started early—can greatly reduce or, in some cases, eliminate the pain associated with the disease.

Section 19.4

FAQs on Paget Disease of Bone

This section includes text excerpted from "Facts a New Patient Needs to Know about Paget's Disease of Bone," NIH Osteoporosis and Related Bone Diseases~National Resource Center (NIH ORBD~NRC), May 2015.

What Is Paget Disease of Bone?

Paget disease of bone causes bones to grow larger and weaker than normal. The disease may affect one or more bones, but does not spread from affected bones to other bones in the body. Paget disease can affect any bone in your body, but most people have it in their pelvis, skull, spine, or leg bones. These bones may become misshapen and, because they are weaker than normal bones, can break more easily. Some people with Paget disease feel pain in these bones, too.

I've Never Heard of Paget Disease before. How Common Is It?

Uncommon in people under age 40, Paget disease grows more common with age. The condition is more common in people of Anglo-Saxon descent in certain geographical areas, including England, the United States, Australia, New Zealand, and Western Europe. It is not common in Scandinavia, China, Japan, or India.

Is Paget Disease a Form of Arthritis?

People with Paget disease often have arthritis at the same time, but they are different diseases. Sometimes Paget disease is confused with arthritis because the pain from Paget disease may be located on the part of the bone closest to a joint. So, it may feel a lot like the joint pain of arthritis. Paget disease can cause arthritis over time when enlarged and misshapen bones put extra stress on nearby joints. Your doctor may use several tests find out if you have Paget disease.

How Did I Get Paget Disease?

Doctors are not sure what causes the disease. Some people have hereditary Paget disease, which means it runs in their family and was passed down by their parents. But most people do not have any relatives with Paget disease. Doctors think a virus may cause Paget disease in some cases. They are studying different kinds of viruses to try to find ones that may cause the disease.

Will My Paget Disease Get Worse? What Should I Expect?

Paget disease does not affect everyone in the same way. Some people have a very mild case with few or no symptoms. Others have symptoms and complications. Pain is the most common symptom. Depending on which of your bones are affected by Paget disease, you might have other symptoms and complications, such as those listed below.

Table 19.1. Symptoms Associated with Paget Disease

If You Have Paget Disease Here:	You May Have Some of These Symptoms and Complications:
Pelvis	Pain or arthritis in the hip joint
Skull	Enlarged head, hearing loss, or headaches
Spine	Curved spine, back pain, or damage to nerves causing problems such as tingling and numbness
Leg	Bowed legs, pain, or arthritis in the hip and knee joints

Although rare, the most serious complication of Paget disease is bone cancer.

Can Paget Disease Be Treated?

Yes, Paget disease can be treated. Finding and treating Paget disease early is best to prevent complications. The U.S. Food and Drug Administration (FDA) has approved several drugs to treat the disease. Doctors most often prescribe drugs called bisphosphonates. These help reduce bone pain and stop or slow down the progress of the disease.

Will These Drugs Also Help Improve the Complications I Have from Paget Disease?

The drugs may help prevent complications from starting or prevent them from getting worse, but they cannot correct problems that have already set in. In some cases, surgery can help. Your doctor can tell you if surgery might be a good idea for you.

How Will the Doctor Know If the Drug I Take Is Working?

Your doctor will probably monitor your progress using two tests: an X-ray of your bones and a blood test to measure the level of a chemical called serum alkaline phosphatase (SAP) in your blood. The X-rays will show your doctor pictures of how your bones are healing. A decrease in the amount of SAP in your blood will tell your doctor that the disease is less active and you are getting better.

Is There a Special Diet I Should Follow?

There is no special diet to prevent or help treat Paget disease. For overall bone health, you should eat a balanced diet rich in calcium and vitamin D. The Institute of Medicine (IOM) of the National Academy of Sciences (NAS) recommends 1,000 mg (milligrams) of calcium daily for adults age 19–50. Women over age 50 and men over age 70 should increase their intake to 1,200 mg daily. To help your body use the calcium, the IOM recommends 600 International Units (IU) of vitamin D up to age 70 and 800 IU after 70.

What about Exercise? Can I Still Be Active?

Exercise is important for people with Paget disease. Being active can help you maintain healthy bones, control your weight, and keep your joints moving. But, you should talk with your doctor before starting an exercise program to make sure what you plan to do is safe and will not put too much stress on the bones that are affected by Paget disease. For example, your doctor might advise you to try walking instead of jogging if you have Paget disease in your legs.

Do I Need to See a Special Doctor? What Kinds of Doctors Specialize in This Disease?

The doctor who diagnosed your Paget disease may be a specialist in the disease. If not, he or she can refer you to someone who is. Doctors who are the most experienced in treating patients with Paget disease are:

- endocrinologists, who treat hormonal and metabolic disorders

- rheumatologists, who treat joint and muscle disorders

Sometimes other doctors may be needed, such as orthopaedists; neurologists; and ear, nose, and throat specialists. Your doctor will help you find the specialists you need.

Will My Children Get This Disease, Too?

Paget disease does not always run in families; however, research suggests that a close relative of someone with Paget disease is seven times more likely to develop the disease than someone without an affected relative. Finding and treating Paget disease early is important, so some doctors recommend that children and siblings of a person with Paget disease be tested for the disease every 2–3 years after the age of 40.

To screen for Paget disease, a doctor uses the SAP test. If the SAP level is high, suggesting that there might be Paget disease, the doctor can perform a test called a bone scan to learn which bones may be affected. The doctor will typically order an X-ray of the affected bones to make sure the diagnosis of Paget disease is correct.

Chapter 20

Polymyalgia Rheumatica and Giant Cell Arteritis

Polymyalgia Rheumatica

What Is It?

Polymyalgia rheumatica (PMR) causes muscle pain and stiffness in the neck, shoulder, and hip. The pain and stiffness usually occur in the morning or when you haven't been moving for a while. It typically lasts longer than 30 minutes. For most people, the condition develops over time. But for some people it can start quickly—even overnight. In addition to stiffness, you may have a fever, weakness, and weight loss.

PMR usually goes away within one year, but it could last several years.

People with PMR often have giant cell arteritis (GCA) a disorder associated with inflammation of arteries located on each side of the head.

This chapter contains text excerpted from the following sources: Text under heading "Polymyalgia Rheumatica" is excerpted from "Polymyalgia Rheumatica," National Institute of Arthritis and Musculoskeletal and Skin Diseases (NIAMS), May 30, 2016; Text under heading "Giant Cell Arteritis" is excerpted from "Giant Cell Arteritis," National Institute of Arthritis and Musculoskeletal and Skin Diseases (NIAMS), May 30, 2016.

Who Gets It

Women are more likely than men to develop PMR. This disease mostly affects people over the age of 50, with highest rates at 70–80 years of age.

What Are the Symptoms

Symptoms of PMR can include:

• Pain and stiffness in the neck, shoulder, and hip area

• Flu-like symptoms, including fever, weakness, and weight loss

What Causes It

Researchers don't know what causes PMR. It is associated with:

• Immune system problems

• Genes

• Environmental triggers, such as an infection

• Aging processes

Is There a Test?

There is no single test to tell if you have PMR. The doctor usually bases the diagnosis on:

• Medical history

• Symptoms

• Physical exam

• Blood tests

How Is It Treated?

PMR is treated by medications including:

• **Corticosteroids** such as prednisone. You will start with a low daily dose that is increased as needed until symptoms disappear. Your doctor may then gradually reduce the dose, and you will probably stop taking the medication after six months to two years. Your doctor will put you back on the medicine if symptoms come back. You will stop taking the medicine when symptoms completely go away.

- **Nonsteroidal anti-inflammatory drugs (NSAIDs),** such as aspirin and ibuprofen. The medication must be taken daily, and long-term use may cause stomach problems. For most patients, NSAIDs by themselves do not make symptoms go away.

Giant Cell Arteritis (GCA)

What Is It?

Giant cell arteritis (GCA) causes the arteries of the scalp and neck to become red, hot, swollen, or painful. The arteries most affected are those in the temples on either side of the head. These arteries narrow, so not enough blood can pass through.

It is important that you get treatment right away. Otherwise, the arteries could be permanently damaged. There is also a risk of blindness or stroke.

If you have GCA, your doctor should also look for signs of another disorder, polymyalgia rheumatica (PMR). These conditions often occur together.

Who Gets It

GCA mainly affects people over 50, especially women. Men with the disorder are more likely to develop blindness.

What Are the Symptoms?

Signs of GCA can include:

- Flu-like symptoms early in the disease, such as feeling tired, loss of appetite, and fever

- Headaches

- Pain and tenderness over the temples

- Double vision or vision loss

- Dizziness

- Problems with coordination and balance

- Pain in the jaw and tongue, especially when eating

- Difficulty in opening the mouth wide

- Scalp scores (rare cases)

Is There a Test?

To diagnose you with GCA, your doctor will:

- Ask you about your medical history

- Give you a physical exam to see if the arteries in your temples are swollen, tender to the touch, and have a reduced pulse

- Take a small section of the artery in your temple to examine it under a microscope

How Is It Treated?

GCA is treated with medications, such as prednisone. You will probably take high doses of the medicine for about one month. Your doctor will slowly reduce the dose, which may cause some symptoms to come back. After a while, symptoms usually go away completely, and the doctor can stop the prednisone altogether.

You should report any symptoms to your doctor so that you can be treated early. This will help prevent serious problems such as permanent vision loss and stroke.

Chapter 21

Psoriasis and Psoriatic Arthritis

Chapter Contents

Section 21.1—Psoriasis... 250
Section 21.2—Psoriatic Arthritis 253

Section 21.1

Psoriasis

This section includes text excerpted from "Psoriasis,"
National Institute of Arthritis and Musculoskeletal and Skin
Diseases (NIAMS), March 30, 2017.

Psoriasis is a skin disease that causes red, scaly skin that may feel painful, swollen or hot.

If you have psoriasis, you are more likely to get some other conditions, including:

- Psoriatic arthritis, a condition that causes joint pain and swelling

- Cardiovascular problems, which affect the heart and blood circulation system

- Obesity

- High blood pressure

- Diabetes

Some treatments for psoriasis can have serious side effects, so be sure to talk about them with your doctor and keep all your appointments.

Who Gets Psoriasis

Anyone can get psoriasis, but it is more common in adults. Certain genes have been linked to psoriasis, so you are more likely to get it if someone else in your family has it.

Types of Psoriasis

There are several different types of psoriasis. Here are a few examples:

- **Plaque psoriasis,** which causes patches of skin that are red at the base and covered by silvery scales.

- **Guttate psoriasis,** which causes small, drop-shaped lesions on your trunk, limbs, and scalp. This type of psoriasis is most often triggered by upper respiratory infections, such as strep throat.

- **Pustular psoriasis,** which causes pus-filled blisters. Attacks or flares can be caused by medications, infections, stress, or certain chemicals.

- **Inverse psoriasis,** which causes smooth, red patches in folds of skin near the genitals, under the breasts or in the armpits. Rubbing and sweating can make this type of psoriasis worse.

- **Erythrodermic psoriasis,** which causes red and scaly skin over much of your body. This can be a reaction to a bad sunburn or taking certain medications, such as corticosteroids. It can also happen if you have a different type of psoriasis that is not well controlled. This type of psoriasis can be very serious, so if you have it, you should see a doctor immediately.

Symptoms of Psoriasis

Psoriasis usually causes patches of thick, red skin with silvery scales that itch or feel sore. These patches can show up anywhere on your body, but they usually occur on the elbows, knees, legs, scalp, lower back, face, palms, and soles of feet. They can also show up on your fingernails and toenails, genitals, and inside your mouth. You may find that your skin gets worse for a while, which is called a flare, and then improves.

Causes of Psoriasis

Psoriasis is an autoimmune disease, which means that your body's immune system—which protects you from diseases—starts overacting and causing problems. If you have psoriasis, a type of white blood cells (WBCs) called the T cells become so active that they trigger other immune system responses, including swelling and fast turnover of skin cells.

Your skin cells grow deep in the skin and rise slowly to the surface. This is called cell turnover, and it usually takes about a month. If you have psoriasis, though, cell turnover can take only a few days. Your skin cells rise too fast and pile up on the surface, causing your skin to look red and scaly. Some things may cause a flare, meaning your psoriasis becomes worse for a while, including:

- Infections

- Stress

- Changes in the weather that dry out your skin

- Certain medicines

- Cuts, scratches or sunburns

Certain genes have been linked to psoriasis, meaning it runs in families.

Diagnosis of Psoriasis

Psoriasis can be hard to diagnose because it can look like other skin diseases. Your doctor may look at a small sample of your skin under a microscope to help them figure out if psoriasis is causing your skin condition.

Treating Psoriasis

There are several different types of treatment for psoriasis. Your doctor may recommend that you try one of these or a combination of them:

- **Topical treatment,** which means putting creams on your skin.

- **Light therapy,** which involves a doctor shining an ultraviolet light on your skin or getting more sunlight. It's important that a doctor controls the amount of light you are getting from this therapy, because too much ultraviolet light may make your psoriasis worse.

- **Systemic treatment,** which can include taking prescription medicines or getting shots of medicine.

Healthcare Team

Several types of healthcare professionals may treat you, including:

- Dermatologists, who treat skin problems

- Internists, who diagnose and treat adults

Living with It

Psoriasis is a chronic disease, which means it lasts a long time. You can take an active role in treating your psoriasis. Besides going to your doctor regularly, here are some things you can try to help manage your symptoms:

- Keeping your skin well moisturized

- Staying healthy overall

- Joining support groups or counseling to help you realize you are not alone in dealing with psoriasis and to share ideas for coping with the disease

Section 21.2

Psoriatic Arthritis

This section includes text excerpted from "Psoriatic Arthritis," National Institute of Arthritis and Musculoskeletal and Skin Diseases (NIAMS), March 30, 2017.

Psoriatic arthritis can occur in people who have psoriasis (scaly red and white skin patches). It affects the joints and areas where tissues attach to the bone.

The joints most often affected are:

- The outer joints of the fingers or toes

- Wrists

- Knees

- Ankles

- Lower back

Who Gets Psoriatic Arthritis

Anyone with psoriasis (scaly red and white skin patches) can have psoriatic arthritis.

It is more common in Caucasians than African Americans or Asian Americans. The disease typically begins between the ages of 30–50, but can begin in childhood.

Symptoms of Psoriatic Arthritis

Symptoms of psoriatic arthritis include:

- Joint pain and swelling that may come and go. Joints may also be red and warm
- Tenderness in the heel and bottom of the foot
- Pain and stiffness in the neck and lower back
- Joint stiffness, especially in the morning
- Painful, sausage-like swelling of the fingers and/or toes
- Thickness and reddening of the skin with flaky, silver-white patches called scales
- Pitting of the nails or separation from the nail bed
- Tiredness
- Pink eye or other eye infections

Causes of Psoriatic Arthritis

No one knows what causes psoriatic arthritis. Researchers believe that both genes and environment are involved.

Is There a Test?

If you have psoriasis and start to develop joint pain, it's important to see your doctor. Early diagnosis and treatment of psoriatic arthritis can help prevent joint damage.

Although there is no test for psoriatic arthritis, your doctor may do the following to diagnose your condition:

- Ask you about your medical and family history
- Give you a physical exam
- Take samples of blood or joint fluid for a laboratory test
- Take X-rays

Treatment of Psoriatic Arthritis

Psoriatic arthritis is treated by medications. The type of medication depends on how severe the disease is.

Healthcare Team

Doctors who diagnose and treat psoriatic arthritis include:

- A general practitioner, such as your family doctor
- A rheumatologist, who treats arthritis and other diseases of the bones, joints, and muscles

Chapter 22

Scleroderma

Scleroderma is the name for a group of diseases that cause patches of tight, hard skin. Some forms of scleroderma can also damage your blood vessels and internal organs.

Who Gets Scleroderma

Anyone can get scleroderma, but it is more common in adults and women.

Some types of scleroderma are more common in different groups. Most localized types show up before age 40. They are also more common in people of European descent. Systemic types are more common in people ages 30–50 and in African Americans.

Types of Scleroderma

Scleroderma's main types are localized and systemic. Localized means the disease affects only certain parts of the body. Systemic means it can affect the whole body.

The localized type often affects only your skin. It does not harm major organs. It may get better or go away without help. But it can be severe in some people and can leave skin damage.

The systemic type affects your skin, tissues under it, blood vessels, and major organs.

This chapter includes text excerpted from "Scleroderma," National Institute of Arthritis and Musculoskeletal and Skin Diseases (NIAMS), August 30, 2016.

Symptoms of Scleroderma

Scleroderma causes your tissues to get hard and thick. Depending on what type of scleroderma you have, you may find that your skin gets hard and tight, or you may have problems with your blood vessels and major organs, such as your heart, lungs, and kidneys.

Causes of Scleroderma

Doctors don't know what causes scleroderma, but they do know you can't catch it from other people. It is probably an autoimmune disease, which means your immune system is attacking your own body.

Diagnosis of Scleroderma

Scleroderma can be hard to diagnose, since other diseases have similar symptoms. To figure out if you have scleroderma, your doctor may ask questions about your health and symptoms and do a physical exam. Your doctor may also do some lab tests and take a sample of your skin to look at under a microscope.

Treatment of Scleroderma

The treatment for scleroderma depends on what part of your body it is affecting. Your doctor may recommend stretching exercises for your joints, creams for your skin, dietary changes, or treatments to make the red patches on your skin less apparent. Scleroderma has no cure, but symptoms and damage can be reduced.

Healthcare Team

Several types of healthcare professionals may treat you, including:

- **Rheumatologists,** who treat diseases of the bones, joints, and muscles

- **Internists,** who diagnose and treat adults

- **Dermatologists,** who treat skin problems

- **Orthopaedists,** who treat and perform surgery for bone and joint diseases

- **Pulmonologists,** who treat lung problems

Living with It

You can take an active part in treating your scleroderma. Be sure to take your medications as prescribed, keep your physical therapy appointments, and call your doctor if you notice new symptoms. Here are some ways to take care of your skin:

- **Skin problems.** With scleroderma, collagen builds up in the skin. Too much of it can make your skin dry and stiff. To help, you can:

  - Use oil-based creams and lotions after every bath

  - Use sunscreen

  - Use a humidifier at home

  - Avoid hot baths or showers

  - Avoid strong soaps, cleaners, and chemicals. Wear rubber gloves if you have to use those products

  - Exercise regularly

- **Cosmetic problems.** Scleroderma can damage your skin and change how it looks. These skin changes can affect your self-image. Ways to fix skin damage include:

  - Lasers that take away red spots on the hands and face

  - Plastic surgery in areas where the disease is not active

If you have systemic scleroderma, the disease may affect other parts of your body, besides just your skin. Here are some common treatments and things to watch for if you have systemic scleroderma:

- **Raynaud phenomenon.** Most people with scleroderma have Raynaud phenomenon. It can affect the fingers, feet, and hands. It makes them change color if you are too cold or anxious. To help, you can:

  - Not smoke

  - Dress warm, and keep hands and feet warm

  - Do exercises that relax the body

  - Ask about medicines that open small blood vessels and help with blood flow

  - Ask about medicines that treat skin sores and ulcers

- **Stiff, painful joints.** Stiffness and pain come from hard skin around joints and joint swelling. To help, you can:

  - Do stretching exercises that help with joint motion

  - Exercise regularly (swimming is best)

  - Take medicine to help ease pain or swelling. Ask your doctor which are the best for you to take.

  - Learn to do daily tasks in ways that put less stress on the joints

- **Dry mouth and dental problems.** If you have tight skin on your face, you may have trouble caring for your teeth. Dry mouth speeds up tooth decay. Harm to tissues in the mouth can loosen teeth. To avoid problems:

  - Brush and floss your teeth each day

  - Have frequent dental checkups

  - See your dentist if you have mouth sores, mouth pain, or lose teeth

  - Ask your dentist about special rinses and toothpaste

  - Learn ways to keep your mouth and face flexible

  - Keep your mouth moist. You can drink lots of water or suck on ice chips. You can also chew gum or suck on hard candy that has no sugar added.

  - Avoid mouthwash that has alcohol

  - If dry mouth still bothers you, ask your doctor about helpful medicines

- **Gastrointestinal problems.** Digestive problems can include heartburn, trouble swallowing, feeling full as soon as you start eating, diarrhea, constipation, and gas. To help, you can:

  - Eat small, frequent meals

  - Stand or sit for 1–3 hours after eating

  - Use blocks to raise the head of your bed

  - Avoid late-night meals, spicy or fatty foods, alcohol, and caffeine

  - Eat moist, soft foods, and chew them well

- Ask your doctor about medicines for diarrhea, constipation, and heartburn

- **Lung damage.** Lung problems with systemic scleroderma can include loss of lung function, severe lung disease, lung tissue scarring, and high blood pressure in the artery that carries blood from your heart to your lungs. Watch for signs of lung disease, such as:

  - Fatigue

  - Shortness of breath

  - Problems with breathing

  - Swollen feet

  - As soon as your skin starts to thicken, see your doctor. Get regular flu and pneumonia shots.

- **Heart problems.** Systemic scleroderma can sometimes cause scarring and weakness in your heart, as well as swelling of the heart muscle and a heartbeat that isn't normal. These problems can all be treated with help from your doctor.

- **Kidney problems.** Scleroderma can cause very high blood pressure and kidney failure in some people. Talk to your doctor about what symptoms to look for so you can spot problems right away. You should:

  - Check your blood pressure often

  - Check your blood pressure if you have new symptoms

  - Call your doctor if your blood pressure is higher than normal

  - Take the medicines your doctor prescribes

Chapter 23

Sjögren Syndrome

Sjögren syndrome is an autoimmune disease, which means that your immune system turns against the body's own cells. Normally, the immune system works to protect us from disease by destroying harmful invading organisms like viruses and bacteria. In the case of Sjögren syndrome, disease-fighting cells attack various organs, usually in the glands that produce tears and saliva. Damage to these glands reduces both the quantity and quality of their secretions.

Sjögren syndrome is also a rheumatic disease, which primarily affect:

- Joints
- Tendons
- Ligaments
- Bones
- Muscles

The signs and symptoms of rheumatic diseases can include:

- Redness or heat
- Swelling

This chapter includes text excerpted from "Sjögren's Syndrome," National Institute of Arthritis and Musculoskeletal and Skin Diseases (NIAMS), September 30, 2016.

- Pain

- Loss of function

Who Gets Sjögren Syndrome

Sjögren syndrome can affect people of either sex and of any age, but most cases occur in women. The average age of onset is the late forties, but in rare cases, Sjögren syndrome is diagnosed in children.

Types of Sjögren Syndrome

Doctor's classify Sjögren syndrome as either primary or secondary. You have primary Sjögren syndrome if you do not have other rheumatic diseases. You have secondary Sjögren syndrome if you already have another rheumatic disease, such as rheumatoid arthritis (RA) or systemic lupus erythematosus (SLE), scleroderma, or polymyositis.

Symptoms of Sjögren Syndrome

Sjögren syndrome can cause many symptoms, the most common symptoms include:

- **Dry eyes.** If you have Sjögren syndrome your eyes may burn or itch. Some people say it feels like they have sand in their eyes. You may have trouble with blurry vision, or bright lights, especially fluorescent lighting.

- **Dry mouth.** If you have Sjögren syndrome your mouth may feel chalky or like your mouth is full of cotton. It may be difficult to swallow, speak, or taste. Because you lack the protective effects of saliva, you may develop more dental decay (cavities) and mouth infections.

Sjögren syndrome can also affect other parts of your body, causing symptoms such as:

- Multiple sites of joint and muscle pain

- Prolonged dry skin

- Skin rashes on the extremities

- Chronic dry cough

- Vaginal dryness

- Numbness or tingling in the extremities

- Prolonged fatigue that interferes with daily life.

A small number of people with Sjögren syndrome may develop lymphoma. A form of cancer, lymphoma can affect the salivary glands, lymph nodes, the gastrointestinal tract, or the lungs. If you have enlargement of a salivary gland, you should contact your doctor. Other symptoms may include the following:

- Unexplained fever

- Night sweats

- Constant fatigue

- Unexplained weight loss

- Itchy skin

- Reddened patches on the skin

Many of these can be symptoms of other problems, including Sjögren syndrome itself. Nevertheless, it is important to see your doctor if you have any of these symptoms.

Causes

Researchers think Sjögren syndrome is caused by a combination of genetic and environmental factors. Several different genes appear to be involved, but scientists are not certain exactly which ones are linked to the disease, because different genes seem to play a role in different people.

Scientists think that the trigger may be a viral or bacterial infection. The possibility that the endocrine and nervous systems play a role in the disease is also under investigation.

Diagnosis

Your doctor will diagnose Sjögren syndrome using your:

- **Medical history.** Because there are many causes of dry eyes and dry mouth (including many common medications, other diseases, or previous treatment such as radiation of the head or neck), your doctor needs a thorough history.

- **A physical exam.** During the exam, your doctor will check for clinical signs of Sjögren syndrome, such as indications of mouth dryness or signs of other connective tissue diseases.

265

- **Results from clinical or laboratory tests.** Depending on what your doctor finds during the history and exam, he or she may want to perform some tests or refer you to a specialist to establish the diagnosis of Sjögren syndrome, including:

  - Blood tests to determine the presence of antibodies common in Sjögren syndrome, including anti-Sjögren-syndrome-related antigen A (SSA) and anti-Sjögren syndrome type B (SSB) antibodies or rheumatoid factor.

  - Other tests can identify decreases in tear and saliva production.

  - Biopsy of the saliva glands and other specialized tests can also help to confirm the diagnosis.

Treatment

Treatment can vary from person to person, depending on what parts of your body are affected.

Treatments for Dry Eyes

There are many treatments you can try or your doctor can prescribe for dry eyes. Here are some that might help:

- **Eye drops** to keep your eyes moist by replacing the natural tears. These products are available by prescription or over the counter under many brand names. Eye drops come in different thicknesses, so you may have to experiment to find the right one. Some drops contain preservatives that might irritate your eyes. Drops without preservatives usually don't bother the eyes.

- **Ointments** are thicker than eye drops. Because they moisturize and protect the eye for several hours, and may blur your vision, they are most effective during sleep.

- **Other therapies,** such as plugging or blocking the tear ducts, anti-inflammatory medication, or surgery may be needed in more severe cases.

Treatments for Dry Mouth

There are many remedies for dry mouth. You can try some of them on your own. Your doctor may prescribe others. Here are some many people find useful:

- **Chewing gum and hard candy.** If your salivary glands still produce some saliva, you can stimulate them to make more by chewing gum or sucking on hard candy. However, gum and candy must be sugar-free, because dry mouth makes you extremely prone to progressive dental decay (cavities).

- **Taking sips of water or another sugar-free, noncarbonated drink** throughout the day to wet your mouth, especially when you are eating or talking. Note that drinking large amounts of liquid throughout the day will not make your mouth any less dry and will make you urinate more often. You should only take small sips of liquid, but not too often. If you sip liquids every few minutes, it may reduce or remove the mucus coating inside your mouth, increasing the feeling of dryness.

- **Using an oil or petroleum-based lip balm or lipstick** can soothe dry, cracked lips. If your mouth hurts, your doctor may give you medicine in a mouth rinse, ointment, or gel to apply to the sore areas to control pain and inflammation.

- **Using other therapies,** such as saliva substitutes or medications that stimulate the salivary glands to produce saliva, is sometimes indicated.

Treatments for Symptoms in Other Parts of the Body

If you have extraglandular involvement, which means a problem that extends beyond the moisture-producing glands of your eyes and mouth, your doctor may treat those problems using nonsteroidal anti-inflammatory drugs (NSAIDs) or immune-modifying drugs.

Healthcare Team

The symptoms of Sjögren syndrome usually develop gradually and are similar to those of many other diseases. This means it can take time to get a diagnosis. You may see a number of doctors, any of whom could diagnose the disease and help with your treatment, including:

- A rheumatologist, a doctor who specializes in diseases of the joints, muscles, and bones

- A primary care physician

- An internist

- An ophthalmologist, a doctor who specializes in caring for the eyes

- An otolaryngologist, a doctor who specializes in caring for the ears, nose, and throat

Usually, a rheumatologist will coordinate your treatment among a number of specialists.

Living with It

Living with Sjögren's syndrome can be easier by following some tips for:

- Eye care

- Mouth care

- Protecting your voice

- Understanding medicines that cause dryness

General Tips for Eye Care

- Don't use eye drops that irritate your eyes. If one brand or prescription bothers you, try another. Eye drops that do not contain preservatives are usually essential for long-term use.

- Practice blinking. You tend to blink less when reading or using the computer. Remember to blink 5–6 times a minute.

- Protect your eyes from drafts, breezes, and wind.

- Put humidifiers in the rooms where you spend the most time, including the bedroom, or install a humidifier in your heating and air conditioning unit.

- Don't smoke, and stay out of smoky rooms.

- Apply mascara only to the tips of your lashes so it doesn't get in your eyes. If you use eyeliner or eyeshadow, put it only on the skin above your lashes, not on the sensitive skin under your lashes, close to your eyes. Avoid facial creams on the lower lid skin at bedtime if you are awakening with eye irritation.

- Ask your doctor whether any medications that you are taking contribute to dryness. If they do, ask how the dryness can be reduced.

Importance of Mouth Care

Natural saliva contains substances that help get rid of bacteria that can cause cavities and mouth infections. Good oral hygiene or mouth care is extremely important when you have dry mouth. Here's what you can do to prevent cavities and infections:

Visit a dentist regularly, at least twice a year, to have your teeth examined and cleaned.

- Rinse your mouth with water several times a day.

- Don't use mouthwash that contains alcohol, because alcohol is drying.

- Use toothpaste that contains fluoride to gently brush your teeth, gums, and tongue after each meal and before bedtime. Nonfoaming toothpaste is less drying. Floss your teeth every day.

- Avoid sugar between meals. That means choosing sugar-free gum, candy, and soda. If you do eat or drink sugary foods, brush your teeth immediately afterward.

- See a dentist right away if you notice anything unusual or have continuous burning or other oral symptoms.

- Ask your dentist whether you need to take fluoride supplements, use a fluoride gel at night, or have a varnish put on your teeth to protect the enamel.

Protect Your Voice

You can develop hoarseness if their vocal cords become inflamed or become irritated from throat dryness or coughing. To prevent further strain on your vocal cords, try not to clear your throat before speaking. Clearing your throat is hard on the vocal cords. To avoid irritating your vocal cords:

- Sip water

- Chew sugar-free gum

- Suck on sugar-free candy

- Make an "h" sound, hum, or laugh to gently bring the vocal cords together

Medicines and Dryness

Some medicines can cause eye and mouth dryness. If you are taking one of the drugs listed below, talk to your doctor about adjusting the dose or finding a different medicine. Don't stop taking any medicine without asking your doctor. These can include medicines that you take for:

- Allergies and colds (antihistamines and decongestants)
- Getting rid of extra fluids in your body (diuretics)
- Diarrhea
- High blood pressure

Some type of medicines that can cause dryness include:

- Antipsychotic medicines
- Tranquilizers
- Antidepressants

Chapter 24

Work-Related Arthritis and Ergonomics

The term arthritis is used to describe more than 100 rheumatic diseases and conditions that affect joints, the tissues which surround the joint and other connective tissue. The pattern, severity, and location of symptoms can vary depending on the specific form of the disease. Forty-six million Americans report that a doctor told them they have arthritis or other rheumatic conditions. Arthritis is the most common cause of disability in the United States. Arthritis limits the activities of nearly 19 million adults. Two-thirds of individuals with arthritis are under age 65.

The National Arthritis Data Working Group estimates that 27 million adults have osteoarthritis. Nine million adults report symptomatic knee osteoarthritis, and 13 million reports symptomatic hand osteoarthritis. Persons are considered to have symptomatic osteoarthritis if they have frequent pain in a joint (e.g., pain in a joint on most days of a recent month) and radiographic (e.g., X-ray) evidence of osteoarthritis in that joint, although sometimes this pain may not actually emanate from arthritis seen on the radiograph. Other forms of arthritis include rheumatoid arthritis and gout. Arthritis is a concern in the workplace both because it may develop from work-related conditions

This chapter includes text excerpted from "Work-Related Musculoskeletal Disorders and Ergonomics," Centers for Disease Control and Prevention (CDC), February 1, 2018.

271

and because it may require worksite adaptations for employees with limitations or disabilities.

Certain occupations are associated with increased prevalence of arthritis, specifically osteoarthritis, most often of the knee and/or hip. These occupations include mining, construction, agriculture, and sectors of the service industry. Common features of these occupations are physically demanding/heavy labor tasks, lifting or carrying heavy loads, exposure to vibration, high risk of joint or tissue injury, and prolonged periods of working in awkward or unnatural postures such as kneeling and crawling.

- In 2003, the total cost for arthritis conditions was $128 billion—$81 billion in direct costs and $47 billion in indirect costs

- Persons who are limited in their work by arthritis are said to have Arthritis-attributable work limitations (AAWL). AAWL affects one in 20 working-age adults (aged 18–64) in the United States and one in three working-age adults with self-reported, doctor-diagnosed arthritis

- The National Business Group on Health (NBGH) recommends that employers address arthritis by encouraging workers to avoid obesity and providing ergonomically appropriate workplace design.

Early diagnosis and appropriate management of arthritis can help people with arthritis decrease pain, improve function, stay productive, and lower healthcare costs. Appropriate management includes consulting with a doctor and self-management education programs to help teach people with arthritis techniques to manage arthritis on a day-to-day basis. Physical activity and weight management programs are also important self-management activities for persons with arthritis.

Developing and Implementing Workplace Controls

Engineering controls, administrative controls and use of personal protective.

A three-tier hierarchy of controls is widely accepted as an intervention strategy for reducing, eliminating, or controlling workplace hazards, including ergonomic hazards. The three tiers are:

- Use of engineering controls

  - The preferred approach to prevent and control WMSDs is to design the job to take account of the capabilities and limitations of the workforce using engineering controls. Some examples include:

- Changing the way materials, parts, and products can be transported. For example, using mechanical assist devices to relieve heavy load lifting and carrying tasks or using handles or slotted hand holes in packages requiring manual handling.

- Changing workstation layout, which might include using height-adjustable workbenches or locating tools and materials within short reaching distances

- Use of administrative controls (changes in work practices and management policies)

  - Administrative control strategies are policies and practices that reduce WMSD risk but they do not eliminate workplace hazards. Although engineering controls are preferred, administrative controls can be helpful as temporary measures until engineering controls can be implemented or when engineering controls are not technically feasible. Some examples include:

  - Reducing shift length or limiting the amount of overtime

  - Changes in job rules and procedures such as scheduling more breaks to allow for rest and recovery

  - Rotating workers through jobs that are physically tiring

  - Training in the recognition of risk factors for WMSDs and instructions in work practices and techniques that can ease the task demands or burden (e.g., stress and strain)

- Use of personal protective equipment (PPE)

  - PPE generally provides a barrier between the worker and hazard source. Respirators, ear plugs, safety goggles, chemical aprons, safety shoes, and hard hats are all examples of PPE.

  - Whether braces, wrist splints, back belts, and similar devices can be regarded as offering personal protection against ergonomic hazards remains an open question. Although these devices may, in some situations, reduce the duration, frequency or intensity of exposure, evidence of their effectiveness in injury reduction is inconclusive. In some instances, these devices may decrease one exposure but increase another because the worker has to "fight" the device to perform the work. An example is the use of wrist splints while engaging in work that requires wrist bending.

Ergonomics

Ergonomics is the science of fitting workplace conditions and job demands to the capability of the working population. The goal of ergonomics is to reduce stress and eliminate injuries and disorders associated with the overuse of muscles, bad posture, and repeated tasks. A workplace ergonomics program can aim to prevent or control injuries and illnesses by eliminating or reducing worker exposure to WMSD risk factors using engineering and administrative controls. PPE is also used in some instances but it is the least effective workplace control to address ergonomic hazards. Risk factors include awkward postures, repetition, material handling, force, mechanical compression, vibration, temperature extremes, glare, inadequate lighting, and duration of exposure. For example, employees who spend many hours at a workstation may develop ergonomic-related problems resulting in musculoskeletal disorders (MSDs).

Chapter 25

Arthritis-Related to Other Disorders

Chapter Contents

Section 25.1—Comorbidities 276

Section 25.2—Arthritis and Human
Immunodeficiency Virus 280

Section 25.3—Arthritis and Inflammatory Bowel
Disease 282

275

Section 25.1

Comorbidities

This section includes text excerpted from
"Comorbidities," Centers for Disease Control and
Prevention (CDC), November 28, 2017.

What Does "Comorbidity" Mean?

Comorbidity means more than one disease or condition is present in the same person at the same time. Conditions described as comorbidities are often chronic or long-term conditions. Other names to describe comorbid conditions are coexisting or co-occurring conditions and sometimes also "multimorbidity" or "multiple chronic conditions."

Comorbidities are common among adults with rheumatic diseases like arthritis.

The Centers for Disease Control and Prevention (CDC) Arthritis Program examines comorbidities in two ways:

- **Comorbidities among people with arthritis**. Everyone in this group has arthritis and at least one other chronic condition.

- **Arthritis among people with other chronic conditions**. People with other chronic conditions, such as heart disease or diabetes, who also have arthritis.

Arthritis Is Common among People with Other Chronic Conditions

In the total U.S. population, 22.7 percent of adults have arthritis. Arthritis is even more common among people with other chronic conditions. In 2013–2015, the unadjusted prevalence of arthritis among adults had:

- Obesity was 31 percent

- Diabetes was 47 percent

- Heart disease was 49 percent

Figure 25.1 shows the age-adjusted estimates for obese, diabetes, and heart disease among adults with arthritis. Age-adjusted prevalence estimates were standardized to the projected 2000 U.S. standard population to allow for comparisons between different groups by accounting for variations in age-distribution. After age-adjustment, adults who were obese, had diabetes, or heart disease were approximately 1.5, 1.7, and 1.9 times more likely than those without the corresponding condition to have arthritis, respectively.

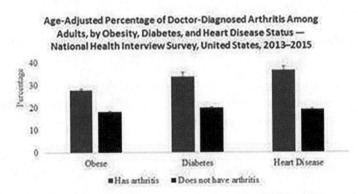

Figure 25.1. *Arthritis Prevalence by Chronic Disease Status, National Health Interview Survey (NHIS) 2013–2015*

Arthritis and Heart Disease

Arthritis may be a barrier to physical activity among adults with heart disease. Being physically active, for example, through aerobic exercise or strength training, can benefit people with arthritis or heart disease and especially those with both conditions.

What Are the Benefits of Increased Physical Activity for People with Heart Disease and Arthritis?

People with heart disease who are inactive can experience many benefits from becoming more physically active. Benefits of physical activity for people with heart disease can include:

- Lower blood pressure
- Better physical function
- Lower low-density lipoprotein cholesterol levels

Physical inactivity is more common in adults who have both arthritis and heart disease compared with people who only have one or neither condition. Physical inactivity puts people at greater risk for complications from chronic conditions.

Arthritis and Diabetes

Arthritis may be a barrier to physical activity among adults with diabetes. Being physically active, for example, through aerobic exercise or strength training, can benefit people with arthritis or diabetes and especially those with both conditions.

What Are the Benefits of Increased Physical Activity for People with Diabetes and Arthritis?

People with diabetes who are inactive can experience many benefits from becoming more physically active. Benefits of physical activity for people with diabetes can include:

- Lower blood glucose levels
- Better weight control
- Lower blood pressure
- Improved mood

Being physically inactive is an even bigger problem for people with diabetes who also have arthritis. Physical inactivity is more common in adults who have both arthritis and diabetes compared with people who only have one or neither condition. Physical inactivity puts people at greater risk for complications from chronic conditions.

Arthritis and Obesity

Arthritis may be a barrier to physical activity among adults who are obese. Being physically active, for example, through aerobic exercise or strength training, can benefit people with arthritis or obesity and especially those with both conditions.

What Are the Benefits of Increased Physical Activity for People Who Are Obese?

People who are obese and physically inactive can experience many benefits from becoming more physically active. Benefits of physical activity for obese people include:

- Better weight control
- Reduce your risk of diabetes, heart disease, and other comorbidities
- Improved mood
- Strengthen muscles and bones

Physical inactivity is more common in adults who have both arthritis and obesity compared with people who only have one or neither condition. Physical inactivity puts people at greater risk for complications from chronic conditions.

What Can People Who Have Arthritis and Comorbidities Do?

The CDC Arthritis Program recommends self-management education programs and physical activity programs for all people with arthritis. These programs teach people skills to take charge of their conditions and engage in effective, joint-friendly physical activity. These programs also have proven benefits for other chronic conditions.

Public Health Chronic Disease Management Strategies

Self-Management Education Programs Are a Proven Approach

Comorbidities can complicate disease management and treatment. Fortunately, there are evidence-based strategies that address the effects of arthritis and other chronic diseases. These strategies help individuals and health professionals with comprehensive disease management.

Healthcare providers can also help improve patients' quality-of-life by referring them to chronic disease self-management education programs that address the effects of arthritis and other chronic conditions.

Keeping People with Arthritis and Comorbidities Physically Active

Being physically active is an essential part of preventing and managing many chronic conditions, including arthritis, heart disease, diabetes, and obesity. However, most adults face the following common barriers to physical activity:

- Lack of time
- Competing responsibilities

- Lack of motivation

- Difficulty finding an enjoyable activity

Adults with arthritis may face the following additional, disease-specific barriers:

- Concerns about making arthritis pain worse

- Fear about causing further joint damage

- Uncertainty about which types and amounts of activity are safe for their joints

Healthcare providers can help people overcome arthritis-specific barriers to physical activity by providing appropriate advice and referrals to evidence-based physical activity programs that are designed for adults with arthritis.

Section 25.2

Arthritis and Human Immunodeficiency Virus

"Arthritis and Human Immunodeficiency Virus," © 2015
Omnigraphics. Reviewed April 2018.

The Human Immunodeficiency Virus (HIV) is a retrovirus that attacks the immune system, leaving the body more vulnerable to various infections and cancers. HIV is transmitted by direct contact with an infected person's bodily fluids—such as blood, semen, or breast milk—through unprotected sex, contaminated blood transfusions, sharing of hypodermic needles, or childbearing.

Although there is no cure for HIV infection, it can be successfully treated using highly active antiretroviral therapy (HAART), a combination of medications that work together to slow the replication of the virus and restore the immune system. HAART enables many patients to manage HIV as a long-term, chronic health condition, and it reduces the death rate from HIV infection by 80 percent. Left untreated, however, HIV can lead to Acquired Immunodeficiency Syndrome (AIDS), a series of complications that are eventually terminal.

HIV-Related Rheumatic Diseases

The relationship between HIV and arthritis is complicated. Since HIV weakens the immune system, it actually reduces a patient's risk of developing some types of rheumatic diseases, including rheumatoid arthritis and lupus (systemic lupus erythematosus). These autoimmune disorders occur when the immune system attacks the body's own joints or tissues, which is less likely to happen in people with compromised immune systems. Yet many people with HIV experience symptoms of arthritis—including pain, swelling, and weakness in the joints—and research indicates that HIV infection increases a person's risk of developing other types of rheumatic diseases. Some of the arthritic conditions that can be HIV-related include:

- **Psoriatic arthritis.** This type of arthritis is usually related to psoriasis, an autoimmune disorder that causes red, scaly skin rashes. It develops when the immune system attacks large joints in the body, causing inflammation and pain. Psoriatic arthritis is fairly common in the early stages of HIV infection. Although it is not necessarily caused by HIV, some doctors believe a link is so likely that they routinely order HIV tests for patients who develop psoriatic arthritis.

- **Reactive arthritis.** This type of arthritis is typically triggered by a bacterial infection, such as food poisoning or Chlamydia. After responding to the bacteria, the immune system goes on to attack the joints, causing pain and swelling. HIV infection can also trigger reactive arthritis, which affects up to 10 percent of HIV patients.

- **Septic arthritis.** The compromised immune systems of HIV patients can make them susceptible to infections of the joints (septic arthritis), as well as the muscles (myositis) and bones (osteomyelitis).

HIV Treatment and Rheumatic Diseases

HAART, the drug cocktail commonly used to treat HIV, works by rebuilding a patient's compromised immune system. As the immune

function is restored; however, some people with HIV develop rheumatoid arthritis and other autoimmune disorders. Researchers believe
that HIV treatment may trigger inflammatory responses in some
patients. The tendency for the newly restored immune system to overreact and attack the joints and other parts of the body is known as
immune reconstitution syndrome (IRS).

Studies have shown a relationship between HIV infection and gout,
a type of arthritis that is caused by a buildup of uric acid in the joints.
An estimated 0.5 percent of HIV patients develop gout each year. Some
researchers attribute the elevated urate levels in these patients to
HAART treatments, and particularly to a certain class of antiretroviral
drugs known as protease inhibitors.

References

1. Espinoza, Luis R. "HIV and Rheumatic Disease," American
    College of Rheumatology (ACR), June 2015.

2. Legge, Adam. "Rheumatoid Arthritis Can Be a Side Effect of
    HIV Therapy," NAM Aidsmap, November 20, 2006.

3. Vann, Madeline. "The HIV-Rheumatic Disease Connection,"
    Everyday Health, 2009.

Section 25.3

Arthritis and Inflammatory Bowel Disease

This section includes text excerpted from "What Is
Inflammatory Bowel Disease (IBD)?" Centers for Disease
Control and Prevention (CDC), June 21, 2017.

Inflammatory Bowel Disease (IBD)

Inflammatory bowel disease (IBD) is a term for two conditions
(Crohn's disease and ulcerative colitis (UC)) that are characterized
by chronic inflammation of the gastrointestinal (GI) tract. Prolonged
inflammation results in damage to the GI tract.

Crohn's Disease

- Can affect any part of the GI tract (from the mouth to the anus)—Most often it affects the portion of the small intestine before the large intestine/colon.

- Damaged areas appear in patches that are next to areas of healthy tissue

- Inflammation may reach through the multiple layers of the walls of the GI tract

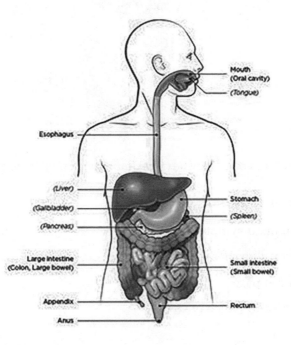

Figure 25.2. *Parts of Gastrointestinal Tract Affected by Crohn's Disease*

Ulcerative Colitis (UC)

- Occurs in the large intestine (colon) and the rectum

- Damaged areas are continuous (not patchy)—usually starting at the rectum and spreading further into the colon

- Inflammation is present only in the innermost layer of the lining of the colon

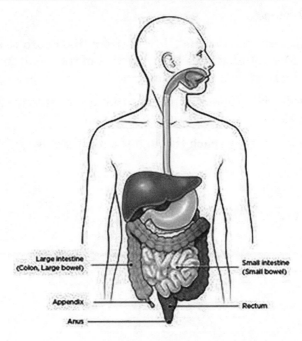

Figure 25.3. *Parts of Gastrointestinal Tract Affected by Ulcerative Disease*

What Are the Symptoms of IBD?

Some common symptoms are:

- Persistent diarrhea
- Abdominal pain
- Rectal bleeding/bloody stools
- Weight loss
- Fatigue

What Causes IBD

The exact cause of IBD is unknown, but IBD is the result of a defective immune system. A properly functioning immune system attacks foreign organisms, such as viruses and bacteria, to protect the body. In IBD, the immune system responds incorrectly to environmental triggers, which causes inflammation of the GI tract. There also appears to be a genetic component—someone with a family history of IBD is more likely to develop this inappropriate immune response.

How Is IBD Diagnosed?

IBD is diagnosed using a combination of endoscopy (for Crohn's disease) or colonoscopy (for UC) and imaging studies, such as contrast radiography, magnetic resonance imaging (MRI), or computed tomography (CT). Physicians may also check stool samples to make sure symptoms are not being caused by an infection or run blood tests to help confirm the diagnosis.

How Is IBD Treated?

Several types of medications may be used to treat IBD: aminosalicylates, corticosteroids (such as prednisone), immunomodulators, and the newest class approved for IBD—the "biologics." Several vaccinations for patients with IBD are recommended to prevent infections. Severe IBD may require surgery to remove damaged portions of the GI tract, but advances in treatment with medications mean that surgery is less common than it was a few decades ago. Since Crohn's disease and UC affect different parts of the GI tract, the surgical procedures are different for the two conditions.

What IBD Is Not

IBD is not irritable bowel syndrome (IBS). IBD should not be confused with IBS. Although people with IBS may experience some similar symptoms to IBD, IBD and IBS are very different. Irritable bowel syndrome is not caused by inflammation and the tissues of the bowel are not damaged the way they are in IBD. Treatment is also different.

IBD is not celiac disease. Celiac disease is another condition with similar symptoms to IBD. It is also characterized by inflammation of the intestines. However, the cause of celiac disease is known and is very specific. It is an inflammatory response to gluten (a group of proteins found in wheat and similar grains). The symptoms of celiac disease will go away after starting a gluten-free diet, although it usually will be months before the full effects of the new diet will be reached.

Part Three

Medical and Surgical Treatments for Arthritis

Chapter 26

Your Arthritis Healthcare Provider

Chapter Contents

Section 26.1—Choosing a Doctor 290

Section 26.2—Talking with Medical Specialists:
Tips for Patients.. 293

Section 26.3—For People with Osteoporosis:
How to Find a Doctor 295

Section 26.1

Choosing a Doctor

This section includes text excerpted from "How to Choose a Doctor
You Can Talk To," National Institute on Aging (NIA), National
Institutes of Health (NIH), May 17, 2017.

Finding the main doctor (often called your primary doctor or primary care doctor) with whom you feel comfortable talking is the first step in good communication. It is also a way to ensure your good health. This doctor gets to know you and what your health is normally like. He or she can help you make medical decisions that suit your values and daily habits and can keep in touch with the other medical specialists and healthcare providers you may need.

If you don't have a primary doctor or are not at ease with the one you currently see, now may be the time to find a new doctor. Whether you just moved to a new city, changed insurance providers, or had a bad experience with your doctor or medical staff, it is worthwhile to spend time finding a doctor you can trust.

People sometimes hesitate to change doctors because they worry about hurting their doctor's feelings. But doctors understand that different people have different needs. They know it is important for everyone to have a doctor with whom they are comfortable.

Primary care physicians frequently are family practitioners, internists, or geriatricians. Here are some suggestions that can help you find a doctor who meets your needs.

Decide What You Are Looking for in a Doctor

A good first step is to make a list of qualities that matter to you.

- Do you care if your doctor is a man or a woman?

- Is it important that your doctor has evening office hours, is associated with a specific hospital or medical center, or speaks your language?

- Do you prefer a doctor who has an individual practice or one who is part of a group so you can see one of your doctor's partners if your doctor is not available?

After you have made your list, go back over it and decide which qualities are most important and which are nice, but not essential.

Identify Several Possible Doctors

Once you have a general sense of what you are looking for, ask friends and relatives, medical specialists, and other health professionals for the names of doctors with whom they have had good experiences. Rather than just getting a name, ask about the person's experiences. For example, say: "What do you like about Dr. Smith?" and "Does this doctor take time to answer questions?" A doctor whose name comes up often may be a strong possibility.

If you belong to a managed care plan—a health maintenance organization (HMO) or preferred provider organization (PPO)—you may be required to choose a doctor in the plan or else you may have to pay extra to see a doctor outside the network. Most managed care plans will provide information on their doctors' backgrounds and credentials. Some plans have websites with lists of participating doctors from which you can choose.

It may be helpful to develop a list of a few names you can choose from. As you find out more about the doctors on this list, you may rule out some of them. In some cases, a doctor may not be taking new patients and you may have to make another choice.

Consult Reference Sources

The American Medical Association's (AMA) DoctorFinder website and the American Board of Medical Specialties' (ABMS) Certification Matters database can help you find doctors in your area. These websites don't recommend individual doctors, but they do provide a list of doctors you may want to consider. MedlinePlus, a website from the U.S. National Library of Medicine (NLM) at National Institutes of Health (NIH), has a comprehensive list of directories, which may also be helpful.

Don't forget to call your local or state medical society to check if complaints have been filed against any of the doctors you are considering.

Learn about Doctors You Are Considering

Once you have narrowed your list to two or three doctors, call their offices. The office staff is a good source of information about the doctor's education and qualifications, office policies, and payment procedures.

Pay attention to the office staff—you will have to communicate with them often!

You may want to set up an appointment to meet and talk with a doctor you are considering. He or she is likely to charge you for such a visit. After the appointment, ask yourself if this doctor is a person with whom you could work well. If you are not satisfied, schedule a visit with one of your other candidates.

When learning about a doctor, consider asking questions like:

- Do you have many older patients?

- How do you feel about involving my family in care decisions?

- Can I call or email you or your staff when I have questions? Do you charge for telephone or email time?

- What are your thoughts about complementary or alternative treatments?

Make a Choice

When making a decision about which doctor to choose, you might want to ask yourself questions like:

- Did the doctor give me a chance to ask questions?

- Was the doctor really listening to me?

- Could I understand what the doctor was saying? Was I comfortable asking him or her to say it again?

Once you've chosen a doctor, make your first actual care appointment. This visit may include a medical history and a physical exam. Be sure to bring your medical records, or have them sent from your former doctor. Bring a list of your current medicines or put the medicines in a bag and take them with you. If you haven't already met the doctor, ask for extra time during this visit to ask any questions you have about the doctor or the practice.

Section 26.2

Talking with Medical Specialists: Tips for Patients

This section includes text excerpted from
"Talking with Medical Specialists: Tips for Patients,"
National Institute on Aging (NIA), May 18, 2017.

Your doctor may send you to a specialist for further evaluation, or you may request to see a specialist yourself. Your insurance plan may require you to have a referral from your primary doctor. A visit to the specialist may be short. Often, the specialist already has seen your medical records or test results and is familiar with your case. If you are unclear about what the specialist tells you, ask questions.

For example, if the specialist says you have a medical condition that you aren't familiar with, you may want to say something like: "I don't know much about that condition. Could you explain what it is and how it might affect me?" or "I've heard that is a painful problem. What can be done to prevent or manage the pain?"

You also may ask for written materials to read, or you can call your primary doctor to clarify anything you haven't understood.

Ask the specialist to send information about any diagnosis or treatment to your primary doctor. This allows your primary doctor to keep track of your medical care. You also should let your primary doctor know at your next visit how well any treatments or medications the specialist recommended are working.

Questions to Ask Your Specialist

- What is my diagnosis?

- What treatment do you recommend? How soon do I need to begin the new treatment?

- Will you discuss my care with my primary doctor?

If You Need Surgery

In some cases, surgery may be the best treatment for your condition. If so, your doctor will refer you to a surgeon. Knowing more about the operation will help you make an informed decision about how to proceed. It also will help you get ready for the surgery, which makes for a better recovery.

Ask the surgeon to explain what will be done during the operation and what reading material, videos, or websites you can look at before the operation.

Find out if you will have to stay overnight in the hospital or if the surgery can be done on an outpatient basis. Will you need someone to drive you home? Minor surgeries that don't require an overnight stay can sometimes be done at medical centers called ambulatory surgical centers.

Questions to Ask Your Surgeon

- What is the success rate of the operation? How many of these operations have you done successfully?

- What problems occur with this surgery? What kind of pain or discomfort can I expect?

- What kind of anesthesia will I have? Are there any risks associated with its use in older people?

- Will I have to stay in the hospital overnight? How long is recovery expected to take? What does it involve? When can I get back to my normal routine?

Seeking a Second Opinion

When patients are diagnosed with a serious illness or surgery is recommended, patients often seek a second opinion. Hearing the views of two different doctors can help you decide what's best for you. In fact, your insurance plan may require it. Doctors are used to this practice, and most will not be insulted by your request for a second opinion. Your doctor may even be able to suggest other doctors who can review your case.

Always remember to check with your insurance provider in advance to find out if a second opinion is covered under your policy, if there are restrictions to which doctors you can see, and if you need a referral form from your primary doctor.

Section 26.3

For People with Osteoporosis: How to Find a Doctor

This section includes text excerpted from "For People with Osteoporosis: How to Find a Doctor," NIH Osteoporosis and Related Bone Diseases~National Resource Center (NIH ORBD~NRC), April, 2015.

For many people, finding a doctor who is knowledgeable about osteoporosis can be difficult. There is no physician specialty dedicated solely to osteoporosis, nor is there a certification program for health professionals who treat the disease. A variety of medical specialists treat people with osteoporosis, including internists, gynecologists, family doctors, endocrinologists, rheumatologists, physiatrists, orthopaedists, and geriatricians.

There are a number of ways to find a doctor who treats osteoporosis patients. If you have a primary care or family doctor, discuss your concerns with him or her. Your doctor may treat the disease or be able to refer you to an osteoporosis specialist.

If you are enrolled in a health maintenance organization (HMO) or a managed care health plan, consult your assigned doctor about osteoporosis. This doctor should be able to give you an appropriate referral.

If you do not have a personal doctor or if your doctor cannot help, contact your nearest university hospital or academic health center and ask for the department that cares for patients with osteoporosis. The department will vary from institution to institution. For example, in some facilities, the department of endocrinology or metabolic bone disease treats osteoporosis patients. In other medical centers, the appropriate department may be rheumatology, orthopedics, or gynecology. Some hospitals have a separate osteoporosis program or women's clinic that treats patients with osteoporosis.

Once you have identified a doctor, you may wish to ask whether the doctor has specialized training in osteoporosis, how much of the practice is dedicated to osteoporosis, and whether he or she uses bone mass measurement.

Your own primary care doctor—whether an internist, orthopaedist, or gynecologist—is often the best person to treat you because she or he knows your medical history, your lifestyle, and your special needs.

Medical Specialists Who Treat Osteoporosis

After an initial assessment, it may be necessary to see an endocrinologist, a rheumatologist, or another specialist to rule out the possibility of an underlying disease that may contribute to osteoporosis:

- **Endocrinologists** treat the endocrine system, which comprises the glands and hormones that help control the body's metabolic activity. In addition to osteoporosis, endocrinologists treat diabetes and diseases of the thyroid and pituitary glands.

- **Rheumatologists** diagnose and treat diseases of the bones, joints, muscles, and tendons, including arthritis and collagen diseases.

- **Family doctors** have a broad range of training that includes internal medicine, gynecology, and pediatrics. They place special emphasis on caring for an individual or family on a long-term, continuing basis.

- **Geriatricians** are family doctors or internists who have received additional training on the aging process and the conditions and diseases that often occur among the elderly, including incontinence, falls, and dementia. Geriatricians often care for patients in nursing homes, in patients' homes, or in office or hospital settings.

- **Gynecologists** diagnose and treat conditions of the female reproductive system and associated disorders. They often serve as primary care doctors for women and follow their patients' reproductive health over time.

- **Internists** are trained in general internal medicine. They diagnose and treat many diseases. Internists provide long-term comprehensive care in the hospital and office, have expertise in many areas, and often act as consultants to other specialists.

- Orthopedic **surgeons** are doctors trained in the care of patients with musculoskeletal conditions, such as congenital skeletal malformations, bone fractures and infections, and metabolic problems.

- **Physiatrists** are doctors who specialize in physical medicine and rehabilitation. They evaluate and treat patients with impairments, disabilities, or pain arising from various medical problems, including bone fractures. Physiatrists focus on restoring the physical, psychological, social, and vocational functioning of the individual.

Chapter 27

Diagnosing and Treating Rheumatoid Arthritis

Rheumatoid arthritis, or RA, is an autoimmune and inflammatory disease, which means that your immune system attacks healthy cells in your body by mistake, causing inflammation (painful swelling) in the affected parts of the body.

RA mainly attacks the joints, usually many joints at once. RA commonly affects joints in the hands, wrists, and knees. In a joint with RA, the lining of the joint becomes inflamed, causing damage to joint tissue. This tissue damage can cause long-lasting or chronic pain, unsteadiness (lack of balance), and deformity (misshapenness).

RA can also affect other tissues throughout the body and cause problems in organs such as the lungs, heart, and eyes.

Risk Factors for RA?

Researchers have studied a number of genetic and environmental factors to determine if they change person's risk of developing RA.

This chapter contains text excerpted from the following sources: Text in this chapter begins with text excerpted from "Rheumatoid Arthritis (RA)," Center for Disease Control and Prevention (CDC), July 7, 2017; Text beginning with the heading "Diagnosing Rheumatoid Arthritis (RA)" is excerpted from "Rheumatoid Arthritis—Treatment," National Institute of Arthritis and Musculoskeletal and Skin Diseases (NIAMS), April 30, 2017.

Characteristics That Increase Risk

- **Age.** RA can begin at any age, but the likelihood increases with age. The onset of RA is highest among adults in their sixties.

- **Sex.** New cases of RA are typically two-to-three times higher in women than men.

- **Genetics/inherited traits.** People born with specific genes are more likely to develop RA. These genes, called HLA (human leukocyte antigen) class II genotypes, can also make your arthritis worse. The risk of RA may be highest when people with these genes are exposed to environmental factors like smoking or when a person is obese.

- **Smoking.** Multiple studies show that cigarette smoking increases a person's risk of developing RA and can make the disease worse.

- **History of live births.** Women who have never given birth may be at greater risk of developing RA.

- **Early Life Exposures.** Some early life exposures may increase risk of developing RA in adulthood. For example, one study found that children whose mothers smoked had double the risk of developing RA as adults. Children of lower income parents are at increased risk of developing RA as adults.

- **Obesity.** Being obese can increase the risk of developing RA. Studies examining the role of obesity also found that the more overweight a person was, the higher his or her risk of developing RA became.

Characteristics That Can Decrease Risk

Unlike the risk factors above which may increase risk of developing RA, at least one characteristic may decrease risk of developing RA.

- **Breastfeeding**. Women who have breastfed their infants have a decreased risk of developing RA.

Diagnosing RA

Rheumatoid arthritis (RA) can be difficult to diagnose in its early stages for several reasons:

- There is no single test for the disease.

- Symptoms differ from person to person and can be more severe in some people than in others.

- Symptoms can be similar to those of other types of arthritis and joint conditions, and it may take some time for other conditions to be ruled out.

- The disease develops over time, and only a few symptoms may be present in the early stages.

As a result, doctors use a variety of the following tools to diagnose the disease and to rule out other conditions.

Medical History

The doctor will begin by asking you to describe your symptoms, when and how they started, and how they have changed over time. The doctor will also ask about any other medical problems you and close family members have and about any medications you're taking. Answers to these questions can help the doctor make a diagnosis and understand the impact the disease has on your life.

Physical Examination

The doctor will:

- Check your reflexes and general health, including muscle strength.

- Examine bothersome joints and watch how you walk, bend, and carry out activities of daily living.

- Look at your skin for a rash.

- Listen to your chest for signs of inflammation in the lungs.

Laboratory Tests

A number of lab tests may be useful in confirming a diagnosis of RA. Some of the common tests include:

- **Rheumatoid factor (RF):** This blood test checks for RF, an antibody most people with RA eventually have in their blood. (An antibody is a special protein made by the immune system that normally helps fight invaders in the body.) Not all people with RA test positive for RF and some people test positive for RF but never develop the disease. RF also can be positive for some other diseases. However, a positive RF in a person who has symptoms consistent with RA can be useful in confirming a diagnosis. Also, high levels of RF are associated with more severe RA.

- **Anti-cyclic citrullinated peptide (CCP) antibodies:** This blood test detects antibodies to CCP. This test is positive in most people with RA and can even be positive years before RA symptoms develop. When used with the RF, this test's results are very useful in confirming an RA diagnosis.

- **Others:** Other common blood tests include:

  - White blood cell (WBC) count.

  - Blood test for anemia, which is common in RA.

  - Erythrocyte sedimentation rate (often called the sed rate), which measures inflammation in the body.

  - C-reactive protein, another common test for inflammation that is useful both in making a diagnosis and monitoring disease activity and response to anti-inflammatory therapy.

Imaging Tests

Doctors use X-rays to see the degree of joint damage. They are not useful in the early stages of RA before damage is evident. Doctors may use them to rule out other causes of joint pain. X-rays may also be used later to monitor the progression of the disease. Magnetic resonance imaging (MRI) and ultrasound may be useful in identifying the early stages of RA and can help determine the severity of the disease.

Treatment for RA

Doctors use a variety of approaches to treat RA. They may be used in combination and at different times during the course of the disease. Your doctor will choose treatments based on your situation.

No matter which treatment is chosen, the goals are the same:

- Relieve pain

- Reduce inflammation

- Slow down or stop joint damage

- Improve well-being and ability to function

To treat RA, doctors may suggest:

- Medications

- Surgery

- Routine monitoring and ongoing care

- Complementary therapies

Medications

Most people who have RA take medications. Studies show that early treatment with powerful drugs and drug combinations instead of one medication alone may be more effective in reducing or preventing joint damage than beginning with aspirin or other pain relievers. If you have persistent RA symptoms, see a doctor familiar with the disease and its treatment to reduce the risk of damage.

Many of the drugs used to treat RA reduce the inflammation that can cause pain and joint damage. However, inflammation is also one way the body fights infection and disease. But the level of risk is hard to judge because infections and cancer can occur in people with RA who are not on treatment. It is important to talk with your doctor about these risks.

Pain Relief and Anti-Inflammatory Drugs

Your doctor may prescribe some medications (analgesics) that only help with pain relief. Others, such as corticosteroids and nonsteroidal anti-inflammatory drugs (NSAIDs), can reduce inflammation.

Disease-Modifying Antirheumatic Drugs (DMARDs)

Disease-modifying antirheumatic drugs (DMARDs) may slow the course of the disease. Common DMARDs your doctor may prescribe include:

- Hydroxychloroquine

- Leflunomide

- Methotrexate

- Sulfasalazine

Other DMARDs, called biologic response modifiers (BRM), may be used if your disease is more severe. These are genetically engineered medications that help reduce inflammation and damage to the joints by interrupting the inflammatory process. Currently, several biologic response modifiers are approved for RA, including:

- Abatacept

- Adalimumab

- Anakinra

- Certolizumab

- Etanercept

- Golimumab

- Infliximab

- Rituximab

- Tocilizumab

Another DMARD, tofacitinib, is from a new class of drugs called jak kinase (JAK) inhibitors. It fights inflammation from inside the cell.

Surgery

The primary purpose of surgery is to reduce pain, improve the affected joints' function, and improve your ability to perform daily activities.

Surgery is not for everyone. Talk with your doctor and together decide what is the right choice for you. Discuss:

- Your overall health

- The condition of the joint or tendon that will be operated on

- The reason for, and the risks and benefits of the surgery

Routine Monitoring and Ongoing Care

Regular medical care is important to monitor the course of the disease, determine the effectiveness and any negative effects of medications, and change therapies as needed.

Monitoring typically includes regular visits to the doctor. It also may include blood, urine, and other lab tests and X-rays.

Good communication between you and your doctor is necessary for effective treatment. Talking to the doctor regularly can help ensure that you receive:

- Necessary exercise and pain management programs
- Necessary and appropriate medications
- Information about surgical options if necessary

Another factor to discuss with your doctor is the risk of osteoporosis, which is a condition in which bones become weakened and fragile. Having RA increases your risk of developing osteoporosis, particularly if you take corticosteroids. You may want to discuss with your doctor the potential benefits of calcium and vitamin D supplements or other osteoporosis treatments.

Complementary Therapies

Special diets, vitamins, and other complementary therapies are sometimes suggested to treat RA.

Research shows that some of these approaches, such as taking fish oil supplements, may help reduce inflammation. However, few, if any controlled scientific studies have been conducted on complementary approaches, and some studies have found no definite benefit to these therapies.

As with any therapy, you should discuss the benefits and risks with your doctor before beginning any complementary or new type of therapy. However, it is important not to neglect regular healthcare.

Chapter 28

Osteoarthritis Medicines

Understanding Your Condition

Osteoarthritis (OA) is a painful condition in which joints become swollen and stiff.

- Cartilage is the soft tissue between the bones that meet at a joint. It acts as a cushion and allows your connecting bones to move smoothly without rubbing against each other.

- In people with OA, the cartilage between bones begins to break down and the bones start grinding together.

- OA causes pain, joint swelling, and damage.

- OA can be very painful and may get worse over time.

- OA can make it hard to move, work, or enjoy activities.

Prevalence of OA

- OA is the most common form of arthritis.

- It affects about 27 million people in the United States.

- It is a leading cause of disability.

This chapter includes text excerpted from "Managing Osteoarthritis Pain with Medicines—A Review of the Research for Adults," Effective Health Care Program, Agency for Healthcare Research and Quality (AHRQ), January 2012. Reviewed April 2018.

- OA is more common in people who are older, overweight or have injured a joint.

Understanding Your Options

What Does It Mean to Manage the Pain?

There is no cure for OA. However, your doctor may suggest one or more of the following to help you manage your pain:

- Taking medicines called analgesics to help with pain and swelling

- Keeping your weight at a healthy level to lessen the impact on your joints

- Exercising to reduce pain and make it easier to do daily tasks

What Are Analgesics?

Analgesics are a type of medicine that helps relieve pain and swelling. Analgesics come in different forms:

- **Acetaminophen:** Most people know this medicine by the brand name Tylenol®.

- **Nonsteroidal anti-inflammatory drugs (NSAIDs):** Some of the brand names of these medicines may be familiar to you, like Advil®, Motrin®, Aleve®, and Celebrex®.

- **Skin creams:** Common brand names include BenGay®, Aspercreme®, or Theragen®.

- **Supplements:** Some people use the nutritional supplements glucosamine and chondroitin to reduce OA pain.

Table 28.1. Types of Analgesics

Acetaminophen	
What are the generic and brand names?	Acetaminophen is the generic name for this medicine. The brand name is Tylenol®.
Is this medicine available without a prescription?	This medicine is available without a prescription.
How well does this medicine help pain and swelling?	• Research says this medicine does not reduce pain as well as NSAIDs do. • This medicine does not reduce swelling.

Table 28.1. Continued

What are the possible side effects of this medicine?	• This medicine can cause liver damage if too much is taken or if it is taken with alcohol.
NSAIDs	

What are the generic and brand names?	These medicines go by many generic and brand names:
	• Ibuprofen
	  • Motrin®
	  • Advil®
	• Diclofenac
	  • Cambia®
	  • Cataflam®
	  • Voltaren®
	  • Voltarol®
	  • Zipsor®
	• Naproxen
	  • Aleve®
	  • Naprosyn®
	• Celecoxib
	  • Celebrex®
	• Etodolac
	  • Lodine®
	• Meloxicam
	  • Mobic®

Are any of these medicines available without a prescription?	Ibuprofen and naproxen are available without a prescription.
How well do these medicines help pain and swelling?	• All these medicines relieve pain and swelling about the same as each other. • Research says that all these medicines reduce pain better than acetaminophen. • Diclofenac skin cream works as well as NSAID pills.

What are the possible side effects of these medicines?	• All of these medicines can cause serious stomach problems like bleeding or ulcers. More people had these problems with these NSAIDs:
	  • Naproxen
	  • Ibuprofen
	  • Diclofenac
	• More people had stomach bleeding after taking naproxen than people taking ibuprofen.
	• All NSAIDs except for naproxen can increase your chances of having heart problems.

Table 28.1. Continued

Skin Creams	
What are the generic and brand names?	NSAIDs • Diclofenac (Voltaren®) • Ibuprofen • Capsaicin • Theragen® • Zostrix® • Capsagel® • Salonpas-Hot® • Salicylate • Aspercreme® • BenGay® • Sportscreme®
Are any of these medicines available without a prescription?	Capsaicin and salicylate creams are available without a prescription.
How well do these medicines help pain and swelling?	• People who used NSAID skin creams instead of pills had less risk of having serious stomach problems, but had a higher risk of having dry skin, rash, and itching. • Diclofenac skin cream works as well as NSAID pills. • Some research says that capsaicin may relieve pain as well as NSAIDs, and salicylate may not, but there is not enough research to know for sure.
What are the possible side effects of these medicines?	• NSAID skin creams may cause dry skin, rash, and itching. • Capsaicin might cause a slight burning feeling the first few times it is used.
Supplements	
What are the generic and brand names?	The generic names for these supplements are glucosamine and chondroitin. These are sold under many brand names and are sometimes sold together as one pill.
Are these supplements available without a prescription?	These supplements are available without a prescription and can be found in grocery stores, drug stores, and natural food stores.
How well do these supplements help pain and swelling?	• They may work as well as NSAID pills to relieve pain, but there is not enough research to know for sure.

Table 28.1. Continued

What are the possible side effects of these supplements?	• There is not enough research to say if these supplements cause side effects. • Supplements sold in the United States are not regulated by the U.S. Food and Drug Administration (FDA). This means that the quality of the glucosamine and chondroitin may vary and their contents may be different from what is listed on the bottle. The supplements that have been studied were prescriptions that are 99 percent pure with no added ingredients and are not available in the United States. This means that the supplements you buy may not be the same as the ones that were researched.

Possible Serious Side Effects from Taking NSAIDs

Stomach problems. Researchers found that:

• More people taking naproxen, ibuprofen, or diclofenac developed ulcers (open sores in the stomach) than people taking celecoxib, meloxicam, or etodolac.

• More people taking naproxen had serious stomach problems like stomach bleeding and ulcers than people taking ibuprofen.

• People taking NSAIDs who have had stomach bleeding in the past are more likely to have stomach bleeding caused by NSAIDs than people who have not had stomach bleeding in the past.

• People who take blood thinners (like Coumadin® or warfarin) or other medicines to block clotting (such as aspirin) while taking naproxen, ibuprofen, or diclofenac are 3–6 times more likely to have stomach bleeding than people who take blood thinners alone.

• People who take a low dose (amount) of aspirin while taking celecoxib, naproxen, ibuprofen, or diclofenac increase their risk of getting an ulcer by about 6 percent.

• People who take higher doses of naproxen, ibuprofen, or diclofenac are more likely to have stomach bleeding than people who take lower doses.

• The risk of stomach problems from NSAIDs increases as you get older.

- Adding a medicine that reduces acid in the stomach (called a proton pump inhibitor, or PPI) to celecoxib could reduce the risk of ulcers and the problems caused by ulcers, including bleeding.

Heart problems. Researchers found that:

- Taking celecoxib, ibuprofen, or diclofenac increases your chances of having heart problems

- Naproxen does not increase your risk of heart attack.

- People who take higher doses of celecoxib have a higher risk of having a heart attack than people taking lower doses.

The risk of having heart problems from NSAIDs increases as you get older. All NSAIDs can worsen blood pressure, heart function, and kidney function. However, there are no clear differences between naproxen, ibuprofen, diclofenac, etodolac, meloxicam, or nabumetone in the risk of high blood pressure, heart failure, or poor kidney function.

What Are the Costs of Analgesics?

The cost to you for analgesics depends on:

- The type of health insurance that you have.

- The dose (amount) you need.

- Whether the medicine is available in generic form or is sold without a prescription "over-the-counter (OTC)." Some NSAIDs are available OTC, but your insurance may not cover the cost of these medicines if you buy them this way.

The cost of OTC analgesics depends on the pharmacy, the brand, and how much you buy at one time. When you shop around for the best price, you should also consider the quality of the product.

Ask Your Doctor

- Which analgesic do you think is safest for me but will still help control my pain?

- Am I at risk for stomach or heart problems if I take an NSAID?

- How long will it take for my pain to be under control?

- What side effects should I watch for?

- Could my other health conditions or medicines affect which medicine I take for my OA pain?

- What are my other options if these medicines do not help?

- Is there anything else I can do to help manage my OA pain?

Chapter 29

Rheumatoid Arthritis Medicines

Learning about Rheumatoid Arthritis (RA)

What Causes RA

No one knows for sure what causes RA. It's an auto-immune problem. That means the body's defense system (called the immune system) attacks its own joints and organs. This can cause swelling of the synovium, the tissue that lines the joint.

What Happens without Treatment?

Without treatment, RA can slowly destroy the joints. The swelling of the synovium damages the cartilage, bone, and tendons. The joints become more and more painful, swollen, and stiff. This can make it hard to do everyday tasks. RA can also affect the eyes, blood vessels, and the lining of the heart. It can also cause low red blood cell counts, weak bones, and scarring in the lungs.

This chapter includes text excerpted from "Rheumatoid Arthritis Medicines," Agency for Healthcare Research and Quality (AHRQ), U.S. Department of Health and Human Services (HHS), April 9, 2008. Reviewed April 2018.

Learning about Medicines for RA

Medicines are the main treatment for RA. They reduce joint swelling and relieve pain. Most people need to keep taking RA medicines for life. This guide talks about two kinds of RA medicines, DMARDs and steroids.

DMARDs

The drugs that work best for RA are called DMARDs. DMARD stands for Disease-Modifying AntiRheumatic Drug. These medicines don't just relieve pain. They slow or stop the changes in your joints.

DMARDs come in two groups. Some are pills. The others are given by shot or IV. Both suppress the immune system. That means they slow down the body's attack on itself.

Table 29.1. DMARDs for Rheumatoid Arthritis (RA)

DMARDs	
Generic Name	**Brand Name**
Pills	
Hydroxychloroquine	Plaquenil®
Leflunomide	Arava®
Methotrexate	Rheumatrex®
	Trexall®
Sulfasalazine	Azulfidine®
	Sulfazine®
Shots (under the skin)	
Adalimumab	Humira®
Anakinra	Kineret®
Etanercept	Enbrel®
Given by IV	
Abatacept	Orencia®
Infliximab	Remicade®
Rituximab	Rituxan®

Steroids

Steroids help with joint pain and swelling, but it is not known if they can slow down the disease. Prednisone is the name of a steroid often used for RA.

Table 29.2. Steroids for Rheumatoid Arthritis (RA)

Steroids	
Generic Name	**Brand Name**
Prednisolone (liquid)	Various brand names
Prednisone (pills)	Various brand names

Learning about the Benefits

Research shows that DMARDs work. They can slow down the disease and relieve pain. But it's hard to predict which drug will work best for any one person. About 65 out of 100 people need to change their RA drug. Some people switch because their drug isn't working well enough. Others switch because of side effects.

Some of the medicines have been compared with each other in research studies. Here's what we know from this research.

Starting Your First RA Drug

- Methotrexate (Rheumatrex®, Trexall®) is a DMARD pill that is often used. It works as well as a DMARD given by shot or IV.

- Two other DMARD pills, leflunomide (Arava®) and sulfasalazine (Azulfidine®, Sulfazine®), work as well as methotrexate (Rheumatrex®, Trexall®).

- Adalimumab (Humira®), etanercept (Enbrel®), and infliximab (Remicade®) all work about the same.

Changing and Combining RA Drugs

- If methotrexate (Rheumatrex®, Trexall®) isn't working well enough, you have options. Adding a DMARD given by shot or IV works better than methotrexate by itself.

- Combining prednisone with hydroxychloroquine (Plaquenil®), methotrexate (Rheumatrex®, Trexall®), or sulfasalazine (Azulfidine®, Sulfazine®) works better than any of these DMARD pills by themselves.

Some Do Not Work as Well

- Anakinra (Kineret®) is a DMARD shot that does not work as well as the other shots.

317

- Combining methotrexate (Rheumatrex®, Trexall®) and sulfasalazine (Azulfidine®, Sulfazine®) does not work any better than either DMARD pill by itself.

Talking with Your Doctor or Nurse about RA Drugs

Benefits

DMARDs reduce swelling and make it easier to do everyday tasks. They also help prevent joint damage and long-term disability. Most people can find a DMARD that works for them. Ask your doctor or nurse these questions.

Do I Need a Shot or Can I Take a Pill?

- Most people can start with a DMARD pill. Many people get good results when they start with methotrexate (Rheumatrex®, Trexall®). It can work as well as the DMARDs given by shot or IV.

How Long Before I Feel Better?

- DMARDs do not start working right away. They can take weeks or months to start working.

- Your doctor or nurse may prescribe a pain reliever until the DMARD starts to work.

What If the First Drug Does Not Work or Stops Working?

- Switching to another DMARD can help.

- Adding a second kind of DMARD may work for you. If you are taking methotrexate (Rheumatrex®, Trexall®), adding a DMARD given by shot or IV can help.

- Adding prednisone to a DMARD pill is also an option.

Learning about Risks

Infections

- RA drugs weaken the body's defenses. That means that serious infections, like pneumonia, are more likely with these drugs. A serious infection needs antibiotics and often must be treated in a hospital.

Other Serious Problems

- Methotrexate (Rheumatrex®, Trexall®) can cause liver and kidney problems. It can also cause low red blood cell counts and painful mouth sores.

- Steroids like prednisone can weaken bones, raise blood sugar, and cause weight gain. That is why steroids are often prescribed in low doses and for a short time.

Needle Reactions

- DMARD shots can cause redness, itching, rash, and pain at the spot where the shot is given. More people taking anakinra (Kineret®) have these reactions than people taking other DMARD shots.

- About half of the people getting DMARDs by IV have a reaction. They get chills, dizzy, or sick to the stomach. But only about 2 out of 100 people stop their medicine because of reactions.

- It's rare, but DMARDs given by IV can also cause a serious reaction, like a seizure.

Risks of Serious Birth Defects

- Methotrexate (Rheumatrex®, Trexall®) and leflunomide (Arava®) can cause serious birth defects.

- Both men and women taking these DMARD pills should talk with their doctor or nurse before planning a pregnancy.

- Be sure to use two forms of birth control while taking these DMARD pills. For example, you could use birth control pills and a condom each time you have sex.

Reducing Your Risks

See your doctor or nurse for regular checkups and blood tests

- Checkups and blood tests will help catch infections and other problems early.

Stay away from people who are sick

- Call your doctor or nurse right away if you have signs of infection, like fever or a cough.

Make sure your flu shot and pneumonia shot are up to date

- These shots can help you fight off infections. Check with your doctor or nurse before getting any other vaccines.

Be sure to get enough calcium and vitamin D

- RA weakens the bones. You can help keep your bones healthy by getting enough calcium and vitamin D. Milk, yogurt, and green leafy vegetables are high in calcium. You can also take calcium and vitamin D pills.

Chapter 30

Help Your Arthritis Treatment Work

Chapter Contents

Section 30.1—Treating and Managing Arthritis 322

Section 30.2—Heat and Cold Therapies for Arthritis.............. 324

Section 30.3—Long-Term Benefit of Steroid
Injections for Knee Osteoarthritis
Challenged... 326

Section 30.1

Treating and Managing Arthritis

This section includes text excerpted from "Arthritis—Frequently Asked Questions (FAQs)," Centers for Disease Control and Prevention (CDC), October 19, 2017.

What Should I Do If I Think I Have Arthritis?

Talk to your doctor if you have arthritis symptoms such as pain, stiffness, or swelling in or around one or more of your joints. Doctors usually diagnose arthritis using the patient's medical history, physical examination, X-rays, and blood tests. It is possible to have more than one form of arthritis at the same time. There are many forms of arthritis, and diagnosing the specific type you have can help your doctor determine the best treatment. The earlier you understand your arthritis, the earlier you can start managing your disease, reducing pain, and making healthy lifestyle changes.

How Is Arthritis Treated?

The focus of arthritis treatment is to control pain, minimize joint damage, and improve or maintain physical function and quality of life. In inflammatory types of arthritis, it is also important to control inflammation. According to the American College of Rheumatology (ACR), arthritis treatment can include medications, nondrug therapies such physical therapy or patient education, and sometimes surgery. Managing your arthritis symptoms is very important as well.

How Can I Manage My Arthritis?

Properly managing your arthritis can help to decrease pain, improve function, retain productivity, and lower healthcare costs. Self-management is what you do day-to-day to manage your condition and stay healthy. Practice proven self-management strategies to reduce arthritis pain so you can pursue the activities that are important to you.

Is Exercise Good for People Who Have Arthritis?

Research shows that arthritis-friendly physical activity is good for people with arthritis. Moderate physical activity 5 or more days a week can help to relieve arthritis pain and stiffness and give you more energy. Regular physical activity can also lift your mood and make you feel more positive.

What Should I Do If I Have Pain When I Exercise?

It's normal to have pain, stiffness, and swelling after starting a new physical activity program. It may take 6–8 weeks for your joints to get used to your new activity level, but sticking with your activity program will result in long-term pain relief. Here are some tips to help you manage pain during and after exercise

- Until your pain improves, modify your physical activity program by exercising less frequently (days per week) or for shorter periods of time (amount of time each session) or with less intensity.

- Try a different type of exercise to reduce pressure on the joints— for example, switch from walking to water aerobics.

- Do proper warm-up and cool-down before and after exercise.

- Exercise at a comfortable pace—you should be able to carry on a conversation while exercising.

- Make sure you have good fitting, comfortable shoes.

See your doctor if you experience any of the following:

- Pain that is sharp, stabbing, and constant

- Pain that causes you to limp

- Pain that lasts more than 2 hours after exercise or gets worse at night

- Pain or swelling that does not get better with rest, medication, or hot or cold packs

- Large increases in swelling or if your joints feel "hot" or are red

How Does Being Overweight Affect Arthritis?

It's important for people with arthritis to maintain a healthy weight. For people who are overweight or obese, losing weight reduces pressure on joints, particularly weight-bearing joints like the hips and knees. In fact, losing as little as 10–12 pounds can reduce pain and improve function for people with arthritis.

At any age, low-impact, arthritis-friendly physical activity, and diet changes can help you lose weight.

Section 30.2

Heat and Cold Therapies for Arthritis

"Heat and Cold Therapies for Arthritis,"
© 2015 Omnigraphics. Reviewed April 2018.

Thermotherapy (heat treatment) and cryotherapy (cold treatment) rank among the simplest and least expensive methods of pain management used in the treatment of arthritis. Both of these therapies work by stimulating the natural healing capacity of the body.

Heat dilates the blood vessels, increases blood flow, and relaxes the muscles. It is effective in helping people loosen up before exercise or soothe tired muscles and stiff joints afterward. Cold, on the other hand, constricts blood vessels, decreases blood flow, and numbs the affected area. It is effective in relieving acute pain and reducing inflammation.

Many doctors recommend using a combination of heat and cold treatments, depending on the patient's symptoms and preferences, since both therapies can help alleviate the pain, redness, swelling, and stiffness associated with arthritis. In general, ice is considered best for treating recent injuries, while heat is the preferred method of treating pain that lasts longer than 48 hours.

Types of Heat Treatment

To relieve pain and stiffness, moist heat should be applied at least twice per day for ten to twenty minutes at a time. Some of the possible types of heat treatment include:

- Taking a warm shower

- Soaking in a warm bath or whirlpool tub

324

- Applying a moist heating pad or a damp towel that has been heated in a microwave

- Using a warm paraffin wax treatment

- Sleeping under an electric blanket

- Warming clothes in a dryer before putting them on

- Getting a deep-heating ultrasound treatment from a physical therapist

Types of Cold Treatment

Cold treatment should be applied for ten to twenty minutes at a time, 2–3 times per day. Some of the possible types of cold treatment include:

- Applying ice or a bag of frozen vegetables wrapped in a moist towel

- Applying a store-bought gel cold pack

- Using topical pain-relieving gels, ointments, or sprays containing menthol, camphor, or other ingredients that produce a superficial cooling effect

References

1. Arthritis Foundation. "Using Heat and Cold for Pain Relief," n.d.

2. "Heat and Cold Therapy for Arthritis Pain," WebMD, 2013.

3. University Health System. "Treating Arthritis," 2015.

Section 30.3

Long-Term Benefit of Steroid Injections for Knee Osteoarthritis Challenged

This section includes text excerpted from "Long-term
Benefit of Steroid Injections for Knee Osteoarthritis Challenged,"
National Institute of Arthritis and Musculoskeletal and
Skin Diseases (NIAMS), October 12, 2017.

Among people with osteoarthritic knees, repeated steroid injections over two years brought no long-term improvement in reducing pain, according to a study funded in part by the NIH's National Institute of Arthritis and Musculoskeletal and Skin Diseases (NIAMS). Rather than showing any benefit, the results revealed that the injections sped the loss of the cartilage that cushions the knee joint. The study appeared in the Journal of the American Medical Association (JAMA).

Osteoarthritis (OA) is a common chronic condition of the joints that involves a breakdown of the cartilage and the ends of the bones, and inflammation of the joint lining. The disease tends to affect heavily used joints, such as those in the hands and spine, and the weight-bearing joints in the knees and hips. It has been estimated that knee OA affects more than 9 million Americans, and it is a leading cause of disability and medical costs.

Many treatments for OA target inflammation to reduce pain. Direct injection of corticosteroids into the joint is a standard treatment for knee OA. However, the treatment is somewhat controversial with regard to the benefit of both single and repeated injections; evidence that they are beneficial comes from small studies that showed only modest improvements.

To address the procedure's effectiveness, Timothy E. McAlindon, M.D., M.P.H., of Tufts Medical Center, Boston, led a team of investigators who enrolled 140 patients with symptomatic knee OA and joint inflammation into a 2-year study. The patients, whose average age was 58 years, were divided into two groups and injected with a corticosteroid called triamcinolone or saline every three months.

During quarterly visits, researchers evaluated participants for overall knee pain, stiffness and the impact these symptoms had on their daily activities. They underwent magnetic resonance imaging (MRI) scans each year so investigators could monitor their knee cartilage. The study was a double-blind trial, meaning that neither the investigators nor the patients knew who was in the steroid or saline group.

The results revealed no differences between the two groups in terms of knee pain, function or stiffness at any of the 3-month visits. However, the injections' short-term impacts were not assessed. Because of the timing for participant visits, these results cannot be compared with studies reporting short-term benefits between one and four weeks following injection.

MRI measurements revealed thinning of knee cartilage in both groups by the end of the study. But loss of cartilage in the steroid group was significantly greater than in controls, with the average change in cartilage thickness being -0.21 mm and -0.10 mm, respectively. This more rapid thinning may be due to the known effects of corticosteroids on tissue breakdown. While the faster loss of cartilage in the steroid-treated group did not correlate with more pain over the 2-year period, it may have a long-term negative impact on the health of the joint.

"Use of corticosteroid injections to treat knee OA is based on the medicine's capacity to reduce inflammation, but corticosteroids have also been reported to have destructive effects on cartilage," said Dr. McAlindon. "We now know that these injections bring no long-term benefit, and may, in fact, do more harm than good by accelerating damage to the cartilage."

Chapter 31

Surgical Procedures Used to Treat Arthritis

Chapter Contents

Section 31.1—Arthroscopic Surgery 330
Section 31.2—Bone Fusion Surgery.. 333

Section 31.1

Arthroscopic Surgery

"Arthroscopic Surgery," © 2015 Omnigraphics.
Reviewed April 2018.

Arthroscopy is a minimally invasive surgical technique used to evaluate, diagnose, and treat or repair a variety of joint-related conditions. Literally translated, arthroscopy means "looking into the joint." Surgeons insert a tiny, fiberoptic camera through a small incision and use it to examine the interior structure of the joint. Images are greatly magnified and displayed on a television screen.

Initially used as a diagnostic tool prior to performing traditional open surgery, arthroscopy has rapidly gained popularity as a stand-alone medical procedure. Since it is most often performed on an outpatient basis, it is less stressful for patients and offers faster recovery times than traditional surgeries. In addition, advancements in medical instrumentation and fiberoptic technology have enabled surgeons to use it to treat an expanding array of conditions.

Indications for Arthroscopy

Arthroscopy is one of the final steps in the process of diagnosing and treating joint injuries and diseases. The process begins with a complete medical history and physical examination of the patient, and then it involves noninvasive imaging tests such as X-rays, magnetic resonance imaging (MRI), or computed tomography (CT). After reviewing the results of these tests, an orthopedic surgeon may recommend an arthroscopic procedure for one of the following problems:

- **Unexplained joint pain.** Arthroscopy can be used to determine the causes of joint pain that cannot be explained using conventional diagnostic tools.

- **Synovitis.** This condition, which is characterized by inflammation of the synovial membrane lining the cavities of joints, can often be treated through arthroscopy.

- **Removal of loose pieces of bone or cartilage.** Fragments arising from arthritis, injury, or other causes can be easily removed through arthroscopy.

- **Arthritis.** Arthroscopy cannot completely cure arthritis, but it may be used to repair damaged joints and relieve symptoms associated with it.

- **Biopsies.** Arthroscopy can be used to collect samples and analyze the characteristics of synovial fluid in order to diagnose joint disease. Arthroscopy is also used to obtain cartilage tissue for use in cartilage transplant procedures.

- **Meniscal injury.** The meniscus is a crescent-shaped cartilage that distributes weight and reduces friction in the knee, wrist, and other joints. Damage to the meniscus—which can occur suddenly from a traumatic injury or gradually from normal wear and tear—can result in pain, swelling, and impaired joint function. Meniscal repair is one of the most common types of arthroscopic procedures, and it leads to improvement in symptoms for many patients.

- **Ligament repair.** Arthroscopy is often used to diagnose, repair, or reconstruct torn or damaged ligaments.

The Arthroscopic Procedure

Arthroscopy may be performed under general, spinal, or local anesthesia, depending on the joint being treated and the type of problem being investigated. The orthopedic surgeon makes a small incision in the skin of the affected joint and inserts a pencil-sized instrument called an arthroscope. The arthroscope is fitted with a small lens and a light source to illuminate the interior structure of the joint. The arthroscope is also equipped with a fiber-optic camera that transmits images onto a screen. If the initial examination of the joint reveals the need for a corrective procedure, the surgeon makes additional incisions as needed to insert other miniature medical instruments.

Recovery after Arthroscopy

As a minimally invasive procedure, arthroscopic surgery causes significantly less trauma to the soft tissues of the joint than traditional open surgery. As a result, it offers a faster recovery time. The small arthroscopic incisions heal quickly, and the operative dressing is usually removed within a couple of days. The joint itself may take several weeks to recover, depending on the overall health of the patient and the procedure involved. In patients who require complex surgical procedures to correct extensive damage to cartilage and ligaments, recovery may take several months. Prior to discharge from the hospital, the healthcare provider generally provides the patient with explicit instructions on the type of activities to avoid, as well as the rehabilitative activities to undertake in order to speed recovery and improve postoperative joint function.

Risks Involved in Arthroscopy

Arthroscopy is generally considered a safe and effective medical procedure. Although most people who undergo it will experience some discomfort and swelling, these symptoms are typically short-lived. Many patients can return to work and resume normal activities within a few weeks. Serious complications are rare, affecting less than 1 percent of cases, and may include the following:

- **Postoperative infection.** If an infection develops within the joint, the patient will experience swelling, pain, and fever.

- **Nerve damage.** When an arthroscopic procedure damages a nerve, the patient may experience numbness and tingling sensations around the joint.

- **Hemorrhage.** A small amount of bleeding is normal in arthroscopic procedures, but excessive bleeding may require treatment in a hospital setting.

- **Equipment or implant failure.** Arthroscopic instruments are tiny and fragile, and they occasionally break during surgery. In these instances, the procedure may be extended, or a second surgery may be required. Likewise, the implants and components the surgeon uses to hold the joint in place (including pins, screws, rods, plates, and suture anchors) may break, leaving loose pieces floating around inside the joint. Since these fragments can rub against and damage surrounding tissues, they may need to be removed in a second surgery.

- **Deep-vein thrombosis (DVT).** DVT occurs when a blood clot forms in a vein following surgery. In rare cases, the blood clot may break away and pass through the bloodstream to the lungs, where it can obstruct the blood supply and create a dangerous condition called pulmonary embolism. Most surgeons take precautions to reduce the risk of DVT, such as administering blood thinners and getting the patients up and moving as soon as possible after surgery.

References

1. NHS Choices. "Arthroscopy," Gov.UK, 2015.

2. Waller, C.S. "Knee Arthroscopy," May 2010.

3. Wilkerson, Rick. "Arthroscopy," American Academy of Orthopaedic Surgeons, May 2010.

Section 31.2

Bone Fusion Surgery

"Bone Fusion Surgery,"
© 2018 Omnigraphics. Reviewed April 2018.

What Is Bone Fusion Surgery?

Bone fusion surgery, also known as spinal fusion surgery, is performed to join two or more vertebrae that are causing pain into a single bone. When the bones heal, they no longer move as they once did. Spinal fusion surgery alters the movement of the spine, thereby preventing pressure on the nearby nerves, ligaments, and muscles.

The surgeon places bones or metal plates, screws, and rods between two vertebrae to fuse them together. This surgery is only recommended by a doctor when the source of pain has been accurately located. The doctor may use X-ray, computed tomography (CT), and magnetic resonance imaging (MRI) to identify the source. Spinal fusion surgeries usually involve only a fragment of the spine and may not restrict much motion, though it may limit complete spinal movement.

Who Needs It

Spinal fusion surgery may be recommended for the following conditions:

- When a broken vertebra has destabilized your spinal column

- When a spinal deformity has caused a sideways curvature of the spine (scoliosis) or abnormal changes in the upper spine (kyphosis)

- When there is an abnormality or excessive movement between two vertebrae

- In the case of back pain or nerve crowding caused by spondylolisthesis

- To stabilize the spine after the removal of a damaged (herniated) disk

- For arthritis of the spine (spinal stenosis)

How to Prepare Yourself

Prior to the surgery, your doctor may take blood tests and order spinal X-rays. Your doctor wants you to be prepared, so don't hesitate to ask questions. The healthcare team will brief you about the procedures. Remind your doctor about the medicines you are taking. There may be medicines you are not supposed to take before the surgery. Always follow your doctor's instructions.

Before the Surgery

- Be prepared to have someone drive you to the surgery center.

- Continue regular medications as per your doctor's advice.

- In the case of diabetes, heart disease, or other medical problems, you may be asked to visit a regular doctor prior to the surgery.

- Keep your doctor informed if you've consumed alcohol.

- Smoking prevents quick recovery from the surgery. It is important to talk to your doctor about this.

- Your doctor may ask you to stop medications such as aspirin, ibuprofen (Advil, Motrin), naproxen (Aleve, Naprosyn), and other drugs as these slow down blood clotting prior to surgery.

- If you have a cold, the flu, a fever, herpes, or other illnesses, you need to talk to your doctor.

- Make sure to carry food with you if you are allowed to eat or drink before the surgery.

- Prepare your home for your return after the surgery.

After the Surgery

- Plan ahead and keep your loved ones informed as you might stay in the hospital for 3–4 days after the surgery.

- Pain medications may be given orally or intravenously in the hospital.

- Your food will be given to you intravenously as you may not be able to eat for 2–3 days.

- You will be required to wear a back brace or a cast when you leave the hospital.

- Your healthcare provider will instruct you on how to sit, stand, walk, and get out of bed without hurting your spine.

- Aftercare at home upon completion of surgery will be briefed by the surgeon. Make sure to follow these directions at home.

How the Surgery Is Done

After putting you to sleep with general anesthesia, the surgeon will examine your spine. Once this examination is complete, your surgeon will carry out the procedure:

- An incision will be made on either of these three locations: on your neck or over your spine from the back, from the sides of the spine, or from the front of the spine through the abdomen or throat.

- In the case of a bone graft, your surgeon will fuse two of your vertebrae together. Your surgeon may use a bone from the bone bank or may use a bone from your own body, usually taken from the pelvis.

- Using metal plates, screws or rods, your surgeon will fuse the vertebrae together permanently so that the bone graft can heal.

In other instances, your surgeon might use a synthetic substance in place of a bone graft. This is to enhance bone growth and speed up the fusion of the vertebrae.

Bone Grafting

In this procedure, fragments of bone are placed between the vertebrae to be fused. A bone graft is usually taken from a patient's hip and fused into the vertebrae. For additional support to the vertebrae, larger pieces of bone are used. This procedure is called autograft. In the case of an allograft, the bone is taken from a genetically nonidentical donor or a bone bank. Synthetic bone graft materials have been largely used since the development of this procedure.

Some bone grafting techniques are:

- **Demineralized bone matrices** (DBMs). Protein and calcium are extracted from cadaver bone to create DBMs. DBMs are largely used to heal bones.

- **Bone morphogenetic proteins (BMPs).** As approved by the U.S. Food and Drug Administration (FDA), autografts may not be necessary when BMPs are used. BMPs promote fusion of bones by bone-building synthetic proteins.

- **Ceramics.** Ceramics are synthetic calcium/phosphate materials that mimic an autograft bone, while maintaining similarity in shape, size, and consistency.

Based on your need, your surgeon will discuss the type of bone graft that will best suit your condition.

Immobilization

The vertebrae fuse together after bone grafting. To prevent damage to the spine and speed up recovery, your surgeon will suggest you to wear a brace. In most cases, the use of plates, screws, and rods speed up the healing process. This is called internal fixation and patients are usually able to exercise and increase mobility after surgery.

Risk Factors

Any surgery involves a certain risk and spinal fusion has its list of complications:

- Infection in the wound or vertebral bones

- The vertebrae above and below the fusion are more likely to wear away, leading to more problems later.

- Damage to a spinal nerve may cause weakness, pain, loss of sensation, and problems with your bowels or bladder.

- Pain at the site from which the bone graft was taken

- Leakage of spinal fluid that may require more surgery

- Slow wound healing

- Blood clots

- Headaches

After spinal fusion surgery, pressure is shifted from the fused vertebrae to other areas of the spine. This additional stress increases the wear and tear of the joints and often results in chronic pain. However, this pain can be prevented by watching out for the following signs:

- Increased pain

- Excessive swelling, redness, or drainage from the wound

- Shaking chills

- Fever over 100° F

Other complications are prone to occur and it is important to watch out for signs of blood clots and other infections as these might take place within a few weeks after the surgery. Possible signs of blood clots may include the following:

- Pain in the calf muscles

- Tenderness or redness, which may extend above or below the knee

- Swelling in the calf, ankle, or foot

Contact your doctor immediately if you have any of these symptoms.

Prognosis

Spinal fusion surgery is an effective treatment for spine-related problems and the source of most of these problems remain unknown. Imaging scans may not always reveal the source of your problems. Patients experience relief from troublesome symptoms following most spinal fusion surgery. However, the fused portion of the spine may cause additional stress to the surrounding areas and result in spine degeneration. This may require another spinal surgery. Below are signs that may require further treatment:

- You are more likely to have pain after the surgery if you've had chronic back pain before.

- Spinal fusion surgery does not always remove all the pain and other symptoms.

- Relief from pain after surgery cannot be guaranteed as it is difficult for a surgeon to predict which people will improve despite MRI scans and other tests.

- Losing weight and getting exercise increase your chances of feeling better.

- Spinal problems may occur in the future even after the surgery as the fused area of the spine exerts pressure on the surrounding areas and results in further problems.

Pain Management

Feel pain after the surgery is natural and is an essential part of the healing process. Your doctor will help reduce the pain by administering medications such as opioids, nonsteroidal anti-inflammatory drugs (NSAIDs), and local anesthetics, which will speed up the process of recovery.

It is important to take directions from your doctor. Stop the intake of opioids when pain begins to reduce, as these narcotics can be addictive. An overdependence on opioids can become a critical health issue. However, if you do not see any considerable improvement after the surgery, contact your doctor for further directions.

Recovering from Spinal Fusion

The first few days after surgery are critical for recovery. Your doctor will determine how soon to discharge you based on your level of fitness. You will be attached to machines that monitor your heart. There will be tubes connected to you. An intravenous (IV) tube will feed you fluids, antibiotics, and pain medicines as required. Sometimes an epidural catheter may be attached through a tube in your back to administer pain medicines. A catheter may help urine leave your body. These are to help you remain in the same state so that your back can heal quickly. It might feel unpleasant for a few days, but these are important for a speedy recovery.

Before returning home, your doctor will order spinal X-rays to confirm that the bone fusion is successful. Moreover, a physical therapist will instruct you how to get out of bed, sit in a chair, and walk. Within 10 days, you might have to visit your doctor to have your stitches removed. You will have follow-up appointments in about 4–6 weeks, and within the following 6 months, 12 months, and 24 months. Your physical therapist will teach you exercises to strengthen your back. Stick to the instructions and make sure to rest, as recovering from a spinal fusion surgery takes commitment and determination.

References

1. "Spinal Fusion," U.S. National Library of Medicine (NLM), September 7, 2017.

2. "Spinal Fusion," Mayo Foundation for Medical Education and Research (MFMER), March 21, 2018.

3. "Spinal fusion," American Academy of Orthopaedic Surgeons, June 2010.

4. "What Is Spinal Fusion?" WebMD LLC., January 8, 2018.

Chapter 32

Understanding Joint Replacement Surgery

Joint replacement surgery is removing a damaged joint and putting in a new one. The doctor may suggest a joint replacement to improve how you live. Replacing a joint can relieve pain and help you move and feel better.

Hips and knees are replaced most often. Other joints that can be replaced include the shoulders, fingers, ankles, and elbows.

The new joint can be made of plastic, metal, or ceramic parts. Sometimes, the surgeon will not remove the whole joint, but will only replace or fix the damaged parts. Types of new joints include:

- **Cemented joints:** Used more often in older people who do not move around as much and in people with "weak" bones. The cement holds the new joint to the bone.

- **Uncemented joints:** Often recommended for younger, more active people and those with good bone quality. It may take longer to heal, because it takes longer for bone to grow and attach to it.

- **Hybrid replacements:** Use both methods to keep the new joint in place.

This chapter includes text excerpted from "Joint Replacement Surgery," National Institute of Arthritis and Musculoskeletal and Skin Diseases (NIAMS), August 30, 2016.

Why It May Be Needed

Pain, stiffness, and swelling may be due to joint damage caused by:

- Arthritis

- Years of use

- Disease

To see if you need a joint replaced, your doctor may:

- Look at your joint with an X-ray or another machine

- Put a small, lighted tube (arthroscope) into your joint to look for damage

- Take a small sample of your tissue for testing

After looking at your joint, the doctor may recommend:

- Exercise

- Walking aids, such as braces or canes

- Physical therapy

- Medicines and vitamin supplements

- Osteotomy, which involves cutting and lining up bone. This may be simpler than replacing a joint, but it may take longer to recover. However, this operation has become less common.

If you still have constant pain and have trouble with things such as walking, climbing stairs, and taking a bath, your doctor may recommend joint replacement.

During the Surgery

During joint replacement surgery your doctors will:

- Give you medicine so you won't feel pain. The medicine may block the pain only in one part of the body, or it may put your whole body to sleep.

- Replace the damaged joint with a new artificial joint.

- Move you to a recovery room until you are fully awake or the numbness goes away.

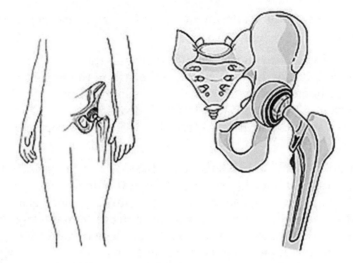

Figure 32.1. *Hip Replacement Location*

After the Surgery

With knee or hip surgery, you will probably need to stay in the hospital for a few days. If you are elderly or have additional disabilities, you may then need to spend several weeks in an intermediate-care facility before going home. You and your team of doctors will determine how long you stay in the hospital.

After hip or knee replacement, you will often stand or begin walking the day of surgery. At first, you will walk with a walker or crutches. You may have some temporary pain in the new joint because your muscles are weak from not being used. Also, your body is healing. The pain can be helped with medicines and should end in a few weeks or months.

Physical therapy can begin the day after surgery to help strengthen the muscles around the new joint and help you regain motion in the joint. If you have your shoulder joint replaced, you can usually begin exercising the same day of your surgery! A physical therapist will help you with gentle, range-of-motion exercises. Before you leave the hospital, your therapist will show you how to use a pulley device to help bend and extend your arm.

Complications

New technology and advances in surgical techniques have greatly reduced the complications involved with joint replacements.

343

When problems do occur, most are treatable. Possible problems include:

- **Infection.** Areas in the wound or around the new joint may get infected. It may happen while you're still in the hospital or after you go home. It may even occur years later. Minor infections in the wound are usually treated with drugs. Deep infections may need a second operation to treat the infection or replace the joint.

- **Blood clots.** If your blood moves too slowly, it may begin to form lumps of blood parts called clots. If pain and swelling develop in your legs after hip or knee surgery, blood clots may be the cause. The doctor may suggest drugs to make your blood thin or special stockings, exercises, or boots to help your blood move faster. If swelling, redness, or pain occurs in your leg after you leave the hospital, contact your doctor right away.

- **Loosening.** The new joint may loosen, causing pain. If the loosening is bad, you may need another operation to reattach the joint to the bone.

- **Dislocation.** Sometimes after hip or other joint replacement, the ball of the prosthesis can come out of its socket. In most cases, the hip can be corrected without surgery. A brace may be worn for a while if a dislocation occurs.

- **Wear.** Some wear can be found in all joint replacements. Too much wear may help cause loosening. The doctor may need to operate again if the prosthesis comes loose. Sometimes, the plastic can wear thin, and the doctor may just replace the plastic and not the whole joint.

- **Nerve and blood vessel injury.** Nerves near the replaced joint may be damaged during surgery, but this does not happen often. Over time, the damage often improves and may disappear. Blood vessels may also be injured.

As you move your new joint and let your muscles grow strong again, the pain will lessen, flexibility will increase, and movement will improve.

Chapter 33

Knee Replacement

Your knee joint is made up of bone, cartilage, ligaments, and fluid. Muscles and tendons help the knee joint move. When any of these structures is hurt or diseased, you have knee problems. Knee problems can cause pain and difficulty walking.

Knee problems are very common, and they occur in people of all ages. Knee problems can interfere with many things, from participation in sports to simply getting up from a chair and walking. This can have a big impact on your life.

The most common disease affecting the knee is osteoarthritis (OA). The cartilage in the knee gradually wears away, causing pain and swelling. Injuries to ligaments and tendons also cause knee problems. A common injury is to the anterior cruciate ligament (ACL). You usually injure your ACL by a sudden twisting motion. ACL and other knee injuries are common sports injuries.

Treatment of knee problems depends on the cause. In some cases, your doctor may recommend knee replacement.

This chapter contains text excerpted from the following sources: Text in this chapter begins with excerpts from "Knee Injuries and Disorders," MedlinePlus, National Institutes of Health (NIH), August 25, 2016; Text under the heading "Who Needs a Knee Replacement?" is excerpted from "Who Needs a Knee Replacement?" *NIH News in Health*, National Institutes of Health (NIH), January 2014. Reviewed April 2018; Text under the heading "Knee Replacement" is excerpted from "Knee Replacement," MedlinePlus, National Institutes of Health (NIH), March 15, 2016.

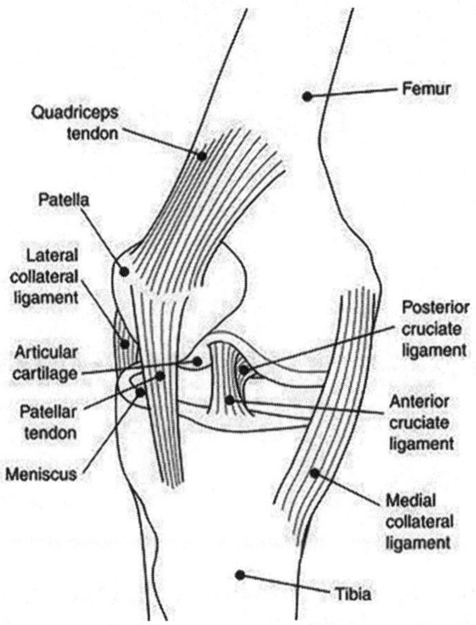

Figure 33.1. *Lateral View of the Knee* (Source: "Knee Problems," National Institute of Arthritis and Musculoskeletal and Skin Diseases (NIAMS).)

Who Needs a Knee Replacement?

Knee replacement involves removing parts of your natural knee joint and replacing them with artificial parts. Knee replacement is the most common type of joint replacement surgery.

Several forms of arthritis can damage knees and cause so much pain and disability that knees need to be replaced. Certain knee deformities—such as bowed legs or knock knees—can wear down cartilage and create difficulties. Knee damage can also result from a problem called avascular necrosis, or osteonecrosis, in which the bones lose their blood supply, die, and eventually collapse.

If other treatments haven't helped, your doctor may suggest knee replacement when pain and stiffness begin to interfere with your everyday activities.

If you'd like to consider knee replacement, ask your doctor to refer you to an orthopedic surgeon, a doctor specially trained to treat problems of the bones and joints.

Knee Replacement

Knee replacement is surgery for people with severe knee damage. Knee replacement can relieve pain and allow you to be more active.

Your doctor may recommend it if you have knee pain and medicine and other treatments are not helping you anymore.

When you have a total knee replacement, the surgeon removes damaged cartilage and bone from the surface of your knee joint and replaces them with a manufactured surface of metal and plastic. In a partial knee replacement, the surgeon only replaces one part of your knee joint. The surgery can cause scarring, blood clots, and, rarely, infections. After a knee replacement, you will no longer be able to do certain activities, such as jogging and high-impact sports.

Chapter 34

Other Types of Joint Surgery

Chapter Contents

Section 34.1—Hip Replacement.. 350

Section 34.2—Shoulder Replacement....................................... 356

Section 34.3—Joint Fusion Surgery (Arthrodesis)................... 363

Section 34.1

Hip Replacement

This section includes text excerpted from "Hip Replacement Surgery," National Institute of Arthritis and Musculoskeletal and Skin Diseases (NIAMS), July 30, 2016.

The hip joint is located where the upper end of the femur (thigh bone) meets the pelvis (hip bone). A ball at the end of the femur, called the femoral head, fits in a socket (the acetabulum) in the pelvis to allow a wide range of motion.

Hip replacement, or arthroplasty, is a surgical procedure in which the diseased parts of the hip joint are removed and replaced with new, artificial parts. These artificial parts are called the prosthesis.

The goals of hip replacement surgery include increasing mobility, improving the function of the hip joint, and relieving pain.

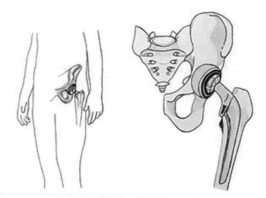

Figure 34.1. *Hip Replacement*

Types

There are two primary types of hip replacement surgery:

Traditional surgery: During a traditional hip replacement, which lasts from 1–2 hours, the surgeon makes a 6–8-inch incision over the side of the hip through the muscles and removes the diseased bone tissue and cartilage from the hip joint while leaving the healthy parts of the joint intact. Then the surgeon replaces the head of the femur and acetabulum with new, artificial parts. The new hip is made of materials that allow a natural gliding motion of the joint.

Minimally invasive surgery: Some surgeons perform what is called a minimally invasive, or mini-incision, hip replacement, which requires smaller incisions and a shorter recovery time than traditional hip replacement. Candidates for this type of surgery are usually age 50 or younger, of normal weight based on body mass index (BMI), and healthier than candidates for traditional surgery. Joint resurfacing is also being used.

Regardless of whether you have traditional or minimally invasive surgery, the parts used to replace the joint are the same and come in two general varieties: cemented and uncemented.

- **Cemented replacements,** which fasten artificial parts to the healthy bone with a special glue or cement. These replacements are typically used for older, less active people and people with weak bones.

- **Uncemented replacements,** which use artificial parts with a porous surface. This allows the bone to grow into the pores to hold the new parts in place. These replacements are typically used for younger, more active people. Because it takes a long time for the natural bone to grow and attach to the prosthesis, the activity must be limited for up to three months to protect the hip joint. Thigh pain may occur while the bone is growing into the prosthesis.

- **Hybrid replacements** use a cemented femur part and uncemented acetabular part.

Why Is This Surgery Needed?

Common reasons for hip replacement surgery include damage to the hip joint from:

- Arthritis

- Disease that breaks down the bone in the joint

- Injuries or fractures

- Bone tumors that break down the hip joint

If hip joint damage causes pain and interferes with daily activities, your doctor may try treatments such as exercise, walking aids (canes and walkers), and medication. If these treatments do not relieve pain and improve joint function, the doctor may suggest either hip replacement surgery or a less complex corrective surgery. One alternative to hip replacement is osteotomy, which involves cutting and realigning bone to shift the weight to a healthier bone surface.

In the past, hip replacement surgery was mostly done in people over 60 years of age. The thinking was that older people are less active, which puts less stress on the artificial hip. However, new technologies have improved artificial parts so that they handle more stress and last longer. This means that hip replacement surgery can also be successful in younger people.

Hip replacement may not be recommended for people with certain health conditions, such as:

- Parkinson disease (PD)

- Conditions that result in severe muscle weakness, which increases the risk of damaging or dislocating an artificial hip

- People at high risk for infections or in poor health, since they are less likely to recover successfully

Preparing for Surgery

You can do a number of things before hip replacement surgery to make everyday tasks easier and help speed your recovery.

- Learn what to expect. Request written information from the doctor, or learn more about the procedure by visiting one of the websites listed near the end of this publication.

- Arrange for transportation to and from the hospital.

- Arrange for someone to help you around the house for a week or two after coming home from the hospital.

- Stock up on kitchen supplies and prepare food in advance, such as frozen casseroles or soups that can be reheated and served easily.

- Set up a "recovery station" at home:

- Place the television remote control, telephone, medicine, tissues, wastebasket, and pitcher and glass next to the spot where you will spend the most time while you recover.

- Place other items you use every day at arm's level to avoid reaching up or bending down.

What to Expect during Surgery

During hip replacement, which lasts from 1–2 hours, your doctors:

- Will give you medicine to put your whole body to sleep so that you won't feel pain

- Makes a 6–8-inch incision over the side of the hip. Your surgeon may recommend a minimally invasive hip replacement, which requires smaller incisions. Candidates for minimally invasive hip replacement surgery are usually:

- Age 50 or younger

- Normal weight based on BMI

- Healthier than candidates for traditional surgery

- Removes the diseased bone tissue and cartilage from the hip joint, while leaving the healthy parts of the joint in place

- Replaces the head of the femur and acetabulum with new, artificial parts

- Move you to a recovery room for 1–2 hours until you are fully awake or the numbness goes away

What to Expect Afterward

Immediate. Usually, people do not spend more than 1–4 days in the hospital after hip replacement surgery. It is important to get instructions from your doctor before leaving the hospital and to follow them carefully once you get home. Doing so will you give you the greatest chance of a successful surgery.

- Immediately after your hip surgery:

  - You will be allowed only limited movement.

  - When you are in bed, pillows or a special device will brace the hip in the correct position.

  - You may receive fluids through an intravenous tube to replace fluids lost during surgery.

- Drains may also be located near the incision to drain fluid, and a catheter may be inserted to remove urine until you can use the bathroom.

- The doctor will prescribe medicine for pain or discomfort.

- The day of or day after surgery:

  - Therapists will teach you exercises to improve recovery.

  - A respiratory therapist may ask you to breathe deeply, cough, or blow into a simple device that measures lung capacity. These exercises reduce the collection of fluid in the lungs after surgery.

- As early as 1–2 days after surgery:

  - You may be able to sit on the edge of the bed, stand, and even walk with assistance.

  - A physical therapist may teach you exercises to strengthen the hip. The physical therapist also will teach you how to perform daily activities without injuring your new hip.

- Once you return home you should:

  - Follow the doctor's instructions.

  - Wear an apron for carrying things around the house. This leaves hands and arms free for balance or to use crutches.

  - Use a long-handled "reacher" to turn on lights or grab things that are beyond arm's length. Hospital personnel may provide one of these or suggest where to buy one.

  - Work with a physical therapist or other healthcare professional to rehabilitate your hip.

Long-term. Full recovery from hip replacement surgery takes about 3–6 months, depending on the type of surgery, your overall health, and the success of your rehabilitation.

You should talk to your doctor or physical therapist about an appropriate exercise program, which can reduce stiffness, increase flexibility, and strengthen muscles. Most of these programs begin with safe range-of-motion activities and muscle-strengthening exercises. The doctor or therapist will decide when you can move on to more demanding activities.

Revision surgery (replacement of an artificial joint) is becoming more common as more people are having hip replacements at a younger age. This is because wearing away of the joint surface becomes a problem after 15–20 years. Doctors consider revision surgery when:

- Medication and lifestyle changes do not relieve pain and disability.
- X-rays show bone loss, wearing of the joint surfaces, or joint loosening.
- Fracture, dislocation of the artificial parts or infection occur.

Possible Complications

New technology and advances in surgical techniques have greatly reduced the risks involved with hip replacements. More common problems that could occur include:

- **Hip dislocation,** in which the ball becomes dislodged from the socket if the hip is placed in certain positions (such as pulling the knees up to the chest). This is the most common problem that may arise soon after hip replacement surgery.
- An **inflammatory reaction** to tiny particles that gradually wear off of the artificial joint surfaces and are absorbed by the surrounding tissues. The inflammation may trigger the action of special cells that eat away some of the bone, causing the implant to loosen. This is the most common later complication of hip replacement surgery.

Less common complications include:

- **Infection:** Warning signs include fever, chills, tenderness, and swelling, or drainage from the wound.
- **Blood clots:** Warning signs include tenderness, redness, and swelling of your calf; or swelling of your thigh, ankle, or foot.
- **Bone growth** beyond the normal edges of bone.

You should call your doctor if you experience any symptoms listed above.

Life after Surgery

For the majority of people who have hip replacement surgery, the procedure results in:

- Reduced pain

- Increased mobility

- Improvements in activities of daily living

- Improved quality of life

Many doctors recommend avoiding high-impact activities, such as basketball, jogging, and tennis. These activities can damage the new hip or cause loosening of its parts. Talk to your doctor about exercises to increase muscle strength and cardiovascular fitness without injuring the new hip. These exercises can include:

- Walking

- Stationary bicycling

- Swimming

- Cross-country skiing

Section 34.2

Shoulder Replacement

"Shoulder Replacement,"
© 2018 Omnigraphics. Reviewed April 2018.

Shoulder replacement is a surgical procedure to replace the bones of the shoulder with an artificial implant. According to the Agency for Healthcare Research and Quality (AHRQ), more than 53,000 people in the United States have shoulder replacement surgeries each year. Shoulder replacement surgery was first performed to treat shoulder fractures; however, it is also used to treat other painful conditions of the shoulder. Shoulder replacement is an effective procedure to remove pain and improve motion, strength, and function in the shoulder.

Causes of Shoulder Pain

There are several causes for shoulder pain, and many reasons why patients should consider a shoulder replacement surgery.

Rheumatoid Arthritis

Rheumatoid arthritis, also called inflammatory arthritis, affects the shoulders. The synovial membrane that lubricates the cartilage becomes inflamed and causes joint stiffness, eventually resulting in loss of cartilage and shoulder pain.

Osteoarthritis (Degenerative Joint Disease)

Osteoarthritis is one of the most common reasons for shoulder replacement surgery. As people age, their chances of developing osteoarthritis are high. The cartilage wears away and causes stiffness in the shoulder bones. As a result, when the bones rub against one another, there is severe shoulder pain.

Rotator Cuff Tear Arthropathy

When the rotator cuff muscles contract, they put pressure on the humerus, resulting in rotator cuff tears. The sudden changes in the shoulder muscles caused by the rotator cuff damages the joint cartilage. This leads to arthritis of the shoulder.

Posttraumatic Arthritis

Arthritis of the shoulder may lead to fractures that cause tears in the shoulder muscles. After a shoulder injury, the ligaments and tendons damage the cartilage and prevent smooth movement of the shoulder.

Severe Fractures

A doctor may recommend a shoulder replacement in the case of a severe fracture. Blood supply to the bone is stopped because of the fracture. When the humerus is fractured, it is not easy to replace the bones, and therefore, a surgeon may recommend shoulder replacement.

Avascular Necrosis (Osteonecrosis)

Osteonecrosis causes shoulder pain when the bone cells die due to a lack of blood supply. This eventually leads to arthritis. Often, this condition is caused by excessive use of alcohol, steroids, shoulder fractures, and sickle cell disease.

Failed Shoulder Replacement Surgery

Sometimes, shoulder replacements fail because of infection, wear and tear, dislocation, or the loosening of the implant. In such cases, another shoulder replacement surgery might be necessary.

Do You Need a Shoulder Replacement Surgery?

When other treatment options have been considered and there is no relief, the doctor may recommend a shoulder replacement surgery. Often in the case of osteoarthritis, rheumatoid arthritis, and severe trauma caused by a shoulder fracture, complete shoulder replacement enables smooth functioning of the shoulder muscles. It is important to discuss this surgery with your loved ones, your doctor, and your surgeon and to be assured of their cooperation as you decide to undergo the surgery.

Your doctor may recommend shoulder replacement surgery for the following reasons:

- Decreased motion or weakness in the shoulder
- Severe pain while resting, to the extent of robbing you of sleep
- Difficulty in performing everyday activities such as reaching into a cabinet, dressing, and washing because of excess strain in the shoulders
- No improvement after treatments with anti-inflammatory medications, cortisone injections, or physical therapy

You may consider shoulder replacement surgery for the following reasons:

- A torn rotator cuff
- A serious shoulder injury like a broken bone
- Severe arthritis

However, your doctor will recommend surgery only after treating you with drugs and physical therapy and determining that they have not helped alleviate your pain.

Types of Shoulder Replacement Surgeries

There are a few types of shoulder replacement surgeries. Your doctor will determine which one is right for you depending on the condition of your shoulder.

Total Shoulder Replacement

Total shoulder replacement surgery is performed by replacing the surface of the affected joint with a metal ball and a plastic socket. They come in all sizes and your surgeon will choose what is necessary for the surgery. Your doctor may use a uncemented humeral component if the quality of the bone is good and bone cement if the bone is soft. However, an all-plastic glenoid substance is inserted with bone cement.

Glenoid component is not recommended when:

- The rotator cuff tendons are torn beyond repair

- The glenoid has good cartilage

- The glenoid bone is severely deficient

Total shoulder replacement surgery is particularly appropriate for patients with osteoarthritis and intact rotator cuff tendons.

Stemmed Hemiarthroplasty

Hemiarthroplasty is the surgical procedure of replacing only the ball in the shoulder. The humeral head is replaced with a metal ball and stem in a traditional hemiarthroplasty, also known as a stemmed hemiarthroplasty.

Hemiarthroplasty is recommended only when the humeral head is damaged but the socket is intact. A hemiarthroplasty also includes:

- Shoulders with considerable damage to the bone in the glenoid

- Torn rotator cuff tendons and arthritis of the shoulders

- Damage to the humeral head but the glenoid has a healthy cartilage surface

However, there are instances when the surgeons decide to make a call whether to proceed with a total shoulder replacement or a hemiarthroplasty during the surgery.

Resurfacing Hemiarthroplasty

As the name suggests, the surface of the humeral head is replaced with a prosthetic cap. Resurfacing hemiarthroplasty is a procedure that increases bone life, offering patients with arthritis of the shoulder an option to choose between the traditional hemiarthroplasty and resurfacing hemiarthroplasty.

You can choose resurfacing hemiarthroplasty if:

- There is no damage to the humeral neck or head
- The cartilage surface of the glenoid is healthy
- The humeral bone has to be preserved

Resurfacing hemiarthroplasty decreases the risk of wear and tear and loosening of the implant and is highly recommended for young patients. If required, later resurfacing hemiarthroplasty can be converted to a total shoulder replacement.

Reverse Total Shoulder Replacement

In a reverse total shoulder replacement, a metal ball is attached to the shoulder bone and to the upper arm bone—a plastic socket. This allows the patient to use the muscles of the upper arm instead of the torn rotator cuff. Reverse total shoulder replacement is recommended only in the case of:

- Severe arthritis and rotator cuff tearing (cuff tear arthropathy)
- A torn rotator cuff with severe arm weakness
- A previously failed shoulder replacement

Sometimes, patients find it difficult to lift their arms and move them sideways. A reverse shoulder replacement provides relief while a traditional total shoulder replacement can still leave them with pain.

Risk Factors

As is the case in most surgeries, your surgeon will describe the potential risks in undergoing a shoulder replacement surgery. Complications can occur after the surgery; however, most of these conditions can be treated:

- Infection or bleeding around the joint
- Allergic reaction to the artificial joint
- Damage to the blood vessel during surgery
- Nerve damage during surgery
- Dislocation of the artificial joint
- Loosening of the implant over time
- Bone break during surgery

Preparing for Surgery

Preparation for a shoulder replacement surgery involves a full physical exam, X-rays, or other imaging tests to confirm the need for surgery. Your orthopedic surgeon will make a thorough examination to determine your fitness level for the surgery.

The medical examination consists of:

- **A medical history.** In addition to the general health checkup, your doctor will examine the functioning of your affected shoulder.

- **A physical examination.** Shoulder motion, strength, and stability are gauged.

- **X-rays.** The level of damage to the shoulder, spaces between the bones, deformities, or any irregularities in the bone or cartilage can be determined by viewing the images generated by the X-ray.

- **Other tests.** Magnetic resonance imaging (MRI) scans and other blood tests help evaluate the condition of bone and soft tissues of the shoulder.

After reviewing the results of your evaluation, your orthopedic surgeon will determine the need for surgery. However, other options for treatment will also be discussed by the doctor, who will consider whether injections, physical therapy, or another type of treatment may be required. If surgery has been confirmed, it will be explained to you ahead of time. This will give you time to prepare yourself for your stay after the surgery, and also allow time to plan for any help required after your discharge from the hospital.

After the Surgery

After you are transported to the postanesthesia recovery unit (PACU), the anesthesiology team will check your vital signs (breathing, pulse, and blood pressure). When you have recovered from the anesthesia, you will be attached to a cooling unit. A large dressing on your shoulder will be covered with an arm sling for protection. After an hour at the PACU, you will be assigned to a hospital room.

- You will stay in the hospital for a few days (1–3) after your surgery.

- A physical therapist will help you keep your shoulder muscles relaxed.

- Active movement of your shoulders will not be allowed until sufficient time has been given for healing your shoulder muscles.

- You will be given instructions on how to care for your shoulder at home. Make sure to follow them.

Pain Management

Pain management is an essential part of your recovery. After surgery, you will feel some pain but, with physical therapy, you will be on the path to recovery soon. The pain gradually reduces as you recover your strength and start exercising your shoulder again. Keep your doctor informed in the event of any complications as you exercise your shoulder muscles. Pain relief medications include opioids, nonsteroidal anti-inflammatory drugs (NSAIDs), and local anesthetics that can help you manage your pain. The doctor may prescribe a combination of medicines and, over time, reduce your need for opioids. The use of opioids is critical and must be taken only under your doctor's approval. However, if the pain does not reduce after the surgery, make sure to inform your doctor.

Rehabilitation

A rehabilitation program is essential to the success of a shoulder replacement. Regular exercises and physical therapy are mandatory after surgery. Your physical therapist will demonstrate exercises to strengthen your shoulder and improve flexibility. The following guidelines will ensure a successful recovery from your surgery:

1. Follow the exercises demonstrated by the physical therapist 2 or 3 times a day.

2. Do not exert pressure on your arm when you get out of bed or up from a chair since this causes additional strain on your shoulder muscles.

3. Overuse of your shoulder may result in excess pain afterward. Try to limit your shoulder movements as much as possible.

4. Ask for assistance at home.

5. Limit your involvement in sports that involve excessive action, as this may cause unnecessary strain on your shoulders.

6. Ask for help when you want to lift something heavy.

7. Keep your arm in the position demonstrated by the physical therapist. Avoid extreme movements such as moving your arms to one side or behind your body for the first weeks after surgery.

Shoulder replacement surgery has greatly improved the quality of life for thousands of patients, improving motion and flexibility. Following the rehabilitation program, you will make several trips to see your doctor and keep him or her informed of your progress.

References

1. "Shoulder Joint Replacement," American Academy of Orthopedic Surgeons (AAOS), December 2011.

2. "Shoulder Replacement," MedlinePlus, April 5, 2018.

3. J. Martin, Laura. "Shoulder Replacement Surgery: What to Know," WebMD, December 21, 2017.

4. "Joint Replacement: Shoulder," The Cleveland Clinic Foundation, August 21, 2009.

Section 34.3

Joint Fusion Surgery (Arthrodesis)

"Joint Fusion Surgery (Arthrodesis),"
© 2018 Omnigraphics. Reviewed April 2018.

Joint fusion surgery, also known as "arthrodesis," is surgical immobilization of a joint by fusion of the bones that make up the joint. This type of intervention is usually indicated in patients with advanced and irreversible arthritic changes that have failed to respond to conservative treatments, including pain-relieving regimens, orthotic management, and lifestyle modifications.

The procedure typically involves stripping out the ligaments, menisci, and the synovial joint which make up the damaged joint and then allowing the bones to "fuse," or "weld." This is followed by fixation of intramedullary rods, plates, or other orthopedic hardware to hold the bones in place. Depending on the condition of the bones and the degree of soft-tissue damage, a bone graft may also be used to help the bones heal together.

Although fusion surgery alleviates pain, restores some degree of stability to the joint, and allows the best possible pain-free motion, it comes at a cost. Primarily, all joint motions are compromised when an arthrodesis is performed. The joint is fixed in the optimal functional position, which is decided by the surgeon based on the patient's specific functional requirements and involvement of associated joints. Arthrodesis may be performed on joints of the hips, wrists, ankles, fingers, thumb, and spine.

Indications for Arthrodesis

While arthrodesis used to be commonly performed on major joints of the body, the surgery has become far less common with the advent of joint-conserving interventions such as arthroplasty and joint placement. This is particularly true of hip and knee fusions. Currently, fusion surgery is only used as a salvage procedure in cases where the joint has been significantly damaged due to trauma or disease, making it impossible to repair or reconstruct. One of the most common indications for an arthrodesis is a flailing joint that arises from paralytic conditions—for instance, poliomyelitis. Arthrodesis is also considered in a failed joint replacement, or for patients who have undergone excision of a malignant joint.

Procedure

A joint is arthrodesed by an orthopedic surgeon assisted by a team of specialized healthcare professionals. The duration of the surgery depends on the type of technique employed. An arthroscopic arthrodesis is less invasive and less invalidating but may be contraindicated in some patients who require correction of significant deformities. The arthroscopic technique involves a small incision on the outer surface of the joint to insert the arthroscope through which the joint is visualized and the procedure performed.

In arthrodesis, one of the following techniques may be used: intra-articular; extra-articular; or a combination of both.

- **Intra-articular arthrodesis** involves debriding the cartilage surface from the opposing bony ends of the joint and exposing the underlying bones prior to fusion. Hip and knee joints may use this technique.

- **Extra-articular arthrodesis** is usually performed when the articular cartilage needs to be preserved, and is of particular use for pediatric patients in whom cartilage forms much of the joint surfaces and may need to be preserved to accommodate future bone growth.

In general, an arthrodesis is performed under general or spinal anesthesia, during which heart rate and blood pressure are closely monitored. A traction may be used for better radiographic visualization of the articular surface. A prophylactic intravenous (IV) antibiotic is administered to control possible infection. The articular surface is debrided and the bones are aligned and secured with orthopedic implants (screws, plates, and others). Other abnormalities, if any, are also corrected before closing the skin and muscle tissues with staples or sutures.

Generally, three types of implants are used, either alone, or in combination, depending on the type of joint and expected functional outcome:

1. **External Fixation:** Orthopedic implants, such as rods and screws are percutaneously inserted into the bone and held in place with clamps. This method helps to immobilize the joint and bring about compression of opposing bone surfaces.

2. **Internal Fixation:** Screws or plates are placed on the inside of the joint to compress the bones and facilitate healing.

3. **Intramedullary Nail/Rods:** A type of internal fixation hardware is inserted into the medullary (central) cavity of the bone shaft; these assist the bones in load-bearing and encourage fusion of the bones.

Bone Grafts

The success of many arthrodesis procedures is determined by successful bone graft fusion. While orthopedic implants can provide initial stabilization, the ultimate goal of an arthrodesis is to prevent long-term failure of the surgical intervention. This is achieved by a bone graft, a piece of bone inserted into the arthrodesed joint to provide a scaffold for the growth of new bone cells. The new bone tissue helps to heal and "weld" the bones together for long-term stability. Bone grafts can be harvested from the patient's own bone (autograft) or from a cadaveric donor (allograft).

Bone graft substitutes are made from a variety of materials, including ceramics or bone morphogenetic proteins (BMPs), which are being increasingly considered for arthrodesed joints as they are associated with fewer risks of infection or rejection. Demineralized bone matrix (DBM) has also emerged as a widely used graft extender when used along with the real bone. Made from allograft bone by a process of demineralization, the DBM is rich in bone-forming protein (collagen) and other growth factors that can stimulate healing. Essentially used to boost bone graft volume, this is available in a variety of forms, such as chip, gel, powder, or putty.

Postoperative Protocol and Physical Therapy

A cast is applied and a period of rest with zero weight-bearing follows surgery. This is important to prevent inflammation and infection. A period of partial weight-bearing follows. If imaging tests and clinical signs indicate a successful fusion, then the patient is allowed to return to full daily activities, although healthcare professionals may advise against full weight-bearing for a few months to ensure that adequate fusion has been achieved.

The primary objective of physical therapy is to educate, assist, and train the patient to perform activities of daily living (ADLs). This is achieved by using compensatory postural adaptations and biomechanisms of the arthrodesed and associated joints. Because immobilization following arthrodesis, particularly in the case of hip, knee, or ankle, is often prolonged, physical therapy usually begins during the immobilization period. It is important to ensure that there is no strain on the arthrodesed joint during nonweight-bearing ambulation. Typically, a range of motion (ROM) and strengthening exercises are initiated within a couple of weeks for all the nonimmobilized, surrounding joints to help improve stability, balance, posture, and other functional outcomes of the fused joint. This is followed by a period of mobilization of the fused joints to achieve optimal function, which should ideally happen four weeks following mobilization.

Complications of Arthrodesis

As with every surgery, arthrodesis carries associated risks that may vary depending on the age and general health conditions of the patient. Low bone density and diabetes, for example, may impact surgical outcomes. While bleeding, infection, damage to adjacent nerves, and blood clots are some of the complications that could arise from the surgical procedure, there may also be significant risks associated with the misalignment of bones and symptomatic hardware problems. Also, the loss of function of the arthrodesed joint may exert more stress on nearby joints, and this could lead to arthritic changes in adjacent joints over time. Studies indicate that one of the most common complications of arthrodesis is nonunion of bones. A nonunion occurs when the bones do not fuse together. Under such circumstances, a second operation to place a bone graft or other hardware may become necessary.

References

1. "Ankle Fusion," The Johns Hopkins University, n.d.

2. "Ankle Arthrodesis versus Ankle Replacement for Ankle Arthritis," U.S. National Library of Medicine (NLM), June 1, 2013.

3. "Arthrodesis of the Wrist in Rheumatoid Arthritis," U.S. National Library of Medicine (NLM), September 18, 2014.

Part Four

Arthritis Self-Management: Strategies to Reduce Pain and Inflammation

Chapter 35

Managing Arthritis

Managing Arthritis: Strive for Five

There are a lot of things you can do to manage your arthritis. The day-to-day things you choose to do to manage your condition and stay healthy are "self-management" strategies and activities. Centers for Disease Control and Prevention's (CDC) arthritis program recommends five self-management strategies for managing arthritis and its symptoms. Practice these simple strategies to reduce symptoms and get relief so that you can pursue the activities that are important to you.

1. Learn New Self-Management Skills

Join a self-management education workshop, which can help you learn the skills to manage your arthritis and make good decisions about your health.

How Can a Self-Management Education Workshop Help Me?

Learning strategies to better manage your arthritis can help you:

- Feel more in control of your health
- Manage pain and other symptoms

This chapter includes text excerpted from "Managing Arthritis," Centers for Disease Control and Prevention (CDC), January 24, 2018.

- Carry out daily activities, like going to work and spending time with loved ones.

- Reduce stress

- Improve your mood

- Communicate better with your healthcare provider(s) about your care

2. Be Active

Physical activity is a simple and effective way to relieve pain from arthritis that does not require medication. Being physically active can reduce pain, improve function, mood, and quality of life for adults with arthritis. Regular physical activity can also reduce your risk of developing other chronic diseases, such as heart disease, and can help you manage these conditions if you already have them. *2008 Physical Activity Guidelines for Americans* recommends that adults be physically active at a moderate intensity for 150 minutes per week.

- For example, walk, swim, or bike 30 minutes a day for 5 days a week.

- These 30 minutes can be broken into three separate 10-minute sessions during the day if needed.

Unsure about What Kind of Activity Is Safe?

Get more information about how to exercise safely with arthritis or find a community program near you. Physical activity community programs—like Enhanced®Fitness, Walk With Ease, and others—help adults with arthritis be healthier and reduce arthritis symptoms. These programs are often held in parks, recreation centers, Ys (Young Men's Christian Associations (YMCAs)), and other community venues.

3. Talk to Your Doctor

Talk to your doctor if you have joint pain and other arthritis symptoms. It's important to get an accurate diagnosis as soon as possible so you can start treatment and work to minimize symptoms and prevent the disease from getting worse.

The focus of arthritis treatment is to:

- Reduce pain

- Minimize joint damage

- Improve or maintain function and quality of life

You can play an active role in controlling your arthritis by attending regular appointments with your healthcare provider and following your recommended treatment plan. This is especially important if you also have other chronic conditions, like diabetes or heart disease.

4. Manage Your Weight

Losing excess weight and maintaining a healthy weight are particularly important for people with arthritis. For people who are overweight or obese, losing weight reduces stress on joints, particularly weight-bearing joints like the hips and knees. In fact, losing as little as 10–12 pounds can improve pain and function for people with arthritis. At any age, low-impact, arthritis-friendly physical activity (like walking) and dietary changes can help you lose weight.

5. Protect Your Joints

Joint injuries can cause or worsen arthritis. Choose activities that are easy on the joints like walking, bicycling, and swimming. These low-impact activities have a low risk of injury and do not twist or put too much stress on the joints.

Sports- or work-related injuries to joints can increase the likelihood of developing osteoarthritis (OA). To reduce the likelihood of developing or worsening OA, take steps to minimize or prevent injuries to joints, such as wearing protective equipment and avoiding repetitive motion.

Chapter 36

Chronic Pain Management

Chronic Pain

Pain is a signal in your nervous system that something may be wrong. It is an unpleasant feeling, such as a prick, tingle, sting, burn, or ache. Pain may be sharp or dull. You may feel pain in one area of your body, or all over. There are two types: acute pain and chronic pain. Acute pain lets you know that you may be injured or a have problem you need to take care of. Chronic pain is different. The pain may last for weeks, months, or even years. The original cause may have been an injury or infection. There may be an ongoing cause of pain, such as arthritis or cancer. In some cases, there is no clear cause. Environmental and psychological factors can make chronic pain worse.

Many older adults have chronic pain. Women also report having more chronic pain than men, and they are at a greater risk for many pain conditions. Some people have two or more chronic pain conditions.

Opioids and Pain Management

Opioids are natural or synthetic chemicals that relieve pain by binding to receptors in your brain or body to reduce the intensity of pain

This chapter contains text excerpted from the following sources: Text under the heading "Chronic Pain" is excerpted from "Chronic Pain," MedlinePlus, National Institutes of Health (NIH), August 17, 2016; Text beginning with the heading "Opioids and Pain Management" is excerpted from "Opioid Overdose," Centers for Disease Control and Prevention (CDC), August 31, 2017.

signals reaching the brain. Opioid pain medications are sometimes prescribed by doctors to treat pain. Common types include:

- Hydrocodone (e.g., Vicodin)

- Oxycodone (e.g., OxyContin)

- Oxymorphone (e.g., Opana), and

- Morphine

Many Americans suffer from chronic pain, a major public health concern in the United States. Patients with chronic pain deserve safe and effective pain management. At the same time, our country is in the midst of a prescription opioid overdose epidemic.

- The amount of opioids prescribed and sold in the United States quadrupled since 1999, but the overall amount of pain reported hasn't changed.

- There is insufficient evidence that prescription opioids control chronic pain effectively over the long-term, and there is evidence that other treatments can be effective with less harm.

Guidelines for Prescribing Opioids for Chronic Pain

Centers for Disease Control and Prevention (CDC) developed the Guideline for Prescribing Opioids for Chronic Pain to:

- Help reduce misuse, abuse, and overdose from opioids

- Improve communication between primary care doctors and patients about the risks and benefits of opioid therapy for chronic pain

The Centers for Disease Control and Prevention's (CDC) *Guideline for Prescribing Opioids for Chronic Pain* provides recommendations to primary care doctors about the appropriate prescribing of opioid pain medications to improve pain management and patient safety:

- It helps primary care doctors determine when to start or continue opioids for chronic pain.

- It gives guidance about medication dose and duration, and on following up with patients and discontinuing medication if needed.

- It helps doctors assess the risks and benefits of using opioids.

Doctors and patients should talk about:

- How opioids can reduce pain during short-term use, yet there is not enough evidence that opioids control chronic pain effectively long term.

- Nonopioid treatments (such as exercise, nonopioid medications, and cognitive behavioral therapy) that can be effective with less harm

- Importance of regular follow-up

- Precautions that can be taken to decrease risks including checking drug monitoring databases, conducting urine drug testing, and prescribing naloxone if needed to prevent fatal overdose.

- Protecting your family and friends by storing opioids in a secure, locked location and safely disposing unused opioids

Nonopioid Treatments for Pain

Patients with pain should receive treatment that provides the greatest benefit. Opioids are not the first-line therapy for chronic pain outside of active cancer treatment, palliative care, and end-of-life care. Evidence suggests that nonopioid treatments, including nonopioid medications and nonpharmacological therapies can provide relief to those suffering from chronic pain, and are safer. Effective approaches to chronic pain should:

- Use nonopioid therapies to the extent possible

- Identify and address coexisting mental health conditions (e.g., depression, anxiety, posttraumatic stress disorder (PTSD))

- Focus on functional goals and improvement, engaging patients actively in their pain management

- Use disease-specific treatments when available (e.g., triptans for migraines, gabapentin/pregabalin/duloxetine for neuropathic pain)

- Use first-line medication options preferentially. Consider interventional therapies (e.g., corticosteroid injections) in patients who fail standard noninvasive therapies.

- Use multimodal approaches, including interdisciplinary rehabilitation for patients who have failed standard treatments, have severe functional deficits, or psychosocial risk factors

Table 36.1. Nonopioid Medications

Medication	Magnitude of Benefits	Harms	Comments
Acetaminophen	Small	Hepatotoxic, particularly at higher doses	First-line analgesic, probably less effective than NSAIDs
NSAIDs	Small-moderate	Cardiac, GI, renal	First-line analgesic, COX-2 selective NSAIDs less GI toxicity
Gabapentin/ pregabalin	Small-moderate	Sedation, dizziness, ataxia	First-line agent for neuropathic pain; pregabalin approved for fibromyalgia
Tricyclic antidepressants and serotonin/ norepinephrine reuptake inhibitors	Small-moderate	TCAs have anticholinergic and cardiac toxicities; SNRIs safer and better tolerated	First-line for neuropathic pain; TCAs and SNRIs for fibromyalgia, TCAs for Headaches
Topical agents (lidocaine, capsaicin, NSAIDs)	Small-moderate	Capsaicin initial flare/ burning, irritation of mucus membranes	Consider as alternative first-line, thought to be safer than systemic medications. Lidocaine for neuropathic pain, topical NSAIDs for localized osteoarthritis, topical capsaicin for musculoskeletal and neuropathic pain

Recommended Treatments for Common Chronic Pain Conditions

Low back pain

Self-care and education in all patients; advise patients to remain active and limit bedrest

Nonpharmacological treatments: Exercise, cognitive behavioral therapy, interdisciplinary rehabilitation

Medications

- First-line: acetaminophen, nonsteroidal anti-inflammatory drugs (NSAIDs)

- Second-line: Serotonin and norepinephrine reuptake inhibitors (SNRIs)/tricyclic antidepressants (TCAs)

Osteoarthritis

Nonpharmacological treatments: Exercise, weight loss, patient education

Medications

- First-line: Acetaminophen, oral NSAIDs, topical NSAIDs

- Second-line: Intra-articular hyaluronic acid, capsaicin (limited number of intra-articular glucocorticoid injections if acetaminophen and NSAIDs insufficient)

Fibromyalgia

Patient education: Address diagnosis, treatment, and the patient's role in the treatment

Nonpharmacological treatments: Low-impact aerobic exercise (e.g., brisk walking, swimming, water aerobics, or bicycling), cognitive behavioral therapy, biofeedback, interdisciplinary rehabilitation

Medications

- FDA-approved: Pregabalin, duloxetine, milnacipran

- Other options: TCAs, gabapentin

Chapter 37

Arthritis and Sleep Deprivation

It is known that osteoarthritis (OA) increases the risk of sleep disturbance and that both pain and sleep problems may trigger functional disability and depression. This chapter examines cross-sectional and longitudinal associations of self-reported sleep disturbance with OA-related pain and disability and depressive symptoms.

Osteoarthritis (OA) in the United States

In the United States, arthritis ranks among the top three health conditions causing disability. Osteoarthritis (OA), the most common form of arthritis, is pervasive and costly, affecting at least 26.9 million Americans and fuelling a $185.5 billion increase in healthcare expenditures between 1996–2005. Of joints commonly affected by OA, the knee ranks high, with symptomatic prevalence rates reaching 16.7 percent.

Sleep Disturbance as Comorbidity

The multifaceted, hyperalgesic nature of OA creates potentially debilitating physical and psychological burdens, making individuals

This chapter includes text excerpted from "Sleep Disturbance in Osteoarthritis: Linkages with Pain, Disability, and Depressive Symptoms," U.S. Department of Health and Human Services (HHS), March 1, 2016.

particularly susceptible to comorbid disorders that may exacerbate OA-associated symptoms. Sleep disturbance is one such comorbidity. Among persons with knee OA, up to 31 percent report significant disturbances initiating sleep, 81 percent have difficulties maintaining nighttime sleep, and up to 77 percent report any sleep problem. Sleep disruption and pain frequently co-occur; both have uniquely been linked with depressed mood and various forms of functional disability.

The relationship between sleep and pain is robust and likely bidirectional. According to Spielman's model of chronic insomnia, pain may serve as a precipitating factor that interacts with certain predisposing factors (e.g., a tendency toward physiological hyperarousal) to fuel onset and maintenance of insomnia. Sleep problems (e.g., sleep fragmentation, difficulty initiating sleep) may disrupt various physiological processes that influence pain perception. According to Smith and colleagues, disrupted sleep may contribute directly to increased central pain processing, exacerbating daily pain—which may then perpetuate sleep disturbances.

What the Research Says

An evidence-based review of the general literature on chronic pain and sleep concluded that pain may be etiologically related to disordered sleep. Analyses from a cross-sectional, nationally representative survey of adults supported this conclusion, indicating that self-reported insomnia symptoms and dissatisfaction with sleep were correlated with pain severity in individuals with and without arthritis. Further, pain partially mediated the relationship of an arthritis diagnosis with sleep outcomes, even when accounting for sociodemographic and lifestyle factors, other chronic conditions, and mental health. Sleep quantity predicted the presence of painful conditions in a cross-sectional, national survey in Spain: persons who reported fewer than 6 hours sleep per day were at increased risk for experiencing a painful condition. Wilcox and colleagues similarly demonstrated that OA-related knee pain was related to sleep disturbance.

Sleep problems may also be associated with functional decline in OA. Conceptually, sleep difficulties may function as a predisposing risk factor for developing impairments or, alternatively, as an intra-individual intervening factor that increases the extent and pace of functional decline. This relationship may be based in part on linkages among sleep, pain, and depression, and particularly on the mediating role of depression and pain in the sleep–disability association. Empirically, poor sleep and diagnosed OA are separately associated with functional impairment in otherwise healthy adults.

The sleep–pain relationship was wholly explained by depressive symptoms; in contrast, depression was significant, independently associated with both pain and sleep problems. Furthermore, sleep disturbance exacerbated effects of pain on depression, such that depressive symptoms were greatest among those with both significant sleep problems and higher-than-average pain. In one-year longitudinal analyses, sleep problems predicted increases in depression and disability, but not pain.

Existing evidence implies that the associations of sleep with both pain and depression are bidirectional; though fewer hard data are available, it is also likely that the three variables interact in complex ways over time. The findings confirm the previously documented associations of sleep with pain and depression. The chronic nature of OA pain, as well as its close linkage with disability, is likely to shape its association with both sleep and emotional well-being beyond dynamics seen in the general population.

A study conducted with older adults with comorbid OA and insomnia showed that short-term improvements in sleep predicted long-term (18 months) improvements in chronic pain and fatigue. The findings also enhance understanding of the linkage between sleep disturbance and depression among persons with OA. Of particular interest here is the obtained interaction of sleep and pain on depressive symptoms at baseline. At low levels of pain, sleep disturbance is unrelated to mood; but where the pain is more severe, sleep problems exacerbate depression. This has important implications for treatment, suggesting that the documented efficacy of analgesic treatment of OA-related pain in reducing sleep disturbance may help relieve pain-related emotional distress as well. At the same time, the analyses suggest that the effects of sleep disturbance on depression may be independent of pain and disability, inasmuch as only sleep was independently associated with increased depression over time. Similarly, changes in pain and disability did not track with the change in depression. This suggests that sleep may be an important mediator of known relationships among pain, disability, and depression.

In sum, this analysis sheds new light on the interrelationships among sleep, pain, disability, and depressive symptoms among older adults with OA. There is the unique role of sleep problems as immediate drivers of pain and depression, and as long-range influences on functional disability and depressed mood. In particular, it appears that poor sleep may interact with severe OA pain to place persons at increased risk of depression and, long range, of functional limitations. Depression represents an important possible mediator of the pain—sleep linkage, highlighting the importance of assessing and treating emotional distress in this very common chronic disorder.

Chapter 38

Weight Management and Arthritis

Obesity is a global health issue, with 315 million adults classified as obese, defined as a body mass index (BMI) of $\geq$ 30 kg/m^2. Both children and the elderly are susceptible to obesity. Significant progress in the medical management of the metabolic symptoms related to obesity has increased the lifespan of the obese individual. There is a trade-off with longevity in the aging obese person, as the musculoskeletal system must bear the burden of carrying excessive weight over the person's lifespan. As BMI values increase, joint pain symptoms and severity increase. Joint pain may reflect the underlying pathological process of osteoarthritis (OA). For every 5-kg (11-pound) weight gain, there is a commensurate 36 percent increase in the risk for developing OA. In obese individuals, pain is most prevalent in the load-bearing joints, including the lower limbs and the low back, but can manifest in upper extremity joints, hand, and digits, thoracic spine, and neck. In addition, cadaveric studies have revealed that obesity is related to greater knee OA severity than in normal weight individuals. Also, obesity is associated with faster OA progression than normal weight. Pain-related physical incapacitation worsens obesity, subsequent gait abnormalities, and muscle weakness. Importantly, pain may mediate

This chapter includes text excerpted from "Weight Loss and Obesity in the Treatment and Prevention of Osteoarthritis," U.S. Department of Health and Human Services (HHS), May 1, 2013. Reviewed April 2018.

obesity-induced impairment of physical functioning and deterioration of the health-related quality of life. Weight loss sets in motion a cascade of events that can prevent OA onset or combat existing OA symptoms and disability. These events include reduction of mechanical and biological stressors. This chapter reviews the evidence of the relationship between obesity and OA, and the effect of weight loss on the prevention and treatment of OA.

Obesity-Specific Mechanisms of OA Pathophysiology

While there are numerous pathways that contribute to OA onset, obesity-specific mechanisms include relative loss of muscle mass and strength over time, mechanical stress and systemic inflammation. Excessive adipose tissue compresses load-bearing joints and creates an inflammatory environment within tissues and joints. Obesity induces abnormal joint loads and leads to adverse changes in the composition, structure, and properties of articular cartilage. With increased body weight, both muscle mass, and fat mass increase; yet the volume of muscle mass remains relatively low and inadequate to match the loads placed upon it.

When strength is normalized for body mass, obese persons have lower muscle strength than normal-weight counterparts, including the quadriceps and lumbar muscle groups. Obese people attempt to compensate for muscle weakness and instability by altering gait patterns and adopting different body transfer patterns to move excessive weight. Less absorption of the impact forces on weight-bearing joints occurs because of their inadequate lower limb strength. Repetitive forces damage articular cartilage. Joint misalignment in the load bearing joints may occur with increased body segment girths, altered posture, skeletal muscle strength imbalance or weakness of muscles that control joint motion.

In obesity, the skeletal muscle becomes laden with intramuscular fat, and this fat is associated with elevated systemic levels of proinflammatory biomarkers. As obesity worsens, these biomarkers induce a feed-forward process of muscle catabolism and loss of strength. Over time, the cumulative effects of excessive body fat, and mechanical loading and aberrant joint motion, contribute to the OA pathophysiology, and the onset of inflammation and pain.

The combined influence of pain and worsening inflammation in untreated obesity likely contribute to an elevated risk for functional impairment in the obese, older adult. Adiponectin is a hormone secreted by adipocytes. Although produced in relatively low concentrations compared to that found in plasma, this hormone could be found in the synovial fluid of osteoarthritic joints likely derived from the infrapatellar fat pad and synovium. Conflicting evidence indicates that adiponectin can be proinflammatory (triggering IL-6 and nitric oxide production) or anti-inflammatory (upregulating inhibitors of metalloproteinases). But what is clear is that there is a link between dysregulation of adiponectin and OA. Therefore, the collective and interrelated effects of relatively low muscle mass and accumulation of adipose tissue in obesity, contribute to joint degeneration and OA onset via joint compressive forces and aberrant biomechanics, hyper-leptinemia, and inflammation.

Functional Disability, Obesity, and OA

Obesity and OA collectively increase the incidence of mobility disability. Activities such as walking, chair rise, and stair climb, and timed up-and-go tasks are performed at slower speeds and are more challenging for the obese individual. Cross-sectional data support that as BMI increases by one standard deviation, the times to complete timed-up-and-go and chair rise tests increase by 5.0 percent and 6.4 percent, respectively. There is a progressive worsening of function and mobility with an increase in BMI. Gait parameters such as stride length and the average daily number of steps taken decreases by 55 percent when BMI exceeds 30 kg/m². Of note, lower limb physical function and disability are not affected by adiposity distribution (assessed by 20-meter walk, knee flexion/extension strength and chair rise time), as demonstrated by a cross-sectional study of a group of older adults with either central or gynoid obesity.

Prospective studies consistently show obesity-related deterioration of walking ability, chair rise, and stair climb ability. Mechanisms for disability include muscle weakness, increased stiffness, and pain. The severity of cartilage defects in obese people with knee OA is moderately associated with stiffness, pain, and subjective and objective assessments of disability.

Kinesiophobia due to Pain

The definition of OA includes the presence of pain symptoms. As such, pain may be a significant factor contributing to mobility impairment in obese individuals. The combined effects of obesity and degenerative joints may induce fear of movement (kinesiophobia) because of weight-bearing activities such as walking, climbing stairs, body transfers, and activities of daily living cause pain. As OA pain worsens over the long term, obese persons disengage from regular weight-bearing activities and weight gain is exacerbated. It has been found that obese persons with low back pain and knee pain rate kinesiophobia higher than nonobese individuals. While higher kinesiophobia scores corresponded to higher perceived disability for tasks such as body transfers (chair rise), climbing stairs, jumping, and running, these higher scores were surprisingly not associated with worse performance during functional tests such as flexibility, range of motion, and muscle strength. These findings suggest that functional impairment in OA may be partly regulated by fear and perceived inability to perform certain tasks. Catastrophizing about pain is associated with severity of pain in obese patients with knee OA. Both catastrophic thought patterns and somatization may foster hypervigilance to OA pain, and lead to avoidance of physical activity. This psychosocial component is commonly overlooked when developing plans of care for the obese patient with OA pain.

Weight loss reduces joint pain and increases physical function. Randomized controlled trials show that knee OA pain reduction is associated with increased mobility and physical function. As weight loss occurs, the compressive forces through the loading bearing joints such as the knee are dramatically reduced by almost fourfold. A reduction of body weight can attenuate the painful symptoms and likely reduces the fear of movement. In obese adults, achieving ~5 percent loss of body weight will relieve some joint pain, but a loss of at least 10 percent of body weight is associated with moderate to large clinical improvements in joint pain. The management of OA pain with weight loss extends past pain reduction, and has powerfully positive ramifications for increased physical capability and independence, increased participation in home and community activities, and overall quality of life.

Weight Loss and Treatment of OA in the Obese Adult

Several options for weight loss exist, ranging from medications, to exercise and dietary modification, and bariatric surgery. The "right choice" of treatment for the obese patient should be tailored to meet individual needs. Depending on the severity of obesity and OA, creative staging of interventions for progressive weight loss in OA may be implemented to minimize pain symptoms and kinesophobia.

Weight-Loss Medications

Medications may be used alone or in concert with other interventions to induce weight loss. Two medications approved by U.S.

Food and Drug Administration (FDA) to treat obesity are Orlistat and Sibutramine. Orlistat is a gastric and pancreatic lipase inhibitor which decreases fat absorption in intestines by roughly 30 percent. Meta-analysis revealed that 120 mg of Orlistat (three times daily) elicits ≥ 5 percent weight loss in 33 percent of patients. Numerous studies have supported the efficacy of Sibutramine when administered for 6–24 months. Around 34 percent of patients achieved a minimum of 5 percent loss of body weight, and 15 percent of patients lost 10 percent or more of body weight over the course of one year. An important finding is that medications may be more effective when coupled with exercise and diet. For example, when Sibutramine is used in conjunction with a lifestyle modification intervention (i.e., exercise and diet), weight loss is greater than that achieved with medication or the intervention alone.

Exercise and Diet

Published randomized controlled trials (RCT) have examined weight loss and functional effects after aerobic exercise and resistance exercise programs, multimodal exercise programs, and multimodal training with or without caloric restriction. Several RCTs were identified that included resistance exercise (RX) and/or aerobic exercise (AX). RX features the use of resistance exercise machines, strengthening exercise using body weight, and home-based strengthening exercise. AX typically involves sustained large muscle activity such as walking, climbing stairs, stationary cycling, or aquatic aerobic exercise. Multimodal training consists of a variety of aerobic, resistive, and flexibility components during a single session. Multimodal activity programs have been implemented for durations lasting three months to one year. Often, the multimodal activity programs are coupled with dietary changes as part of a comprehensive lifestyle overhaul.

Among these RCTs, several have focused on the obese knee OA population. Training periods ranged from 2–6 months with a frequency of 2–3 times a week, and follow-ups up to 18 months. Favorable functional AX changes included an intensity of 50–85 percent heart rate reserve for the land-based exercise or maximal heart rate in aquatic exercise. The intensity of performing RX exercises varied among studies, ranging from body weight or cuff weight resistance to the use of dumbbells. Even simple home-based exercise studies indicate efficacy in reducing OA pain in this population. Studies have featured quadricep contractions and functional tasks (e.g., rising from a chair) for up to 24 months. Compared with education control and diet groups, the exercise group achieved a 30 percent reduction in Western Ontario and McMaster Universities Osteoarthritis Index (WOMAC) pain scores and improvement in WOMAC functional scores.

Benefits of exercise for OA symptoms can include reduction of body weight. When exercise is coupled with diet, greater weight loss can occur. Compressive forces on the joint are significantly reduced in proportion with the degree of weight loss. Comparative studies show that multimodal exercise induces a 3.7 percent loss of body weight, while the diet-only and diet-plus multimodal exercise result in 4.9 percent and 5.7 percent losses of body weight by six months. Knee OA pain can be reduced with exercise or combined intervention, but the largest pain reduction (30.3%) was related to the greatest weight loss. Pain improvement during the exercise intervention is the strongest contributing factor in explaining the association between exercise adherence and decreases in self-reported disability.

The value of exercise for OA in the obese patient is that it can be used to treat the disease and help prevent or delay the onset of the disease. Ideally, the incorporation of AX to stimulate caloric expenditure and RX to strengthen the musculature supporting the joints provides a well-rounded program to treat OA symptoms. Exercise can be applied to this population at any disease stage to help provide pain relief, strengthen muscles that surround the arthritic joint, and help control or reduce body weight (the latter being the main modifiable factor underlying OA). To help overcome kinesiophobia, exercise may need to be supervised initially and periodically thereafter to help ensure that activity is performed at the appropriate training stimulus and not compromised because of fear. Importantly, exercise interventions can be cost effective to treat knee OA in obese adults. Pain severity and functional outcomes such as walking performance and stair climb demonstrate the greatest improvements after exercise alone than after diet programs or exercise plus diet interventions.

Bariatric Surgery

For many obese patients, meaningful weight loss is difficult as lifestyle changes are difficult and long-term adherence is typically low. Bariatric surgery can elicit massive weight loss when postsurgical instructions are followed. Common surgical techniques include laparoscopic adjustable gastric banding, sleeve gastrectomy, and vertical banded gastroplasty. Joint pain can be attenuated or abolished in morbidly obese persons with pain in the hip, knee, ankle, spine, neck, shoulder, elbow, wrist and hand, and knee, ankle, and foot. Although there are methodological inconsistencies in the measurement follow-up times for joint pain between and within studies, the most common postoperative time point was approximately two years. Reductions in BMI values ranged from 6.2–14.7 kg/m² and this corresponded with a resolution of knee and back pain in 5–100 percent of patients, while pain severity was reduced in 31–94 percent, depending on the joint and study.

Knee

Several studies have demonstrated that among patients with knee OA pain, bariatric procedures can predictably provide relief. Dramatic reductions in pain can occur as quickly as three months postsurgery. Studies reported 9–76 percent less prevalence in knee pain by the final study time point as reflected by self-report surveys of joint pain and severity. Average and median WOMAC pain scores for knee pain were reduced by 51 percent and 66 percent, respectively, at follow-up. Another study showed that Knee Society pain subscores are reduced by 14.8 percent while the function subscores improved by almost the same percent after surgery. A mechanism of pain relief underlying these collective findings may be knee joint space widening with weight loss. For example, Abu-Abeid et al. found that when BMI was reduced by an average of 6.3 kg/m² after bariatric surgery, joint space widened from 4.6–5.25 mm. These intriguing findings show that independent of physical activity level or muscle strength, knee pain–related disability could be improved with weight loss alone. Relief from pain may facilitate re-engagement of the individual into regular exercise or activities that were previously unattainable.

Low Back

The lumbar spine is the most researched "joint area" in bariatric populations. In one study, back pain was followed in morbidly obese patients undergoing vertical banded gastroplasty and nonobese counterparts for two years. BMI was reduced by 14.3 kg/m², and improvements occurred in all pain and disability assessments (Visual analog scale for pain, Oswestry Disability Index (ODI), Roland-Morris Disability Questionnaire and the Waddell Disability Index). Uncontrolled studies have revealed that the frequency of back pain was reduced in 83 percent of patients, and lumbar back pain symptoms were reduced in 82–90 percent patients after 6–22 months. In obese persons with chronic debilitating axial back pain, the severity of back pain symptoms was reduced by 44 percent after bariatric surgery. Pain relief was also associated with lower ODI scores.

Other Joint Pain

Weight loss after bariatric surgery may not impact hip OA pain as much as that experienced by other load-bearing joints. While some data indicate that hip pain can improve, most studies do not support favorable changes in hip pain after surgery. Lateral and medial hip pain symptoms were not significantly reduced by one year, and the presence of hip OA pain was not different in bariatric patients at two or six years after surgery. Even if obesity increases the vertical loading stressors and compressive forces with weight-bearing activity, the positioning of the femoral head in the acetabulum may not be affected by increased weight as much as other load-bearing joints. Limited data indicate that the frequency of foot pain is reduced by 42–95 percent after a bariatric surgery procedure. While hand OA pain symptoms moderately decreased after bariatric surgery, shoulder pain did not decrease with palpation or range of motion. The lack of OA pain relief in the shoulder may be due to the low baseline prevalence of shoulder OA or high error within the small sample sizes to detect a surgery related change.

Potential Mechanisms Underlying Relief from OA Symptoms

Weight loss with medications, exercise (with or without diet) and bariatric surgery can favorably alter the mechanical and biochemical profiles of obese adults with OA. Mechanical stress can be reduced as shown by a lowering of maximal knee compressive forces relative to magnitude of weight loss. Surgical weight loss can also substantially lower joint compressive forces, which may increase the joint space width. Reductions in the central deposition of fat on the abdomen and in the girths of lower limb segments may facilitate normalization of joint alignment. The collective benefits of lower joint loading and joint realignment would attenuate cartilage stress and silence one trigger of local joint inflammation. Weight loss reduces the synthesis of IL-6 and TNF-α and increases the production of anti-inflammatory cytokines (IL-10) by subcutaneous adipose. A loss of body fat attenuates systemic levels of inflammatory cytokines such as IL-6 by 25–30 percent. Leptin and CRP levels also decrease with weight loss. Irrespective of the method of weight loss, suppression of the proinflammatory cytokines can occur. These biochemical changes would complement the mechanical benefits of weight loss to reduce OA symptoms.

Prevention

Identification of effective treatments to prevent OA in obese younger populations is lacking. This is partly due to the challenges of long-term prospective research, and the lack of control in documenting processes that may influence OA onset. However, the participation in the regular physical activity and weight management may be critical in avoiding early onset of OA or increased risk of the disease. Some advocates suggest a screening process that begins in adolescence, in which family history is reviewed. If there is a positive family history, the individual can be counseled by the healthcare team on prevention techniques including strengthening exercise (e.g., leg raises, weight-bearing exercise, strengthening exercise [quadriceps, hamstrings]), endurance exercise, and judicious use of resistance exercise. Guidelines to achieve or maintain a healthy weight can include dietary recommendations, healthful living, and management of musculoskeletal pain. Successful disease prevention programs include the family, and therefore, OA risk may be decreased if the entire family adopts healthy behaviors and loses excessive weight. From the physiological perspective, the OA-related states of chronic inflammation and elevated mechanical stress on the joints may be curtailed or avoided if preventative measures are put into place during adolescence. Inflammation is improved with interventions that induce a 5 percent weight loss, regardless of the type or duration of the intervention. The adage "an ounce of prevention is worth a pound of cure" may be directly applicable to the obese person at risk for OA: for every reduction in weight, there is a decrease in the risk of OA onset.

Conclusion

Obesity induces several pathways that predispose an individual to symptomatic OA. Growing evidence indicates that irrespective of weight loss method, reduction of body fat can reduce the mechanical and biochemical stressors that contribute to joint degeneration. A variety of methods can be used treat OA including medications, exercise (with or without diet), and bariatric surgery. Prevention of OA may be achieved in part through screening of children at risk for OA, and education of the whole family to increase the chance of long-term success of disease prevention.

Chapter 39

Exercise and Arthritis

Chapter Contents

Section 39.1—Physical Activity for Arthritis 396

Section 39.2—Yoga Promotes Physical Fitness and
Joint Health 399

Section 39.3—Tai Chi and Qi Gong for Knee
Osteoarthritis 403

Section 39.4—Water Aerobics Can Benefit People
with Arthritis 406

Section 39.1

Physical Activity for Arthritis

This section includes text excerpted from "Arthritis—
Physical Activity for Arthritis," Centers for Disease
Control and Prevention (CDC), February 7, 2018.

Why Is Physical Activity Important for People with Arthritis?

If you have arthritis, participating in joint-friendly physical activity can improve your arthritis pain, function, mood, and quality of life. Joint-friendly physical activities are low impact, which means they put less stress on the body, reducing the risk of injury. Examples of joint-friendly activities include walking, biking, and swimming. Being physically active can also delay the onset of arthritis-related disability and help people with arthritis manage other chronic conditions such as diabetes, heart disease, and obesity. Learn how you can increase your physical activity safely.

How Much Activity Do I Need?

Stay as active as your health allows, and change your activity level depending on your arthritis symptoms. Any physical activity is better than none.

For substantial health benefits, adults with arthritis should follow the 2008 Physical Activity Guidelines for Americans recommendations for Active Adult or Active Older Adult, whichever meets your personal health goals and matches your age and abilities.

How Do I Exercise Safely with Arthritis?

Learn how you can safely exercise and enjoy the benefits of increased physical activity with the S.M.A.R.T. tips below.

Start Low, and Go Slow

When starting or increasing physical activity, start slow and pay attention to how your body tolerates it. People with arthritis may take more time for their body to adjust to a new level of activity. If you are not active, start with a small amount of activity, for example, 3–5 minutes 2 times a day. Add activity a little at a time (at least 10 minutes at a time) and allow enough time for your body to adjust to the new level before adding more activity.

Modify Activity When Arthritis Symptoms Increase, Try to Stay Active

Your arthritis symptoms, such as pain, stiffness, and fatigue, may come and go and you may have good days and bad days. Try to modify your activity to stay as active as possible without making your symptoms worse.

Activities Should Be "Joint Friendly"

Choose activities that are easy on the joints like walking, bicycling, water aerobics, or dancing. These activities have a low risk of injury and do not twist or "pound" the joints too much.

Recognize Safe Places and Ways to Be Active

Safety is important for starting and maintaining an activity plan. If you are currently inactive or you are not sure how to start your own physical activity program, an exercise class may be a good option. If you plan and direct your own activity, find safe places to be active. For example, walk in an area where the sidewalks or pathways are level and free of obstructions, are well lighted, and are separated from heavy traffic.

Talk to a Health Professional or Certified Exercise Specialist

Your doctor is a good source of information about physical activity. Healthcare professionals and certified exercise professionals can answer your questions about how much and what types of activity match your abilities and health goals.

What Types of Activities Should I Do?

Low impact aerobic activities do not put stress on the joints and include brisk walking, cycling, swimming, water aerobics, light gardening, group exercise classes, and dancing.

For major health benefits, do at least:

- 150 minutes (2 hours and 30 minutes) of moderate-intensity aerobic activity, like cycling at less than 10 miles per hour, or

- 75 minutes (1 hour and 15 minutes) of vigorous-intensity aerobic activity, like cycling at 10 mph or faster, each week. Another option is to do a combination of both. A rule of thumb is that 1 minute of vigorous-intensity activity is about the same as 2 minutes of moderate-intensity activity. Aerobic activity can be broken into short periods of 10 minutes or more during the day.

In addition to aerobic activity, you should also do muscle-strengthening activities that involve all major muscle groups two or more days a week.

Muscle-strengthening exercises include lifting weights, working with resistance bands, and yoga. These can be done at home, in an exercise class, or at a fitness center.

Flexibility exercises like stretching and yoga are also important for people with arthritis. Many people with arthritis have joint stiffness that makes daily tasks difficult. Doing daily flexibility exercises helps maintain range of motion so you can keep doing everyday things like household tasks, hobbies, and visiting with friends and family.

Balance exercises like walking backwards, standing on one foot, and tai chi are important for those who are at a risk of falling or have trouble walking. Do balance exercises 3 days per week if you are at risk of falling. Balance exercises are included in many group exercise classes.

How Hard Are You Working?

Measure the relative intensity of your activity with the talk test. In general, if you're doing moderate activity you can talk, but not sing, during the activity. If you are doing vigorous activity, you will not be able to say more than a few words without pausing for a breath.

What Do I Do If I Have Pain during or after Exercise?

It's normal to have some pain, stiffness, and swelling after starting a new physical activity program. It may take 6–8 weeks for your joints to get used to your new activity level, but sticking with your activity program will result in long-term pain relief.

Here are some tips to help you manage pain during and after physical activity so you can keep exercising:

- Until your pain improves, modify your physical activity program by exercising less frequently (fewer days per week) or for shorter periods of time (less time each session).

- Try a different type of exercise that puts less pressure on the joints—for example, switch from walking to water aerobics.

- Do proper warm-up and cool-down before and after exercise.

- Exercise at a comfortable pace—you should be able to carry on a conversation while exercising.

- Make sure you have good fitting, comfortable shoes.

See Your Doctor If You Experience Any of the Following

- Pain that is sharp, stabbing, and constant.

- Pain that causes you to limp.

- Pain that lasts more than 2 hours after exercise or gets worse at night.

- Pain or swelling that does not get better with rest, medication, or hot or cold packs.

- Large increases in swelling or your joints feel "hot" or are red.

Section 39.2

Yoga Promotes Physical Fitness and Joint Health

This section includes text excerpted from "Yoga: In Depth," National Center for Complementary and Integrative Health (NCCIH), June 2013. Reviewed April 2018.

Yoga is a mind and body practice with historical origins in ancient Indian philosophy. Like other meditative movement practices used for health purposes, various styles of yoga typically combine physical postures, breathing techniques, and meditation or relaxation. Yoga in its full form combines physical postures, breathing exercises, meditation, and a distinct philosophy. There are numerous styles of yoga. Hatha yoga, commonly practiced in the United States and Europe, emphasizes postures, breathing exercises, and meditation. Hatha yoga styles include Ananda, Anusara, Ashtanga, Bikram, Iyengar, Kripalu, Kundalini, Viniyoga, and others.

- Recent studies in people with chronic low back pain suggest that a carefully adapted set of yoga poses may help reduce pain and improve function (the ability to walk and move). Studies also suggest that practicing yoga (as well as other forms of regular exercise) might have other health benefits such as reducing heart rate and blood pressure and may also help relieve anxiety and depression. Other research suggests yoga is not helpful for asthma, and studies looking at yoga and arthritis have had mixed results.

- People with high blood pressure, glaucoma, or sciatica, and women who are pregnant should modify or avoid some yoga poses.

- Ask a trusted source (such as a healthcare provider or local hospital) to recommend a yoga practitioner. Contact professional organizations for the names of practitioners who have completed an acceptable training program.

- Tell all your healthcare providers about any complementary health approaches you use. Give them a full picture of what you do to manage your health. This will help ensure coordinated and safe care.

Side Effects and Risks

- Yoga is generally low impact and safe for healthy people when practiced appropriately under the guidance of a well-trained instructor.

- Overall, those who practice yoga have a low rate of side effects, and the risk of serious injury from yoga is quite low. However, certain types of stroke, as well as pain from nerve damage, are among the rare possible side effects of practicing yoga.

- Women who are pregnant and people with certain medical conditions, such as high blood pressure, glaucoma (a condition in which fluid pressure within the eye slowly increases and may damage the eye's optic nerve), and sciatica (pain, weakness, numbing, or tingling that may extend from the lower back to the calf, foot, or even the toes), should modify or avoid some yoga poses.

Use of Yoga for Health in the United States

According to a National Health Interview Survey (NHIS), which included a comprehensive survey on the use of complementary health approaches by Americans, yoga is the sixth most commonly used complementary health practice among adults. More than 13 million adults practiced yoga in the previous year, and between the 2002 and 2007 NHIS, use of yoga among adults increased by 1 percent (or approximately 3 million people). The survey also found that more than 1.5 million children practiced yoga in the previous year.

Many people who practice yoga do so to maintain their health and well being, improve physical fitness, relieve stress, and enhance the quality of life. In addition, they may be addressing specific health conditions, such as back pain, neck pain, arthritis, and anxiety.

What the Science Says about Yoga

Current research suggests that a carefully adapted set of yoga poses may reduce low back pain and improve function. Other studies also suggest that practicing yoga (as well as other forms of regular exercise) might improve quality of life; reduce stress; lower heart rate and blood pressure; help relieve anxiety, depression, and insomnia; and improve overall physical fitness, strength, and flexibility. But some research suggests yoga may not improve asthma, and studies looking at yoga and arthritis have had mixed results.

- One National Center for Complementary and Integrative Health (NCCIH)-funded study of 90 people with chronic low back pain found that participants who practiced Iyengar yoga had significantly less disability, pain, and depression after 6 months.

- In a 2011 study, also funded by NCCIH, researchers compared yoga with conventional stretching exercises or a self-care book in 228 adults with chronic low-back pain. The results showed that both yoga and stretching were more effective than a self-care book for improving function and reducing symptoms due to chronic low-back pain.

- Conclusions from another 2011 study of 313 adults with chronic or recurring low-back pain suggested that 12 weekly yoga classes resulted in better function than usual medical care.

However, studies show that certain health conditions may not benefit from yoga.

A 2011 systematic review of clinical studies suggests that there is no sound evidence that yoga improves asthma.

A 2011 review of the literature reports that few published studies have looked at yoga and arthritis, and of those that have, results are inconclusive. The two main types of arthritis—osteoarthritis and rheumatoid arthritis—are different conditions, and the effects of yoga may not be the same for each. In addition, the reviewers suggested that even if a study showed that yoga helped osteoarthritic finger joints, it may not help osteoarthritic knee joints.

If You Are Considering Practicing Yoga

- Do not use yoga to replace conventional medical care or to postpone seeing a healthcare provider about pain or any other medical condition.

- If you have a medical condition, talk to your healthcare provider before starting yoga.

- Ask a trusted source (such as your healthcare provider or a nearby hospital) to recommend a yoga practitioner. Find out about the training and experience of any practitioner you are considering.

- Everyone's body is different, and yoga postures should be modified based on individual abilities. Carefully selecting an instructor who is experienced with and attentive to your needs is an important step toward helping you practice yoga safely. Ask about the physical demands of the type of yoga in which you are interested and inform your yoga instructor about any medical issues you have.

- Carefully think about the type of yoga you are interested in. For example, hot yoga (such as Bikram yoga) may involve standing and moving in humid environments with temperatures as high as 105°F. Because such settings may be physically stressful, people who practice hot yoga should take certain precautions. These include drinking water before, during, and after a hot yoga practice and wearing suitable clothing. People with conditions that may be affected by excessive heat, such as heart disease, lung disease, and a prior history of heatstroke may want to avoid this form of yoga. Women who are pregnant may want to check with their healthcare providers before starting hot yoga.

- Tell all your healthcare providers about any complementary health approaches you use. Give them a full picture of what you do to manage your health. This will help ensure coordinated and safe care.

Section 39.3

Tai Chi and Qi Gong for Knee Osteoarthritis

This section includes text excerpted from "Tai Chi and Qi Gong: In Depth," National Center for Complementary and Integrative Health (NCCIH), October 2016.

What Are Tai Chi and Qi Gong?

Tai chi and qi gong are centuries-old, related mind and body practices that involve certain postures and gentle movements with mental focus, breathing, and relaxation. The movements can be adapted or practiced while walking, standing, or sitting. In contrast to qi gong, tai chi movements, if practiced quickly, can be a form of combat or self-defense.

What the Science Says about the Effectiveness of Tai Chi and Qi Gong

Research findings suggest that practicing tai chi may improve balance and stability in older people and those with Parkinson disease (PD), reduce pain from knee osteoarthritis (OA), help people cope with fibromyalgia (FM) and back pain, and promote quality of life and mood in people with heart failure and cancer. There's been less research on the effects of qi gong, but some studies suggest it may reduce chronic neck pain (although results are mixed) and pain from FM. Qi gong also may help to improve general quality of life.

There's some evidence that practicing tai chi may help people manage pain associated with knee OA (a breakdown of cartilage in the knee that allows leg bones to rub together), FM (a disorder that causes muscle pain and fatigue), and back pain. Qi gong may offer some benefit for chronic neck pain, but results are mixed.

Knee Osteoarthritis (OA)

Results of a small National Center for Complementary and Integrative Health (NCCIH)-funded clinical trial involving 40 participants with knee OA suggested that practicing tai chi reduced pain and improved function better than an education and stretching program.

An analysis of seven small and moderately-sized clinical studies concluded that a 12-week course of tai chi reduced pain and improved function in people with this condition.

Fibromyalgia (FM)

Results from a small 2010 NCCIH-supported clinical trial suggested that practicing tai chi was more effective than wellness education and stretching in helping people with FM sleep better and cope with pain, fatigue, and depression. After 12 weeks, those who practiced tai chi also had better scores on a survey designed to measure a person's ability to carry out certain daily activities such as walking, housecleaning, shopping, and preparing a meal. The benefits of tai chi also appeared to last longer.

A small 2012 NCCIH-supported trial suggested that combining tai chi movements with mindfulness allowed people with FM to work through the discomfort they may feel during exercise, allowing them to take advantage of the benefits of physical activity.

Results of a 2012 randomized clinical trial with 100 participants suggested that practicing qi gong reduced pain and improved sleep, the ability to do daily activities, and mental function. The researchers also observed that most improvements were still apparent after 6 months.

Chronic Neck Pain

Research results on the effectiveness of qi gong for chronic neck pain are mixed, but the people who were studied and the way the studies were done were quite different.

A 2009 clinical study by German researchers showed no benefit of qi gong or exercise compared with the absence of therapy in 117 elderly adults (mostly women) with, on average, a 20-year history of chronic neck pain. Study participants had 24 exercise or qi gong sessions over 3-month period.

In a 2011 study, some of the same researchers observed that qi gong was just as effective as exercise therapy (and both were more effective than no therapy) in relieving neck pain in the 123 middle-aged adults (mostly women) who had chronic neck pain for an average of 3 years. Exercise therapy included throwing and catching a ball, rowing and climbing movements, arm swinging, and stretching, among other activities. People in the study had 18 exercise or qi gong sessions over 6 months.

Back Pain

In people who had low-back pain for at least 3 months, a program of tai chi exercises reduced their pain and improved their functioning.

More to Consider

Tai chi and qi gong appear to be safe practices. One NCCIH-supported review noted that tai chi is unlikely to result in serious injury but it may be associated with minor aches and pains. Women who are pregnant should talk with their healthcare providers before beginning tai chi, qi gong, or any other exercise program.

Note

- Learning tai chi or qi gong from a video or book does not ensure that you're doing the movements correctly or safely.

- If you have a health condition, talk with your healthcare provider before starting tai chi or qi gong.

- Ask a trusted source (such as your healthcare provider) to recommend a tai chi or qi gong instructor. Find out about the training and experience of any instructor you're considering.

Tell all your healthcare providers about any complementary or integrative health approaches you use. Give them a full picture of what you do to manage your health. This will help ensure coordinated and safe care.

Section 39.4

Water Aerobics Can Benefit People with Arthritis

This section includes text excerpted from "Healthy
Swimming—Health Benefits of Water-Based Exercise,"
Centers for Disease Control and Prevention (CDC), May 4, 2016.

Swimming is the fourth most popular sports activity in the United
States and a good way to get regular aerobic physical activity

1. Just two and a half hours per week of aerobic physical activity,
   such as swimming, bicycling, or running, can decrease the risk
   of chronic illnesses. This can also lead to improved health for
   people with diabetes and heart disease

2. Swimmers have about half the risk of death compared with
   inactive people

3. People report enjoying water-based exercise more than exercising on land

4. They can also exercise longer in water than on land without
   increased effort or joint or muscle pain.

Water-Based Exercise and Chronic Illness

Water-based exercise can help people with chronic diseases. For
people with arthritis, it improves the use of affected joints without
worsening symptoms. People with rheumatoid arthritis (RA) have
more health improvements after participating in hydrotherapy than
with other activities. Water-based exercise also improves the use of
affected joints and decreases pain from osteoarthritis.

Water-Based Exercise and Mental Health

Water-based exercise improves mental health. Swimming can
improve mood in both men and women. For people with fibromyalgia, it can decrease anxiety and exercise therapy in warm water can

decrease depression and improve mood. Water-based exercise can improve the health of mothers and their unborn children and has a positive effect on the mothers' mental health. Parents of children with developmental disabilities find that recreational activities, such as swimming, improve family connections.

Water-Based Exercise and Older Adults

Water-based exercise can benefit older adults by improving the quality of life and decreasing disability. It also improves or maintains the bone health of postmenopausal women.

A Good Choice

Exercising in water offers many physical and mental health benefits and is a good choice for people who want to be more active. When in the water, remember to protect yourself and others from illness and injury by practicing healthy and safe swimming behaviors.

Chapter 40

Herbs, Dietary Supplements, and Arthritis

Chapter Contents

Section 40.1—Glucosamine and Chondroitin............................ 410

Section 40.2—Cat's Claw.. 413

Section 40.3—Evening Primrose Oil.................................... 415

Section 40.4—Flaxseed and Flaxseed Oil.............................. 417

Section 40.5—Ginger 419

Section 40.6—Thunder God Vine...................................... 421

Section 40.7—Turmeric 423

Section 40.8—Dietary Supplements for
           Osteoarthritis 425

Section 40.9—Omega-3 Fatty Acids.................................... 427

Section 40.1

Glucosamine and Chondroitin

This section includes text excerpted from "Glucosamine
and Chondroitin for Osteoarthritis," National Center for
Complementary and Integrative Health (NCCIH),
November 2014. Reviewed April 2018.

What Are Glucosamine and Chondroitin?

Glucosamine and chondroitin are structural components of cartilage, the tissue that cushions the joints. Both are produced naturally
in the body. They are also available as dietary supplements. Researchers have studied the effects of these supplements, individually or in
combination, on osteoarthritis (OA), a common type of arthritis that
destroys cartilage in the joints.

Cartilage is the connective tissue that cushions the ends of bones
within the joints. In OA, the surface layer of cartilage between the
bones of a joint wears down. This allows the bones to rub together,
which can cause pain and swelling and make it difficult to move the
joint. The knees, hips, spine, and hands are the parts of the body most
likely to be affected by OA.

What the Science Says about Glucosamine and Chondroitin for Osteoarthritis (OA)

For the Knee or Hip

Glucosamine

Major studies of glucosamine for OA of the knee have had conflicting results.

- A large National Institutes of Health (NIH) study, called the
  Glucosamine/chondroitin Arthritis Intervention Trial (GAIT),
  compared glucosamine hydrochloride, chondroitin, both supplements together, celecoxib (a prescription drug used to manage
  OA pain), or a placebo (an inactive substance) in patients with
  knee OA. Most participants in the study had mild knee pain.

- Those who received the prescription drug had better short-term pain relief (at 6 months) than those who received a placebo.

- Overall, those who received the supplements had no significant improvement in knee pain or function, although the investigators saw evidence of improvement in a small subgroup of patients with moderate to severe pain who took glucosamine and chondroitin together.

- In several European studies, participants reported that their knees felt and functioned better after taking glucosamine. The study participants took a large, once-a-day dose of a preparation of glucosamine sulfate sold as a prescription drug in Europe.

- Researchers don't know why the results of these large, well-done studies differ. It may be because of differences in the types of glucosamine used (glucosamine hydrochloride in the NIH study versus glucosamine sulfate in the European studies), differences in the way they were administered (one large daily dose in the European studies versus three smaller ones in the NIH study), other differences in the way the studies were done, or chance.

Chondroitin

In general, research on chondroitin has not shown it to be helpful for pain from knee or hip OA.

More than 20 studies have looked at the effect of chondroitin on pain from knee or hip OA. The quality of the studies varied and so did the results. However, the largest and best studies (including the NIH study discussed under the heading "Glucosamine" above) showed that chondroitin doesn't lessen OA pain.

Joint structure. A few studies have looked at whether glucosamine or chondroitin can have beneficial effects on the joint structure. Some but not all studies found evidence that chondroitin might help, but the improvements may be too small to make a difference to patients. There is little evidence that glucosamine has beneficial effects on the joint structure.

Experts' Recommendations

Experts disagree on whether glucosamine and chondroitin may help knee and hip OA. The American College of Rheumatology (ACR) has recommended that people with knee or hip OA not use glucosamine or chondroitin. But the recommendation was not a strong one, and the ACR acknowledged that it was controversial.

For Other Parts of the Body

Only a small amount of research has been done on glucosamine and chondroitin for OA of joints other than the knee and hip. Because there have been only a few relatively small studies, no definite conclusions can be reached.

- **Chondroitin for OA of the hand**

  A 6-month trial of chondroitin in 162 patients with severe OA of the hand showed that it may improve pain and function.

- **Glucosamine for OA of the jaw**

  One study of 45 patients with OA of the jaw showed that those given glucosamine had less pain than those given ibuprofen. But another study, which included 59 patients with OA of the jaw, found that those taking glucosamine did no better than those taking a placebo (pills that don't contain the active ingredient).

- **Glucosamine for chronic low-back pain and OA of the spine**

  A Norwegian trial involving 250 people with chronic low back pain and OA of the lower spine found that participants who received glucosamine fared the same at 6 months as those who received placebo.

What the Science Says about Safety and Side Effects

- No serious side effects have been reported in large, well-conducted studies of people taking glucosamine, chondroitin, or both for up to 3 years.

- However, glucosamine or chondroitin may interact with the anticoagulant (blood-thinning) drug warfarin (Coumadin).

- A study in rats showed that long-term use of moderately large doses of glucosamine might damage the kidneys. Although results from animal studies don't always apply to people, this study does raise concern.

- Glucosamine might affect the way your body handles sugar, especially if you have diabetes or other blood sugar problems, such as insulin resistance or impaired glucose tolerance.

If you use dietary supplements, such as glucosamine and chondroitin, read and follow the label instructions, and recognize that "natural" does not always mean "safe."

The U.S. Food and Drug Administration (FDA) regulates dietary supplements, but the regulations for dietary supplements are different and less strict than those for prescription or over-the-counter (OTC) drugs.

Some dietary supplements may interact with medications or pose risks if you have medical problems or are going to have surgery. Most dietary supplements have not been tested in pregnant women, nursing mothers, or children.

Section 40.2

Cat's Claw

This section includes text excerpted from "Cat's Claw,"
National Center for Complementary and Integrative
Health (NCCIH), September 2016.

Background

- Cat's claw is a woody vine that grows wild in the Amazon rainforest and other tropical areas of Central and South America. Its thorns resemble a cat's claws.

- The two most common species are *U. tomentosa* and *U. guianensis*. Most commercial preparations of cat's claw contain *U. tomentosa*.

- Using cat's claw for health dates back to the Inca civilization. Its historical uses have included for contraception, inflammation, cancer, and viral infections, and to stimulate the immune system.

- Cat's claw is used as a dietary supplement for a variety of health conditions including viral infections (such as herpes and human immunodeficiency virus (HIV)), Alzheimer disease (AD), cancer, arthritis, diverticulitis, peptic ulcers, colitis, gastritis, hemorrhoids, parasites, and leaky bowel syndrome.

- The bark and root of cat's claw are used to make liquid extracts, capsules, tablets, and tea.

How Much Do We Know?

There have been very few high-quality clinical trials (studies done in people) of cat's claw.

What Have We Learned?

There's no conclusive scientific evidence-based on studies in people that support using cat's claw for any health purpose.

What Do We Know about Safety?

- Few side effects have been reported for cat's claw when taken in small amounts.

- Women who are pregnant or trying to become pregnant should avoid using cat's claw because of its past use for preventing and aborting the pregnancy.

Keep in Mind

Tell all your healthcare providers about any complementary or integrative health approaches you use. Give them a full picture of what you do to manage your health. This will help ensure coordinated and safe care.

Section 40.3

Evening Primrose Oil

This section includes text excerpted from "Evening
Primrose Oil," National Center for Complementary and
Integrative Health (NCCIH), September 2016.

Background

- Evening primrose is a plant native to North America, but it grows in Europe and parts of the Southern hemisphere as well. It has yellow flowers that bloom in the evening. Evening primrose oil contains the fatty acid gamma-linolenic acid (GLA).

- Native Americans used the whole plant for bruises and its roots for hemorrhoids. The leaves were traditionally used for minor wounds, gastrointestinal complaints, and sore throats.

- People use evening primrose oil dietary supplements for eczema (a condition involving red, swollen, itchy skin, sometimes caused by allergies), rheumatoid arthritis (RA), premenstrual syndrome (PMS), breast pain, menopause symptoms, and other conditions.

- Evening primrose oil is obtained from the seeds of the evening primrose and is usually sold in capsule form.

How Much Do We Know?

Many studies in people have evaluated evening primrose oil for eczema, PMS, or breast pain. Smaller numbers of studies have evaluated it for other health conditions.

What Have We Learned?

- There's not enough evidence to support the use of evening primrose oil for any health condition.

- According to a comprehensive 2013 evaluation of the evidence, evening primrose oil, taken orally (by mouth), is not helpful for relieving symptoms of eczema.

- Most studies of evening primrose oil for PMS have not found it to be helpful.

- Studies of evening primrose oil for breast pain have had conflicting results.

- A small amount of evidence suggests that evening primrose oil might be helpful for diabetic neuropathy (nerve problems caused by diabetes).

What Do We Know about Safety?

- Evening primrose oil is probably safe for most people when taken for short periods of time. There can be mild side effects, such as stomach upset and headache.

- The safety of long-term use of evening primrose oil has not been established.

- Evening primrose oil may increase the risk of some complications of pregnancy. Talk with your healthcare provider if you're considering using evening primrose oil during pregnancy.

- Evening primrose oil may increase bleeding in people who are taking the anticoagulant (blood thinning) medication warfarin (Coumadin).

Keep in Mind

- Tell all your healthcare providers about any complementary or integrative health approaches you use. Give them a full picture of what you do to manage your health. This will help ensure coordinated and safe care.

Section 40.4

Flaxseed and Flaxseed Oil

This section includes text excerpted from "The Benefits of Flaxseed," Agricultural Research Service (ARS), U.S. Department of Agriculture (USDA), August 13, 2016.

North Dakota is one of the few states in the United States that produce flax. Flax is an annual plant, and it is grown both for its fiber and for its seeds. The ancient Egyptians were probably the first to use flax. They used fiber from the plant to make clothes, fishnets and other products, and they used flaxseed or linseed as food and medicine. Historically, flaxseed is primarily used as a laxative, because it is high in fiber and a gummy material called mucilage. These substances expand when they come in contact with water, so they add bulk to stool and help it move more quickly through the body.

Flaxseed is rich in nutrients. One hundred grams of ground flaxseed supply approximately 450 kilocalories, 41 grams of fat, 28 grams of fiber and 20 grams of protein. Flaxseed oil or linseed oil is rich in alpha-linolenic acid, an omega-3 fatty acid. Omega-3 fatty acids are "good" fats that may be good for heart disease, inflammatory bowel disease (IBD), arthritis and other health problems. Each tablespoon of ground flaxseed contains about 1.8 grams of omega-3 fatty acids. Studies suggest that consumption of flaxseed may be beneficial in improving cardiovascular health.

People who eat a Mediterranean diet tend to have high-density lipoproteins (HDL) ("good") cholesterol levels. The Mediterranean diet has a healthy balance of dietary fatty acids including omega-3 fatty acids. It includes whole grains; green vegetables and fruits; fish and poultry; olive; canola and flaxseed oils; and walnuts. The Mediterranean diet limits the amount of red meat, butter, and cream consumption. In laboratory animal studies, flaxseed and flaxseed oil have been shown to lower cholesterols.

One of the best ways to prevent heart disease is to eat a low-fat diet, avoiding foods rich in saturated fats and trans-fats and eating those that are rich in unsaturated fats, for example, omega-3 fatty acids from flaxseed. Evidence suggests that people who eat an alpha-linolenic acid-rich diet are less likely to have a fatal heart attack. A diet rich in fruits, vegetables, whole grains, nuts or legumes, and omega-3, fatty acid–rich foods may reduce the risk of heart attack and stroke, both as first-time events and after the first heart attack or stroke. Furthermore, several human studies show that diets rich in omega-3 fatty acids (including alpha-linolenic acid) may lower blood pressure in people with hypertension.

In addition to the important omega-3 fatty acids, flaxseed also contains a group of bioactive components called lignans. Emerging evidence suggests that lignans may help protect the body from cancer. Human clinical study involving postmenopausal participants who were newly diagnosed with breast cancer who ate a muffin containing 25 grams of flaxseed for 40 days showed the potential for reduced tumor growth in postmenopausal women who were newly diagnosed with breast cancer. Laboratory studies reported that flaxseed or its bioactive components lignans reduced breast tumor growth and spread in laboratory rodents. Evidence also suggests that flaxseed may benefits men at risk for prostate cancer. In one study, eating a low-fat diet with 30 grams of flaxseed daily lowered prostate-specific antigen levels (a marker of prostate health) in men with a precancerous prostate condition called prostatic intraepithelial neoplasia. However, more clinical studies are needed to understand how flaxseed and lignans may affect cancer in humans.

The optimum intake required to obtain health benefits is not known. However, 1–2 tablespoons of ground flaxseed a day is currently suggested. Flaxseed, when eaten whole, is more likely to pass through the body undigested, which means the body does not get all of the nutrients and bioactive components. The best approach is to buy the whole flaxseed, as the outside shell in the whole seed appears to keep the fatty acids inside well protected, and grind it on an as-needed basis. An electric coffee grinder seems to work the best. Storing ground flaxseed in the freezer will keep the ground seed from oxidizing and losing its nutritional potency. Flaxseed comes in two basic varieties: golden and brown. Golden seed is more visually appealing, but there is very little difference nutritionally between the two.

Eating flaxseed is easy. Top a salad with some ground flaxseed, sprinkle it on top of yogurt, smoothies, or cereal; or stir a teaspoon into your soup. It also can be a substitute for a tablespoon or two of flour in bread, cookies, or muffins. Flaxseed oil works best in cold foods like salad dressings and should not be used for frying because it burns easily.

Section 40.5

Ginger

This section includes text excerpted from "Ginger,"
National Center for Complementary and Integrative
Health (NCCIH), September 2016.

Background

- Ginger is a tropical plant that has green-purple flowers and a fragrant underground stem (called a rhizome). It is widely used as a flavoring or fragrance in foods, beverages, soaps, and cosmetics.

- Ancient Sanskrit, Chinese, Greek, Roman, and Arabic texts discussed the use of ginger for health-related purposes. In Asian medicine, dried ginger has been used for thousands of years to treat stomach ache, diarrhea, and nausea.

- Ginger is used as a dietary supplement for postsurgery nausea; nausea caused by motion, chemotherapy, or pregnancy; rheumatoid arthritis (RA); and osteoarthritis (OA).

- Common forms of ginger include the fresh or dried root, tablets, capsules, liquid extracts, and teas.

How Much Do We Know?

- There's some information from human studies using ginger for nausea and vomiting.

- Much less is known about other human uses of ginger for other health conditions.

What Have We Learned?

- Some evidence indicates that ginger may help relieve pregnancy-related nausea and vomiting.

- Ginger may help to control chemotherapy-related nausea for cancer patients when used in addition to conventional anti-nausea medication.

- It's unclear whether ginger is helpful for postsurgery nausea, motion sickness, RA, or OA.

What Do We Know about Its Safety?

- Ginger, when used as a spice, is believed to be generally safe.

- In some people, ginger can have mild side effects such as abdominal discomfort, heartburn, diarrhea, and gas.

- Some experts recommend that people with gallstone disease use caution with ginger because it may increase the flow of bile.

- Research has not definitely shown whether ginger interacts with medications, but concerns have been raised that it might interact with anticoagulants (blood thinners).

- Although several studies have found no evidence of harm from taking ginger during pregnancy, it's uncertain whether ginger is always safe for pregnant women. If you're considering using ginger while you're pregnant, consult your healthcare provider.

Keep in Mind

- Tell all your healthcare providers about any complementary or integrative health approaches you use. Give them a full picture of what you do to manage your health. This will help ensure coordinated and safe care.

Section 40.6

Thunder God Vine

This section includes text excerpted from "Thunder God Vine," National Center for Complementary and Integrative Health (NCCIH), September 2016.

Background

- Thunder god vine is a perennial grown in China and Taiwan. It has been used for hundreds of years in traditional Chinese medicine to treat swelling caused by inflammation.

- Currently, thunder god vine is used orally (by mouth) as a dietary supplement for autoimmune diseases such as rheumatoid arthritis (RA), multiple sclerosis (MS), and lupus. It is also used topically for RA.

- Extracts are prepared from the roots of thunder god vine.

How Much Do We Know?

- A small number of studies have evaluated oral thunder god vine for RA. Very little research has been done on thunder god vine for other health conditions or on topical use of this herb for RA.

What Have We Learned?

- There have been only a few high-quality studies of oral thunder god vine for RA in people. These studies indicate that thunder god vine may improve some RA symptoms.

- Results from a small 2009 study funded by the National Institute of Arthritis and Musculoskeletal and Skin Diseases (NIAMS), which compared an extract of thunder god vine root with a conventional drug (sulfasalazine) for RA, found that participants' symptoms (e.g., joint pain and swelling, inflammation) improved significantly more with thunder god vine than with the drug.

- A study from China, published in 2014, compared thunder god vine to a conventional drug (methotrexate) and found that both were comparably helpful in relieving RA symptoms and that the combination of the herb and the drug was better than either one alone.

- There is not enough evidence to show whether thunder god vine is helpful for any health conditions other than RA or whether its topical use in RA has any benefits.

What Do We Know about Safety?

- Thunder god vine may have side effects, including decreased bone mineral content (with long-term use), infertility, menstrual cycle changes, rashes, diarrhea, headache, and hair loss. Because some of these side effects are serious, the risks of using thunder god vine may be greater than its benefits.

- Thunder god vine can be extremely poisonous if the extract is not prepared properly.

Keep in Mind

- Tell all your healthcare providers about any complementary or integrative health approaches you use. Give them a full picture of what you do to manage your health. This will help ensure coordinated and safe care.

Section 40.7

Turmeric

This section includes text excerpted from "Turmeric,"
National Center for Complementary and Integrative
Health (NCCIH), September 2016.

Background

- Turmeric, a plant related to ginger, is grown throughout India, other parts of Asia, and Central America. Javanese turmeric (*Curcuma xanthorrhiz*) is a different plant.

- Historically, turmeric has been used in Ayurvedic medicine, primarily in South Asia, for many conditions, including breathing problems, rheumatism, serious pain, and fatigue.

- Turmeric is used as a dietary supplement for inflammation; arthritis; stomach, skin, liver, and gallbladder problems; cancer; and other conditions.

- Turmeric is a common spice and a major ingredient in curry powder. Its primary active ingredients, curcuminoids, are yellow and used to color foods and cosmetics.

- Turmeric's underground stems (rhizomes) are dried and made into capsules, tablets, teas, or extracts. Turmeric powder is also made into a paste for skin conditions.

How Much Do We Know?

There is a lot of research, including human studies conducted in response to a variety of health conditions.

What Have We Learned?

- Claims that curcuminoids found in turmeric help to reduce inflammation aren't supported by strong studies.

- Preliminary studies found that curcuminoids may

  - Reduce the number of heart attacks that heart-bypass patients have after surgery

  - Control knee pain from osteoarthritis (OA) as well as ibuprofen

  - Reduce the skin irritation that often occurs after radiation treatments for breast cancer.

- Other preliminary human studies have looked at curcumin, a type of curcuminoid, for different cancers, colitis, diabetes, surgical pain, and as an ingredient in mouthwash for reducing plaque.

- The National Center for Complementary and Integrative Health (NCCIH) has studied curcumin for Alzheimer disease (AD), rheumatoid arthritis (RA), and prostate and colon cancer.

What Do We Know about Safety?

- Turmeric in amounts tested for health purposes is generally considered safe when taken by mouth or applied to the skin.

- High doses or long-term use of turmeric may cause gastrointestinal problems.

Keep in Mind

- Tell all your healthcare providers about any complementary or integrative health approaches you use. Give them a full picture of what you do to manage your health. This will help ensure coordinated and safe care.

Section 40.8

Dietary Supplements for Osteoarthritis

This section includes text excerpted from "6 Things You
Should Know about Dietary Supplements for Osteoarthritis,"
National Center for Complementary and Integrative
Health (NCCIH), September 24, 2015.

Osteoarthritis (OA) is the most common type of arthritis—affecting 27 million Americans—and is an increasing problem among older adults. Treatments for osteoarthritis address its symptoms, such as pain, swelling, and reduced function in the joints. Nonmedicinal approaches involve lifestyle changes such as exercise, weight control, and rest. Conventional medicinal treatments for OA include nonsteroidal anti-inflammatory drugs (NSAIDS), acetaminophen (a class of pain reliever), and injections of corticosteroids (anti-inflammatory hormones).

Many people with OA report trying various dietary supplements, including glucosamine and chondroitin, alone or in combination, in an effort to relieve pain and improve function. However, there is no convincing evidence that any dietary supplement helps with OA symptoms or the course of the underlying disease. Here are 6 things you should know about dietary supplements for osteoarthritis:

- **The majority of research has found little effect of glucosamine or chondroitin on symptoms or joint damage associated with OA of the knee or hip.** Studies have found that glucosamine and chondroitin supplements may interact with the anticoagulant (blood-thinning) drug warfarin (Coumadin). But overall, studies have not shown any other serious side effects.

- **Dimethyl Sulfoxide (DMSO) and Methylsulfonylmethane (MSM) are two chemically related dietary supplements that have been used for arthritic conditions; however, the evidence does not suggest that DMSO and MSM are helpful for OA symptoms.** Although limited safety data are available, some side effects from topical DMSO have been reported, including upset stomach; skin irritation; and garlic taste; breath, and body odor. Minor side effects associated with MSM in humans include allergic reaction, upset stomach, and skin rashes.

- **S-Adenosyl-L-methionine (SAMe) is a molecule that is naturally produced in the body and is often taken as a dietary supplement; however, there is not enough evidence to support the use of SAMe for OA of the knee or hip.** SAMe is generally considered safe, but common side effects include gastrointestinal (GI) problems, dry mouth, headache, sweating, dizziness, and nervousness.

- **There is preliminary evidence that avocado/soybean unsaponifiables (ASU), supplements made from avocado oil and soybean oil extracts, may have modest beneficial effects on symptoms of osteoarthritis.** Safety information has not been sufficiently available.

- **Although some results suggest that a few herbs may be beneficial for OA symptoms, the overall evidence is weak, and conclusions among reviews of the literature provide conflicting interpretations.** In general, herbs have not been studied or prepared in a consistent way. There is also a general lack of safety data available.

- **If you take or are considering taking, dietary supplements for OA, tell your healthcare providers.** They can do a better job caring for you if they know what dietary supplements you use.

Section 40.9

Omega-3 Fatty Acids

This section includes text excerpted from "Omega-3 Fatty Acids," Office of Dietary Supplements (ODS), National Institutes of Health (NIH), March 2, 2017.

What Are Omega-3 Fatty Acids and What Do They Do?

Omega-3 fatty acids are found in foods such as fish and flaxseed, and in dietary supplements such as fish oil.

The three main omega-3 fatty acids are alpha-linolenic acid (ALA), eicosapentaenoic acid (EPA), and docosahexaenoic acid (DHA). ALA is found mainly in plant oils such as flaxseed, soybean, and canola oils. DHA and EPA are found in fish and other seafood.

ALA is an essential fatty acid, meaning that your body can't make it, so you must get it from the foods and beverages you consume. Your body can convert some ALA into EPA and then to DHA, but only in very small amounts. Therefore, getting EPA and DHA from foods (and dietary supplements if you take them) is the only practical way to increase levels of these omega-3 fatty acids in your body.

Omega-3s are important components of the membranes that surround each cell in your body. DHA levels are especially high in the retina (eye), brain, and sperm cells. Omega-3s also provide calories to give your body energy and have many functions in your heart, blood vessels, lungs, immune system, and endocrine system (the network of hormone-producing glands).

How Much Omega-3s Do I Need?

Experts have not established recommended amounts of omega-3 fatty acids, except for ALA. Average daily recommended amounts for ALA are listed below in grams (g). The amount you need depends on your age and sex.

Table 40.1. Recommended Amount of ALA

Life Stage	Recommended Amount of ALA
Birth to 12 months*	0.5 g
Children 1–3 years	0.7 g
Children 4–8 years	0.9 g
Boys 9–13 years	1.2 g
Girls 9–13 years	1.0 g
Teen boys 14–18 years	1.6 g
Teen girls 14–18 years	1.1 g
Men	1.6 g
Women	1.1 g
Pregnant teens and women	1.4 g
Breastfeeding teens and women	1.3 g

As total omega-3s. All other values are for ALA alone.

What Foods Provide Omega-3s?

Omega-3s are found naturally in some foods and are added to some fortified foods. You can get adequate amounts of omega-3s by eating a variety of foods, including the following:

- Fish and other seafood (especially cold-water fatty fish, such as salmon, mackerel, tuna, herring, and sardines)
- Nuts and seeds (such as flaxseed, chia seeds, and walnuts)
- Plant oils (such as flaxseed oil, soybean oil, and canola oil)
- Fortified foods (such as certain brands of eggs, yogurt, juices, milk, soy beverages, and infant formulas)

What Kinds of Omega-3 Dietary Supplements Are Available?

Omega-3 dietary supplements include fish oil, krill oil, cod liver oil, and algal oil (a vegetarian source that comes from algae). They provide a wide range of doses and forms of omega-3s.

Am I Getting Enough Omega-3s?

Most people in the United States get enough ALA from the foods they eat. They also get small amounts of EPA and DHA. Recommended amounts of EPA and DHA have not been established.

What Happens If I Don't Get Enough Omega-3s?

A deficiency of omega-3s can cause rough, scaly skin and a red, swollen, itchy rash. Omega-3 deficiency is very rare in the United States.

What Are Some Effects of Omega-3s on Health?

Scientists are studying omega-3s to understand how they affect health. People who eat fish and other seafood have a lower risk of several chronic diseases. But it is not clear whether these health benefits come from simply eating these foods or from the omega-3s in these foods. Examples of what the research has shown follow.

Rheumatoid Arthritis (RA)

RA causes chronic pain, swelling, stiffness, and loss of function in the joints. Some clinical trials have shown that taking omega-3 supplements may help manage RA when taken together with standard RA medications and other treatments. For example, people with RA who take omega-3 supplements may need less pain-relief medication, but it is not clear if the supplements reduce joint pain, swelling, or morning stiffness.

Infant Health and Development

During pregnancy and breastfeeding, eating 8–12 ounces of fish and other seafood per week may improve your baby's health. However, it is important to choose fish that are higher in EPA and DHA and lower in mercury. Examples are salmon, herring, sardines, and trout. It is not clear whether taking dietary supplements containing EPA and DHA during pregnancy or breastfeeding affects a baby's health or development. However, some studies show that taking these supplements may slightly increase a baby's weight at birth and the length of time the baby is in the womb, both of which may be beneficial. Breast milk contains DHA. Most commercial infant formulas also contain DHA.

Age-Related Macular Degeneration (AMD)

AMD is a major cause of vision loss among older adults. Studies suggest that people who get higher amounts of omega-3s from the foods they eat may have a lower risk of developing AMD. But once someone has AMD, taking omega-3 supplements does not keep the disease from getting worse or slow vision loss.

Other Conditions

Researchers are studying whether taking omega-3 dietary supplements may help lessen some of the symptoms of attention deficit hyperactivity disorder (ADHD), childhood allergies, and cystic fibrosis (CF), but more research is needed to fully understand the potential benefits of omega-3s for these and other conditions.

Can Omega-3s Be Harmful?

The U.S. Food and Drug Administration (FDA) recommends consuming no more than 3 g/day of EPA and DHA combined, including up to 2 g/day from dietary supplements. Higher doses are sometimes used to lower triglycerides, but anyone taking omega-3s for this purpose should be under the care of a healthcare provider because these doses could cause bleeding problems and possibly affect immune function. Any side effects from taking omega-3 supplements in smaller amounts are usually mild. They include an unpleasant taste in the mouth, bad breath, heartburn, nausea, stomach discomfort, diarrhea, headache, and smelly sweat.

Are There Any Interactions with Omega-3s That I Should Know About?

Omega-3 dietary supplements may interact with the medications you take. For example, high doses of omega-3s may cause bleeding problems when taken with warfarin (Coumadin®) or other anticoagulant medicines.

Talk with your healthcare provider about possible interactions between omega-3 supplements and your medications.

Omega-3s and Healthful Eating

People should get most of their nutrients from food, advises the federal government's *Dietary Guidelines for Americans*. Foods contain vitamins, minerals, dietary fiber, and other substances that benefit health. In some cases, fortified foods and dietary supplements may provide nutrients that otherwise may be consumed in less than recommended amounts.

Chapter 41

Complementary and Alternative Medicine for Arthritis

Chapter Contents

Section 41.1—What Is Complementary and
　　　　　Alternative Medicine? 432

Section 41.2—Complementary Health Approaches
　　　　　for Chronic Pain 435

Section 41.3—Acupuncture 437

Section 41.4—Magnets 439

Section 41.5—Research on Massage Therapy and
　　　　　Arthritis 440

Section 41.1

What Is Complementary and Alternative Medicine?

This section includes text excerpted from
"Complementary, Alternative, or Integrative Health:
What's in a Name?" National Center for Complementary
and Integrative Health (NCCIH), June 2016.

Complementary versus Alternative

Many Americans—more than 30 percent of adults and about 12 percent of children—use healthcare approaches developed outside of mainstream Western, or conventional, medicine. When describing these approaches, people often use "alternative" and "complementary" interchangeably, but the two terms refer to different concepts:

- If a nonmainstream practice is used together with conventional medicine, it's considered "complementary."

- If a nonmainstream practice is used in place of conventional medicine, it's considered "alternative."

True alternative medicine is uncommon. Most people who use non-mainstream approaches use them along with conventional treatments.

Integrative Medicine

There are many definitions of "integrative" healthcare, but all involve bringing conventional and complementary approaches together in a coordinated way. The use of integrative approaches to health and wellness has grown within care settings across the United States. Researchers are currently exploring the potential benefits of integrative health in a variety of situations, including pain management for military personnel and veterans, relief of symptoms in cancer patients and survivors, and programs to promote healthy behaviors.

Chronic pain is a common problem among active-duty military personnel and veterans. The National Center for Complementary and

Integrative Health (NCCIH), the U.S. Department of Veterans Affairs (VA), and other agencies are sponsoring research to see whether integrative approaches can help. For example, NCCIH-funded studies are testing the effects of adding mindfulness meditation, self-hypnosis, or other complementary approaches to pain-management programs for veterans. The goal is to help patients feel and function better and reduce their need for pain medicines that can have serious side effects.

Healthy behaviors, such as eating right, getting enough physical activity, and not smoking, can reduce people's risks of developing serious diseases. Can integrative approaches promote these types of behaviors? Researchers are working to answer this question. Preliminary research suggests that yoga and meditation-based therapies may help smokers quit, and NCCIH-funded studies are testing whether adding mindfulness-based approaches to weight control programs will help people lose weight more successfully.

Types of Complementary Health Approaches

Most complementary health approaches fall into one of two subgroups—natural products or mind and body practices.

Natural Products

This group includes a variety of products, such as **herbs** (also known as botanicals), **vitamins and minerals, and probiotics**. They are widely marketed, readily available to consumers, and often sold as dietary supplements.

According to the 2012 National Health Interview Survey (NHIS), which included a comprehensive survey on the use of complementary health approaches by Americans, 17.7 percent of American adults had used a dietary supplement other than vitamins and minerals in the past year. These products were the most popular complementary health approach in the survey. The most commonly used natural product was fish oil.

Researchers have done large, rigorous studies on a few natural products, but the results often showed that the products didn't work. Research on others is in progress. While there are indications that some may be helpful, more needs to be learned about the effects of these products in the human body and about their safety and potential interactions with medicines and other natural products.

Mind and Body Practices

Mind and body practices include a large and diverse group of procedures or techniques administered or taught by a trained practitioner or teacher. The 2012 NHIS showed that yoga, chiropractic and osteopathic manipulation, meditation, and massage therapy are among the most popular mind and body practices used by adults. The popularity of yoga has grown dramatically in recent years, with almost twice as many U.S. adults practicing yoga in 2012 as in 2002.

Other mind and body practices include acupuncture, relaxation techniques (such as breathing exercises, guided imagery, and progressive muscle relaxation), tai chi, qi gong, healing touch, hypnotherapy, and movement therapies (such as Feldenkrais method, Alexander technique, Pilates, Rolfing Structural Integration (RSI), and Trager psychophysical integration (TPI)).

The amount of research on mind and body approaches varies widely depending on the practice. For example, researchers have done many studies on acupuncture, yoga, spinal manipulation, and meditation, but there have been fewer studies on some other practices.

Other Complementary Health Approaches

The two broad areas discussed above—natural products and mind and body practices—capture most complementary health approaches. However, some approaches may not neatly fit into either of these groups—for example, the practices of traditional healers, Ayurvedic medicine, traditional Chinese medicine (TCM), homeopathy, and naturopathy.

Section 41.2

Complementary Health Approaches for Chronic Pain

This section includes text excerpted from "Complementary Health Approaches for Chronic Pain," National Center for Complementary and Integrative Health (NCCIH), December 14, 2017.

This section summarizes current scientific evidence about the complementary health approaches most often used by people for chronic pain, including fibromyalgia (FM), headache, irritable bowel syndrome (IBS), low-back pain, neck pain, osteoarthritis (OA), and rheumatoid arthritis (RA).

The scientific evidence to date suggests that some complementary health approaches may provide modest effects that may help individuals manage the day-to-day variations in their chronic pain symptoms. Some complementary approaches do show modest benefit depending on the approach and pain condition; in most instances, though, the amount of evidence is too small to clearly show whether an approach is useful.

Pain Conditions and Current Evidence of Complementary Health Approaches

Fibromyalgia (FM)

In general, research on complementary health approaches for FM must be regarded as preliminary. However, recent systematic reviews and randomized clinical trials provide encouraging evidence that practices such as tai chi, qi gong, yoga, massage therapy, acupuncture, and balneotherapy may help relieve some FM symptoms.

Osteoarthritis (OA)

The preponderance of evidence on glucosamine and chondroitin sulfate—taken separately or together—indicates little or no meaningful effect on pain or function. Independent clinical practice guidelines published in 2012 by the American College of Rheumatology (ACR), and in 2010 by the American Academy of Orthopaedic Surgeons (AAOS) recommend not using glucosamine or chondroitin for OA. Recommendations from OA Research Society International (OARSI) published in 2014 conclude that current evidence does not support the use of glucosamine or chondroitin in knee OA for disease-modifying effects, but leave unsettled the question of whether either may provide symptomatic relief.

In 2012, the ACR issued recommendations for using pharmacologic and nonpharmacologic approaches for OA of the hand, hip, and knee. The guidelines conditionally recommend tai chi, along with other nondrug approaches such as self-management programs and walking aids, for managing knee OA. Acupuncture is also conditionally recommended for those who have chronic moderate to severe knee pain and are candidates for total knee replacement but can't or won't undergo the procedure.

Rheumatoid Arthritis (RA)

Omega-3 fatty acids found in fish oil may have modest benefits in relieving rheumatoid arthritis (RA) symptoms; however, omega-3s do not prevent ongoing joint damage or modify disease course. No other dietary supplement has shown clear benefits for RA, but there is preliminary evidence for a few, particularly fish oil, gamma-linolenic acid, and the herb thunder god vine; however, serious safety concerns have been raised about thunder god vine.

Results from clinical trials, however, suggest that some mind and body practices—such as relaxation, mindfulness meditation, tai chi, and yoga—may be beneficial additions to conventional treatment plans, but some studies indicate that these practices may do more to improve other aspects of patients' health than to relieve pain.

Section 41.3

Acupuncture

This section includes text excerpted from "Acupuncture:
In Depth," National Center for Complementary and
Integrative Health (NCCIH), January 2016.

What Is Acupuncture?

Acupuncture is a technique in which practitioners stimulate specific points on the body—most often by inserting thin needles through the skin. It is one of the practices used in traditional Chinese medicine.

What the Science Says about the Effectiveness of Acupuncture

Results from a number of studies suggest that acupuncture may help ease types of pain that are often chronic such as low-back pain, neck pain, and osteoarthritis (OA)/knee pain. It also may help reduce the frequency of tension headaches and prevent migraine headaches. Therefore, acupuncture appears to be a reasonable option for people with chronic pain to consider. However, clinical practice guidelines are inconsistent with recommendations about acupuncture.

The effects of acupuncture on the brain and body and how best to measure them are only beginning to be understood. Current evidence suggests that many factors—like expectation and belief—that are unrelated to acupuncture needling may play important roles in the beneficial effects of acupuncture on pain.

What the Science Says about Safety and Side Effects of Acupuncture

- Relatively few complications from using acupuncture have been reported. Still, complications have resulted from the use of nonsterile needles and improper delivery of treatments.

- When not delivered properly, acupuncture can cause serious adverse effects, including infections, punctured organs, collapsed lungs, and injury to the central nervous system (CNS).

The U.S. Food and Drug Administration (FDA) regulates acupuncture needles as medical devices for use by licensed practitioners and requires that needles be manufactured and labeled according to certain standards. For example, the FDA requires that needles be sterile, nontoxic, and labeled for single use by qualified practitioners only.

More to Consider

- Don't use acupuncture to postpone seeing a healthcare provider about a health problem.

- If you decide to visit an acupuncturist, check his or her credentials. Most states require a license, certification, or registration to practice acupuncture; however, education and training standards and requirements for obtaining these vary from state to state. Although a license does not ensure the quality of care, it does indicate that the practitioner meets certain standards regarding the knowledge and use of acupuncture. Most states require a diploma from the National Certification Commission for Acupuncture and Oriental Medicine (NCCAOM) for licensing.

- Some conventional medical practitioners—including physicians and dentists—practice acupuncture. In addition, national acupuncture organizations (which can be found through libraries or by searching the Internet) may provide referrals to acupuncturists. When considering practitioners, ask about their training and experience.

- Ask the practitioner about the estimated number of treatments needed and how much each treatment will cost. Some insurance companies may cover the costs of acupuncture, while others may not.

- Help your healthcare providers give you better coordinated and safe care by telling them about all the health approaches you use. Give them a full picture of what you do to manage your health.

Section 41.4

Magnets

This section includes text excerpted from "Magnets for Pain," National Center for Complementary and Integrative Health (NCCIH), December 27, 2017.

Magnets are often marketed for different types of pain, such as foot or back pain resulting from arthritis and fibromyalgia (FM). Made from metal or alloys, magnets vary considerably in their strength. Magnets marketed for pain are usually encased in a wrap or sold in a product that is placed against the skin near where the pain is felt. Different types of magnets have been studied for pain.

- **Static or permanent magnets:** Static magnets have magnetic fields that do not change. The activity of electrons in the metal causes it to be magnetic. These magnets usually aren't very strong and are often put in products such as shoe insoles, headbands, bracelets, and more.

- **Electromagnets**: This type of magnet is created when an electrical current charges the metal, making it magnetic. Devices with electromagnets in them are also marketed for health purposes.

Bottom Line

- Research studies don't support the use of **static magnets** for any form of pain.

- **Electromagnets** may help with osteoarthritis (OA) but it's unclear if they can relieve the pain enough to improve quality of life and day-to-day functioning, a 2013 research review concluded. For OA, small machines or mats are used to deliver electromagnetic fields to the whole body or to certain joints.

- In 2013 the U.S. Food and Drug Administration (FDA) approved a device that uses strong electromagnets to treat migraines by stimulating nerve cells in the brain, a process called

transcranial magnetic stimulation (TMS). TMS may help other pain conditions as well.

Safety

- Some magnets may interfere with medical devices, such as pace-makers and insulin pumps.

- Beyond interference with medical devices, there isn't much good information on the possible side effects of magnets, but few problems have been reported.

- Children may swallow or accidentally inhale small magnets, which can be deadly.

- Do not use static magnets or electromagnets that you can buy without a prescription to postpone seeing a healthcare provider about pain or any other medical problem.

Section 41.5

Research on Massage Therapy and Arthritis

This section includes text excerpted from "Pilot Study with 25 Veterans Yields Promising Results on Swedish Massage for Knee Pain," U.S. Department of Veterans Affairs (VA), July 1, 2015.

Put down the pill bottle—get a massage instead.

Lots of people with arthritis pain would be happy to hear this advice from their doctor. But researchers are still testing the benefits of this therapy with ancient roots—whom it helps, for what conditions.

Now, good news from a team at Duke University and the Durham (N.C.), U.S. Department of Veterans Affairs (VA) Medical Center. They showed in a small pilot study that Swedish massage is an acceptable and feasible treatment for VA healthcare users with osteoarthritis (OA) of the knee. Moreover, the Veterans who took part in the study reported, on average, about a 30 percent improvement in pain, stiffness, and function.

Trial Involved 25 Veterans

Dr. Adam Perlman of the Duke Integrative Medicine Center (DIMC), working with VA colleagues, led the trial, involving 25 veterans. The group was mostly white and African American males, with an average age of 57, and an average body mass index (BMI) of around 32, which is above the obesity threshold.

Perlman led an earlier clinical trial that found the therapy effective for knee OA in a general population. But he wanted to put Swedish massage to the test for VA patients.

For one thing, most VA patients are men, who as a group might be somewhat less receptive than women to the idea of massage. Think about who typically goes to spas.

Second, VA patients are more likely than the general population to have multiple health problems—physical or mental. This could complicate how massage is delivered, or its effects.

As it turns out, the idea of Swedish massage sat well with the veterans in the study.

High Retention Rate

Almost all of those who started the study—23 out of 25—completed the eight weekly, one-hour massage sessions, given at Duke Integrative Medicine, about a mile from the Durham VA. More than 90 percent of them said they wanted to continue to receive massage as part of their arthritis treatment plan. Nearly 90 percent said they thought other Veterans would try massage if it were offered in VA.

Dr. Kelli Allen, a VA health services researcher who worked on the study, says recruiting a diverse mix of VA arthritis patients for the study posed no particular challenge.

"We had comparable rates of recruitment, among eligible participants, as those we have seen in clinical trials of other behavioral and lifestyle interventions among Veterans with OA. That was an important aspect of feasibility for us to assess in a pilot study. Our experience suggests there is indeed interest in massage therapy among VA healthcare users."

Swedish massage, introduced in the United States in the mid-1800s, generally uses a whole-body approach, working for all the major muscle groups. Therapists apply firm but gentle pressure to compress and relax muscles, boosting circulation. Patients are typically draped with a sheet, but they can opt to wear clothes during the treatment and have only certain areas worked on.

"Massage need not be full-body, but often is," says Perlman. "Massage therapists see different parts of the body as being connected, and therefore, one might massage the foot as part of an approach to helping someone with low back pain."

Little Improvement on Walking Test

Notwithstanding the encouraging pain results, participants didn't show much improvement in one measure in the study: a timed 50-foot walk.

"We're still learning about the effects of massage for those with knee OA—the different benefits, and the outcomes it may impact the most," explains Allen. "Regarding the walking test, there are many factors that could affect the results, such as muscle endurance and cardiovascular function. So it's not overly surprising that the results of this test, though improved, were not significantly different from baseline."

She says it could be that further gains would be seen with continued treatment. "It's possible that over time, massage therapy would help patients improve their walking ability even more. If their pain were reduced, they might be able to maintain greater daily physical activity, and therefore, build muscle strength and function."

Speaking of pain, the researchers say it's not clear whether massage could eliminate the need for medication. But used as an adjunct treatment, it could conceivably reduce the need.

"Even being able to reduce pain medication use would be a highly valued outcome for many patients," notes Allen. "We know from our prior studies among Veterans with OA that many would like to reduce reliance on medications for many reasons, including side effects and the possibility of longer-term risks."

Allen says the group plans to conduct a larger clinical trial and to also explore whether Veterans could do self-massage at home to help manage their arthritis.

Part Five

Living with Arthritis

Chapter 42

Living with Arthritis and Other Rheumatic Diseases

Almost 15 million U.S. adults live with severe joint pain-related to arthritis. Severe joint pain limits a person's ability to do basic tasks and affects their quality of life. Learning self-management skills and being active can help manage severe joint pain.

New Study on Severe Joint Pain

A new Centers for Disease Control and Prevention (CDC) study looked at severe joint pain among adults aged 18 years or older with arthritis. Study highlights include

- Severe joint pain from arthritis is from the breakdown of cartilage (tissues around a joint) in the body and pain that is not managed well.

- Severe joint pain occurs in more than one-third of 54 million adults with arthritis.

- The number of adults with arthritis and severe joint pain has increased significantly, reaching nearly 15 million in 2014 compared with more than 10 million in 2002.

This chapter contains text excerpted from the following sources: Text in this chapter begins with excerpts "Living with Severe Joint Pain," Centers for Disease Control and Prevention (CDC), March 7, 2017; Text under the heading "Managing Arthritis and Other Rheumatic Diseases" is excerpted from "Rabies," National Institute of Arthritis and Musculoskeletal and Skin Diseases (NIAMS), April 14, 2017.

• Some groups are affected by severe arthritis pain more than others and include African Americans, Hispanics/Latinos, people in fair to poor health, adults with serious psychological distress, people who are unable to work, and people with diabetes or heart disease.

What to Do to Ease Severe Joint Pain

People with severe joint pain related to arthritis have multiple ways to improve how they feel and enjoy life.

• **Get physically active.** CDC recommends that adults with arthritis be moderately physically active (e.g., walking, swimming, biking) for at least 150 minutes per week. CDC also recommends strength training. Further, physical activity has been proven to reduce arthritis pain. You can do low impact physical activity—like walking, biking, and swimming—30 minutes a day for 5 days a week to reduce joint pain. This can be done in ten-minute sessions throughout the day.

• **Go to CDC-recommended physical activity programs.** Particular community-based programs (such as EnhanceFitness and Walk With Ease) are helpful in learning how to exercise safely and reduce joint pain and disability related to arthritis. These programs can improve mood and ability to move as well. Classes take place at local Ys, parks, and community centers and help people with arthritis feel their best.

• **Enroll in proven programs.** Adults living with joint pain can benefit from joining CDC-recommended self-management education classes, which are designed to teach people with arthritis and other chronic conditions how to control their symptoms (like severe joint pain), live well with these conditions, and learn more about how to manage health problems that affect their lives.

Managing Arthritis and Other Rheumatic Diseases

There are many things you can do to help you live with arthritis and other rheumatic diseases, including the following.

• Exercise can reduce joint pain and stiffness and increase flexibility, muscle strength, and endurance. Exercise can help people lose weight, which reduces stress on painful joints. You should speak to your doctor about a safe, well-rounded exercise program.

- Diet is especially important if you have gout. You should avoid alcohol and foods that are high in purines, such as liver, kidney, sardines, anchovies, and gravy.

- Heat and cold therapies can reduce the pain and inflammation of arthritis. Heat therapy increases blood flow, tolerance for pain, and flexibility. Cold therapy numbs the nerves around the joint to reduce pain and may relieve inflammation and muscle spasms.

- Relaxation therapy can help reduce pain by teaching you ways to release muscle tension throughout the body.

- Splints and braces support weakened joints or allow them to rest. You should see your doctor before wearing a splint or brace to ensure proper fit. Otherwise, incorrect use of a splint or brace can cause joint damage, stiffness, and pain.

- Assistive devices, such as a cane to help with walking, can reduce some of the weight placed on a knee or hip affected by arthritis. A shoe insert (orthotic) can ease the pain of walking caused by arthritis of the foot or knee. Other devices can help with activities such as opening jars, closing zippers, and holding pencils.

Chapter 43

Healthy Eating and Arthritis

Studies involving people with arthritis have increasingly found links between their diet and the severity of their pain, inflammation, and other symptoms. Although no food or dietary supplement can cure arthritis, research has shown that some foods can lead to improvement in symptoms while other foods can lead to worsening of symptoms. These results have generated a great deal of interest in developing dietary therapies for the treatment of joint disorders. At the very least, eating a healthy, balanced diet can benefit people with arthritis by improving their general health, reducing inflammation, and strengthening bones.

Maintaining a healthy weight is a particular concern for people with arthritis because carrying extra pounds puts additional stress on weight-bearing joints. Studies have also shown that excess body fat contributes to inflammation. Fat cells release proteins called cytokines that can create a constant state of low-grade inflammation in the body. For arthritis patients who are overweight, therefore, losing weight can significantly reduce symptoms of pain and inflammation.

Diet can also play a role in reducing a person's likelihood of developing heart disease and circulatory problems, which are common side effects of arthritis and some of the medications used to treat it. Research has shown that certain foods help protect the body against heart disease, while other foods help control inflammation. The so-called Mediterranean diet includes many nutrients with powerful anti-inflammatory properties, such as omega-3 fatty acids, antioxidants, and phytochemicals. These nutrients are found in fish, olive oil, fruits and vegetables, nuts and seeds, and beans. Studies have found that consuming a diet rich in these foods can lead to improvements in pain, stiffness, and joint function for people with arthritis.

The Arthritis Diet

Given the impact that proper nutrition can have on arthritis symptoms, experts have developed dietary recommendations for people with arthritis. Many of these recommendations mirror the guidelines for healthy eating that the U.S. government publishes to help all Americans make informed food choices, maintain a healthy weight, reduce their risk of chronic disease, and improve their overall health. The adjustments for people with arthritis are mainly designed to limit foods that contribute to inflammation and increase foods with anti-inflammatory properties.

Foods to Avoid with Arthritis

- **Sodium.** Experts recommend that people with arthritis reduce their daily salt intake to 1,500 mg, which is less than half the daily intake of an average American. Excess sodium contributes to high blood pressure and kidney disease, and the corticosteroids commonly prescribed to treat arthritis cause the body to retain sodium.

- **Saturated fats.** Experts recommend that saturated fats—which are present in red meat, full-fat dairy products, creamy or cheesy pasta dishes, and many desserts—comprise less than ten percent of total calories. Saturated fats not only increase the risk of heart disease but also trigger inflammation in fat cells.

- **Trans fats.** Also known as partially hydrogenated oils, these inflammation-causing fats are found in fried and fast foods, in processed snacks like cookies, crackers, and donuts, and in most stick margarine. Experts recommend limiting consumption as much as possible.

- **Sugars.** The processed sugars found in baked goods, candy, sodas, and other sweetened foods trigger the release of cytokines that cause inflammation. Reducing sugar intake also offers the added benefits of lowering the risk of diabetes and promoting weight loss.

- **Refined carbohydrates.** Research has found links between the consumption of processed grain products (white breads, rolls, crackers, cereals, pastas, and rice) and increased levels of obesity, diabetes, and other chronic conditions. These high-glycemic foods also stimulate the release of chemicals that cause inflammation.

- **Alcohol.** Consumption of alcohol places stress on the liver, disrupts the function of other organs, and causes inflammation. Experts recommend eliminating it from the diet or using it in moderation, which is defined as one drink per day for women and two drinks per day for men.

Foods to Emphasize with Arthritis

- **Vegetables and fruits.** Dark green, leafy vegetables, including broccoli and Brussels sprouts, contain a variety of compounds that can help prevent or slow the progression of arthritis. Many fruits, particularly cherries, strawberries, and apples, also contain chemicals that help reduce inflammation and alleviate pain from arthritis.

- **Whole grains.** Eating whole, unrefined grains, including oatmeal and brown rice, has been associated with lower levels of inflammation indicators in the bloodstream.

- **Dairy products.** Low-fat dairy products, such as milk, yogurt, and cheese, contain calcium and vitamin D to help strengthen bones and boost the immune system.

- **Fish.** Certain types of fish, including salmon, tuna, mackerel, and herring, contain omega-3 fatty acids that help fight inflammation. Experts recommend eating a four-ounce portion twice each week in place of other meats and poultry.

- **Healthy oils.** Many oils offer health benefits, such as reducing inflammation, protecting the heart, and lowering cholesterol. Some of the best options include olive, safflower, avocado, and walnut oils. Experts recommend using these oils to replace solid fats wherever possible.

- **Green tea.** Full of antioxidants, green tea is believed to slow down the process of cartilage and joint damage in people with arthritis.

- **Allium.** Foods in the allium family, which includes onions, garlic, and leeks, contain compounds that limit cartilage damage and slow the progress of arthritis in people who consume them regularly.

Dietary Management of Gout

Gout is a type of arthritis that results from hyperuricemia, the buildup of uric acid in the joints. Uric acid is formed as the body breaks down purine, a naturally occurring organic substance that is found in many foods. Ordinarily, excess uric acid is excreted from the cells and eliminated from the body in urine. People with gout either produce too much uric acid or have trouble eliminating it from the body. The excess uric acid forms crystals in the joints, resulting in inflammation and severe pain.

Studies suggest that gout has a significant dietary component. Eating foods that contain high levels of purine may increase the risk of getting gout, while consuming certain other foods may reduce the frequency of gout attacks or help slow the progression of the disease. Doctors recommend that people with gout maintain a healthy body weight and drink plenty of water to help flush urate crystals from the body. They also suggest increasing consumption of cherries and berries, which contain anthocyanins that help reduce inflammation. Studies have also shown that consuming coffee and low-fat dairy products may help lower uric acid levels.

Foods to Limit with Gout

Doctors recommend that people with gout avoid consuming foods high in purine. Since it may be difficult to completely eliminate purine from the diet, people with gout are generally encouraged to eat a healthy, balanced diet that strictly limits the following foods:

- alcohol, especially beer
- anchovies
- asparagus
- beef kidneys
- brains
- dried beans and peas
- game meats

- gravy
- herring
- liver
- mackerel
- mushrooms
- sardines
- scallops
- sweetbreads

References

1. Arthritis Foundation. "Arthritis Diet," n.d.

2. Arthritis Research UK. "Diet and Arthritis," 2013.

3. National Institute of Arthritis and Musculoskeletal and Skin Diseases. "Questions and Answers about Gout," USA.gov, June 2015.

4. U.S. Department of Agriculture and U.S. Department of Health and Human Services. Dietary Guidelines for Americans, 2010. 7th Edition, Washington, DC: U.S. Government Printing Office, December 2010.

Chapter 44

Arthritis and Mental Health

Having a long-term illness such as arthritis may contribute to stress, depression, and problems with emotions. Adults with arthritis are limited in their everyday activities, have lower employment than those without arthritis, and have other chronic diseases such as diabetes or heart disease. All of these integrated factors may impact their mental and emotional well-being. In addition, poor mental health can exacerbate functional disabilities, affect adherence to treatment, and be a barrier to self-care. Healthcare providers can help by screening all adults with arthritis for depression, anxiety, and other emotional problems. Healthcare providers can also refer those suffering from arthritis and other chronic conditions to appropriate care services and disease management education programs.

This chapter contains text excerpted from the following sources: Text in this chapter begins with excerpts from "Association of Painful Musculoskeletal Conditions and Migraine Headache with Mental and Sleep Disorders among Adults with Disabilities, Spain, 2007–2008," Centers for Disease Control and Prevention (CDC), February 27, 2014. Reviewed April 2018; Text beginning with the heading "Chronic Illness and Higher Risk of Depression" is excerpted from "Chronic Illness and Mental Health," National Institute of Mental Health (NIMH), December 2015; Text under the heading "Self-Management Programs: A Proven Public Health Strategy That Enhances Physical and Psychological Well-Being" is excerpted from "Help Members of Your Community Thrive," Centers for Disease Control and Prevention (CDC), June 19, 2012. Reviewed April 2018; Text under the heading "Arthritis Self-Management Program (ASMP)" is excerpted from "Self-Management Education," Centers for Disease Control and Prevention (CDC), December 4, 2017.

Effect of Mental–Physical Comorbidity on Severe Disability

The association between painful conditions and anxiety or depression has been addressed in clinical settings and population-based studies. In these populations, negative emotional factors play an important role in the perception and experience of pain, and pain intensity is consistently documented as a predictor of physical disability and depression. The relationship between chronic pain and depression or anxiety is complex, and according to some researchers, reciprocal. However, the mechanisms that associate depression and anxiety with increased sensitivity to pain and greater disability remain poorly understood.

A synergistic effect of mental-physical comorbidity on severe disability has been reported, and mechanisms for this synergy have been proposed, including the possibility that depression exacerbates the disabling effect of a chronic physical condition by influencing treatment adherence and healthy behavior. Depression can also interfere with the psychological capacity to adjust to physical conditions, and it can affect the perception and appraisal of pain and the ability to cope with it.

Gender Response to Disability and Pain

The stronger link between depression and disability (both physical and mental) in women than in men further complicates the aforementioned relationships, suggesting that depression may have a greater disabling effect on women who suffer from pain. Anxiety has also been proposed to potentially mediate the sex differences in pain sensitivity; women tend to report higher levels of anxiety and are more likely to have anxiety disorders. However, increasing evidence suggests that anxiety is more strongly associated with pain responses in men than in women, and inconsistent or contradictory results have been reported on the direction of the link between anxiety and chronic pain within sexes and across outcome measures.

Chronic Illness and Higher Risk of Depression

The same factors that increase the risk of depression in otherwise healthy people also raise the risk in people with other medical illnesses. These risk factors include a personal or family history of depression or loss of family members to suicide. Illness-related anxiety and stress can also trigger symptoms of depression. Sometimes, symptoms of depression may follow a recent medical diagnosis but

456

lift as you adjust or as the other condition is treated. In other cases, certain medications used to treat the illness may trigger depression. Depression may persist, even as physical health improves.

Research suggests that people who have depression and another medical illness tend to have more severe symptoms of both illnesses. They may have more difficulty adapting to their co-occurring illness and more medical costs than those who do not also have depression.

It is not yet clear whether treatment of depression when another illness is present can improve physical health. However, it is still important to seek treatment. It can make a difference in day-to-day life if you are coping with a chronic or long-term illness.

Depression Is Treatable Even When Other Illness Is Present

Do not dismiss depression as a normal part of having a chronic illness. Effective treatment for depression is available and can help even if you have another medical illness or condition. If you or a loved one think you have depression, it is important to tell your healthcare provider and explore treatment options.

You should also inform the healthcare provider about all treatments or medications you are already receiving, including treatment for depression (prescribed medications and dietary supplements). Sharing information can help avoid problems with multiple medications interfering with each other. It also helps the provider stay informed about your overall health and treatment issues.

Recovery from depression takes time, but treatment can improve the quality of life even if you have a medical illness. Treatments for depression include:

- **Cognitive behavioral therapy (CBT)**, or talk therapy, that helps people change negative thinking styles and behaviors that may contribute to their depression. Interpersonal and other types of time-limited psychotherapy have also been proven effective, in some cases combined with antidepressant medication.

- **Antidepressant medications**, including, but not limited to, selective serotonin reuptake inhibitors (SSRIs) and serotonin and norepinephrine reuptake inhibitors (SNRIs).

- **While electroconvulsive therapy (ECT)** is generally reserved for the most severe cases of depression, newer brain stimulation approaches, including transcranial magnetic stimulation (TMS), can help some people with depression without the need for general anesthesia and with few side effects.

Self-Management Programs: A Proven Public Health Strategy That Enhances Physical and Psychological Well-Being

Chronic disease takes enormous toll on people's' lives. It causes pain, disability, decreased physical activity, and poor emotional health, which can seriously compromise the quality of daily life. Fortunately, there are community self-help programs that can help people with chronic diseases learn how to manage symptoms and maintain active and fulfilling lives. Self-management education programs have been proven to significantly help people with chronic conditions. As a complement to clinical care, these programs teach participants how to exercise properly and eat healthy, use medications appropriately, solve everyday problems, and communicate effectively with family members and healthcare providers—all positive life skills to enhance well-being. As a result, these interventions help participants reduce pain, depression, fear, and frustration; improve mobility and exercise; increase energy; and boost confidence in their ability to manage their condition.

Arthritis Self-Management Program (ASMP)

ASMP, previously called the Arthritis Foundation Self-Help Program, is an effective self-management education intervention for people with arthritis. Developed by Dr. Kate Lorig of Stanford University, the course helps people learn and practice the different techniques needed to build an individualized self-management program and gain the confidence to carry it out. The 6-week interactive workshop consists of weekly 2-hour sessions guided by two trained instructors, at least one of which has arthritis. This program covers topic such as techniques to deal with problems associated with arthritis, appropriate exercise, appropriate use of medications, communicating effectively with family, friends, and health professionals, nutrition and, how to evaluate new treatments. There is a robust science base that demonstrates the positive impacts of participation in ASMP. One year after participating in the program, people continue to report greater confidence in their ability to manage their arthritis, less fatigue, and less depressed mood, anxiety, and frustration or worry about their health.

Chapter 45

Maintaining Independence

Chapter Contents

Section 45.1—Modifying Your Home for
Independence.. 460

Section 45.2—Avoiding Falls and Fractures 464

Section 45.3—Assistive Devices Can Make Life with
Arthritis Easier 470

Section 45.4—Driving When You Have Arthritis 473

Section 45.1

Modifying Your Home for Independence

This section includes text excerpted from "Aging in Place: Growing
Old at Home," National Institute on Aging (NIA), National Institutes
of Health (NIH), May 1, 2017.

Planning Ahead to Stay in Your Home

Planning ahead is hard because you never know how your needs
might change. The first step is to think about the kinds of help you
might want in the near future. Maybe you live alone, so there is no
one living in your home who is available to help you. Maybe you don't
need help right now, but you live with a spouse or family member who
does. Everyone has a different situation.

One way to begin planning is to look at any illnesses, like diabetes
or emphysema, that you or your spouse might have. Talk with your
doctor about how these health problems could make it hard for someone to get around or take care of him or herself in the future. If you're
a caregiver for an older adult, learn how you can get them the support
they need to stay in their own home.

What Support Can Help Me Stay at Home?

You can get almost any type of help you want in your home—often
for a cost. You can get more information on many of the services listed
here from your local Area Agency on Aging (AAA), local and state offices
on aging or social services, tribal organization, or nearby senior center.

Personal care. Is bathing, washing your hair, or dressing getting
harder to do? Maybe a relative or friend could help. Or, you could hire
a trained aide for a short time each day.

Household chores. Do you need help with chores like house cleaning, yard work, grocery shopping, or laundry? Some grocery stores and
drug stores will take your order over the phone and bring the items
to your home. There are cleaning and yard services you can hire, or
maybe someone you know has a housekeeper or gardener to suggest.

Some housekeepers will help with laundry. Some drycleaners will pick up and deliver your clothes.

Meals. Worried that you might not be eating nutritious meals or tired of eating alone? Sometimes you could share cooking with a friend or have a potluck dinner with a group of friends. Find out if meals are served at a nearby senior center or house of worship. Eating out may give you a chance to visit with others. Is it hard for you to get out? Ask someone to bring you a healthy meal a few times a week. Meal delivery programs bring hot meals into your home; some of these programs are free or low-cost.

Money management. Do you worry about paying bills late or not at all? Are health insurance forms confusing? Maybe you can get help with these tasks. Ask a trusted relative to lend a hand. Volunteers, financial counselors, or geriatric care managers can also help. Just make sure you get the referral from a trustworthy source, like your local AAA. If you use a computer, you could pay your bills online. Check with your bank about this option. Some people have regular bills like utilities and rent or mortgage paid automatically from their checking account.

Be careful to avoid money scams. Never give your Social Security number, bank or credit card numbers, or other sensitive information to someone on the phone (unless you placed the call) or in response to an email. Always check all bills, including utility bills, for charges you do not recognize.

Even though you might not need it now, think about giving someone you trust permission to discuss your bills with creditors or your Social Security or Medicare benefits with those agencies.

Healthcare. Do you forget to take your medicine? There are devices available to remind you when it is time for your next dose. Special pill boxes allow you or someone else to set out your pills for an entire week. Have you just gotten out of the hospital and still need nursing care at home for a short time? The hospital discharge planner can help you make arrangements, and Medicare might pay for a home health aide to come to your home.

If you can't remember what the doctor told you to do, try to have someone go to your doctor visits with you. Ask them to write down everything you are supposed to do or, if you are by yourself, ask the doctor to put all recommendations in writing.

Be Prepared for a Medical Emergency. If you were to suddenly become sick and unable to speak for yourself, you probably would want someone who knows you well to decide on your medical care. To make sure this happens, think about giving someone you trust permission

461

to discuss your healthcare with your doctor and make necessary decisions. Talk with your doctor about whether you should get a medical alert ID bracelet or necklace.

Aging in Place: Common Concerns

If staying in your home is important to you, you may still have concerns about safety, getting around, or other activities of daily life. Find suggestions below to help you think about some of these worries.

Getting around—at home and in town. Are you having trouble walking? Perhaps a walker would help. If you need more, think about getting an electric chair or scooter. These are sometimes covered by Medicare. Do you need someone to go with you to the doctor or shopping? Volunteer escort services may be available. If you are no longer driving a car, find out if there are free or low-cost public transportation and taxis in your area. Maybe a relative, friend, or neighbor would take you along when they go on errands or do yours for you. To learn about resources in your community, contact Eldercare Locator at 800-677-1116 (toll-free) or www.eldercare.gov.

Activities and friends. Are you bored staying at home? Your local senior center offers a variety of activities. You might see friends there and meet new people too. Is it hard for you to leave your home? Maybe you would enjoy visits from someone. Volunteers are sometimes available to stop by or call once a week. They can just keep you company, or you can talk about any problems you are having. Call your local AAA to see if they are available near you.

Safety. Are you worried about crime in your neighborhood, physical abuse, or losing money as a result of a scam? Talk to the staff at your local AAA. If you live alone, are you afraid of becoming sick with no one around to help? You might want to get an emergency alert system. You just push a special button that you wear, and emergency medical personnel are called. There is typically a monthly fee for this service.

Housing. Would a few changes make your home easier and safer to live in? Think about things like a ramp at the front door, grab bars in the tub or shower, nonskid floors, more comfortable handles on doors or faucets, and better insulation. Sound expensive? You might be able to get help paying for these changes. Check with your local AAA, state housing finance agency, welfare department, community development groups, or the federal government.

Help during the day. Do you need care but live with someone who can't stay with you during the day? For example, maybe they work. Adult day care outside the home is sometimes available for older people who need help caring for themselves. The daycare center can pick you up and bring you home. If your caretaker needs to get away overnight, there are places that provide temporary respite care.

Where Can I Look for Help Staying at Home?

Here are some resources to start with:

People you know. Family, friends, and neighbors are the biggest source of help for many older people. Talk with those close to you about the best way to get what you need. If you are physically able, think about trading services with a friend or neighbor. One could do the grocery shopping, and the other could cook dinner, for example.

Community and local government resources. Learn about the services in your community. Healthcare providers and social workers may have suggestions. The local AAA, local and state offices on aging or social services, and your tribal organization may have lists of services. If you belong to a religious group, talk with the clergy, or check with its local office about any senior services they offer.

Geriatric care managers. These specially trained professionals can help find resources to make your daily life easier. They will work with you to form a long-term care plan and find the services you need. Geriatric care managers can be helpful when family members live far apart.

Federal government sources. The federal government offers many resources for seniors. Longtermcare.gov, from the Administration for Community Living (ACL), is a good place to start.

How Much Will It Cost to Get Help at Home?

An important part of planning is thinking about how you are going to pay for the help you need. Some things you want may cost a lot. Others may be free. Some might be covered by Medicare or other health insurance. Some may not. Check with your insurance provider(s). It's possible that paying for a few services out of pocket could cost less than moving into an independent living, assisted living, or long-term care facility. And you will have your wish of still living on your own. Resources like Benefits.gov and BenefitsCheckUp® can help you find out about possible benefits you might qualify for.

Section 45.2

Avoiding Falls and Fractures

This section includes text excerpted from "Preventing
Falls and Related Fractures," NIH Osteoporosis and
Related Bone Diseases~National Resource
Center (NIH ORBD~NRC), April 2015.

Falls are serious at any age and breaking a bone after a fall becomes
more likely as a person ages. Many of us know someone who has fallen
and broken a bone. While healing, the fracture limits the person's
activities and sometimes requires surgery. Often, the person wears a
heavy cast to support the broken bone and needs physical therapy to
resume normal activities. People are often unaware of the frequent
link between a broken bone and osteoporosis. It is known as a silent
disease because it progresses without symptoms, osteoporosis involves
the gradual loss of bone tissue or bone density and results in bones so
fragile they break under the slightest strain. Consequently, falls are
especially dangerous for people who are unaware that they have low
bone density. If the patient and the doctor fail to connect the broken
bone to osteoporosis, the chance to make a diagnosis with a bone density test and begin a prevention or treatment program is lost. Bone
loss continues, and other bones may break.

Even though bones do not break after every fall, the person who
has fallen and broken a bone nearly always becomes fearful of falling again. As a result, she or he may limit activities for the sake of
"safety." Among Americans age 65 and older, fall-related injuries are
the leading cause of accidental death.

This section explores the components of the Fracture Triangle and
offers tips for reducing the chances of fall-related fractures that result
from low bone mass and osteoporosis. If one of the following three factors is modified, the chances of breaking a bone are greatly reduced:

The Fall Itself

Several factors can lead to a fall. Loss of footing or traction is a
common cause of falls. Loss of footing occurs when there is less than

total contact between one's foot and the ground or floor. Loss of traction occurs when one's feet slip on wet or slippery ground or floor. Other examples of loss of traction include tripping, especially over uneven surfaces such as sidewalks, curbs, or floor elevations that result from carpeting, risers, or scatter rugs. Loss of footing also happens from using household items intended for other purposes—for example, climbing on kitchen chairs or balancing on boxes or books to increase height.

A fall may occur because a person's reflexes have changed. As people age, reflexes slow down. Reflexes are automatic responses to stimuli in the environment. Examples of reflexes include quickly slamming on the car brakes when a child runs into the street or quickly moving out of the way when something accidentally falls. Aging slows a person's reaction time and makes it harder to regain one's balance following a sudden movement or shift of body weight.

Improving Balance

- Do muscle-strengthening exercises
- Obtain maximum vision correction
- Practice using bifocal or trifocal glasses
- Practice balance exercises daily

Changes in muscle mass and body fat also can play a role in falls. As people get older, they lose muscle mass because they have become less active over time. Loss of muscle mass, especially in the legs, reduces one's strength to the point where she or he is often unable to get up from a chair without assistance. In addition, as people age, they lose body fat that has cushioned and protected bony areas, such as the hips. This loss of cushioning also affects the soles of the feet, which upsets the person's ability to balance. The gradual loss of muscle strength, which is common in older people but not inevitable, also plays a role in falling. Muscle-strengthening exercises can help people regain their balance, level of activity, and alertness no matter what their age.

Changes in vision also increase the risk of falling. Diminished vision can be corrected with glasses. However, often these glasses are bifocal or trifocal so that when the person looks down through the lower half of her or his glasses, depth perception is altered. This makes it easy to lose one's balance and fall. To prevent this from happening, people who wear bifocals or trifocals must practice looking straight ahead and lowering their head. For many other older people, vision changes cannot be corrected completely, making even the home environment hazardous.

Medications That May Increase the Risk of Falling

- Blood pressure pills
- Heart medicines
- Diuretics or water pills
- Muscle relaxers or tranquilizers

As people get older, they also are more likely to suffer from a variety of chronic medical conditions that often require taking several medications. People with chronic illnesses that affect their circulation, sensation, mobility, or mental alertness as well as those taking some types of medications are more likely to fall as a result of drug-related side effects such as dizziness, confusion, disorientation, or slowed reflexes.

Drinking alcoholic beverages also increases the risk of falling. Alcohol slows reflexes and response time; causes dizziness, sleepiness, or lightheadedness; alters balance, and encourages risky behaviors that can lead to falls.

The Force and Direction of a Fall

The force of a fall (how hard a person lands) plays a major role in determining whether or not a person will break a bone. For example, the greater the distance of the hip bone to the floor, the greater the risk of fracturing a hip, so tall people appear to have an increased risk of fracture when they fall. The angle at which a person falls also is important. For example, falling sideways or straight down is riskier than falling backward.

Protective responses, such as reflexes and changes in posture that break the fall, can reduce the risk of fracturing a bone. Individuals who land on their hands or grab an object on their descent are less likely to fracture their hip, but they may fracture their wrist or arm. Although these fractures are painful and interfere with daily activities, they do not carry the high risks that a hip fracture does.

The type of surface on which one lands also can affect whether or not a bone breaks. Landing on a soft surface is less likely to cause a fracture than landing on a hard surface.

Preliminary research suggests that by wearing trochanteric (hip) padding, people can decrease the chances of fracturing a hip after a fall. The energy created by the fall is distributed throughout the pad, lessening the impact to the hip. Further research is needed to fully evaluate the role of these devices in decreasing the risk of a hip fracture following a fall.

Bone Fragility

Although most serious falls happen when people are older, steps to prevent and treat bone loss and falls can never begin too early. Many people begin adulthood with less than optimal bone mass, so the fact that bone mass or density is lost slowly over time puts them at increased risk for fractures.

Bones that once were strong become so fragile and thin that they break easily. Activities that once were done without a second thought are now avoided for fear that they will lead to another fracture.

Prevention of Falls and Fractures

Safety first to prevent falls: At any age, people can change their environments to reduce their risk of falling and breaking a bone.

Outdoor safety tips:

- In nasty weather, use a walker or cane for added stability.

- Wear warm boots with rubber soles for added traction.

- Look carefully at floor surfaces in public buildings. Many floors are made of highly polished marble or tile that can be very slippery. If floors have plastic or carpet runners in place, stay on them whenever possible.

- Identify community services that can provide assistance, such as 24-hour pharmacies and grocery stores that take orders over the phone and deliver. It is especially important to use these services in bad weather.

- Use a shoulder bag, fanny pack, or backpack to leave hands free.

- Stop at curbs and check their height before stepping up or down. Be cautious at curbs that have been cut away to allow access for bikes or wheelchairs. The incline up or down may lead to a fall.

Indoor safety tips:

- Keep all rooms free from clutter, especially the floors.

- Keep floor surfaces smooth but not slippery. When entering rooms, be aware of differences in floor levels and thresholds.

- Wear supportive, low-heeled shoes, even at home. Avoid walking around in socks, stockings, or floppy, backless slippers.

- Check that all carpets and area rugs have skid-proof backing or are tacked to the floor, including carpeting on stairs.

- Keep electrical and telephone cords and wires out of walkways.

- Be sure that all stairwells are adequately lit and that stairs have handrails on both sides. Consider placing fluorescent tape on the edges of the top and bottom steps.

- For optimal safety, install grab bars on bathroom walls beside tubs, showers, and toilets. If you are unstable on your feet, consider using a plastic chair with a back and nonskid leg tips in the shower.

- Use a rubber bath mat in the shower or tub.

- Keep a flashlight with fresh batteries beside your bed.

- Add ceiling fixtures to rooms lit by lamps only, or install lamps that can be turned on by a switch near the entry point into the room. Another option is to install voice- or sound-activated lamps.

- Use bright light bulbs in your home.

- If you must use a step-stool for hard-to-reach areas, use a sturdy one with a handrail and wide steps. A better option is to reorganize work and storage areas to minimize the need for stooping or excessive reaching.

- Consider purchasing a portable phone that you can take with you from room to room. It provides security because you can answer the phone without rushing to it and you can call for help should an accident occur.

- Don't let prescriptions run low. Always keep at least 1 week's worth of medications on hand at home. Check prescriptions with your doctor and pharmacist to see if they may be increasing your risk of falling. If you take multiple medications, check with your doctor and pharmacist about possible interactions between the different medications.

- Arrange with a family member or friend for daily contact. Try to have at least one person who knows where you are.

- If you live alone, you may wish to contract with a monitoring company that will respond to your call 24 hours a day.

- Watch yourself in a mirror. Does your body lean or sway back and forth or side to side? People with the decreased ability to balance often have a high degree of body sway and are more likely to fall.

Reducing the Force of a Fall

Take steps to lessen your chances of breaking a bone in the event that you do fall:

- Remember that falling sideways or straight down is more likely to result in a hip fracture than falling in other directions. If possible, try to fall forward or to land on your buttocks.

- If possible, land on your hands or use objects around you to break a fall.

- Walk carefully, especially on hard surfaces.

- When possible, wear protective clothing for padding.

- Talk to your doctor about whether you may be a candidate for hip padding.

Decreasing Bone Fragility

Individuals can protect bone health by following osteoporosis prevention and treatment strategies:

- Consume a calcium-rich diet that provides between 1,000 mg (milligrams) daily for men and women up to age 50. Women over age 50 and men over age 70 should increase their intake to 1,200 mg daily from a combination of foods and supplements.

- Obtain 600 IU (International Units) of vitamin D daily up to age 70. Men and women over age 70 should increase their uptake to 800 IU daily.

- Participate in weight-bearing and resistance-training exercises most days, preferably daily.

- Talk with your doctor about having a bone mineral density (BMD) test. The most widely recognized BMD test is called a dual-energy X-ray absorptiometry, or DXA test. It is painless, a bit like having an X-ray, but with much less exposure to radiation. It can measure bone density at your hip and spine.

• Talk with your doctor about possibly beginning a medication approved by the Food and Drug Administration for osteoporosis to stop bone loss, improve bone density, and reduce fracture risk.

People need to know whether they are at risk for developing osteoporosis or whether they have lost so much bone that they already have osteoporosis. Although risk factors can alert a person to the possibility of low bone density, only a BMD test can measure current bone density, diagnose osteoporosis, and determine fracture risk. Many different techniques measure bone mineral density painlessly and safely. Most of them involve machines that use extremely low levels of radiation to complete their readings. Sometimes, ultrasound machines, which rely on sound waves, are used instead.

Individuals may wish to have a BMD test to determine current bone health. Medicare and many private insurance carriers cover bone density tests to detect osteoporosis for individuals who meet certain criteria. Talk with your doctor about whether or not this test would be appropriate for you. Falls are serious, but simple, inexpensive steps can be taken to reduce your risk of falling and of breaking a bone if you do fall.

Section 45.3

Assistive Devices Can Make Life with Arthritis Easier

"Assistive Devices," © 2015 Omnigraphics.
Reviewed April 2018.

The joint pain and stiffness associated with arthritis can make it difficult for people to accomplish everyday self-care tasks, such as bathing, dressing, cooking, cleaning, and move around. A variety of assistive technologies and adaptive devices have been developed to help people accomplish these tasks with less pain and make it easier for them to live independently. Assistive technology can improve or conserve functional capabilities of people with arthritis, enabling them to perform tasks that were once difficult to accomplish. Self-help devices for arthritis can range from simple rubber grippers that help people open jars to sophisticated robots that can process sensory information and compensate for a partial or total loss of function. Since arthritis is a lifelong condition, the most appropriate tools to help manage it may change over time.

Recognizing the Need for Assistive Devices

As people with arthritis experience gradual changes in their ability levels, they sometimes simply give up their favorite activities. They may not be aware that using adaptive equipment could enable them to continue enjoying these activities. Arthritis affects every person differently, so the decision about when to use assistive devices is an individual one. Recognizing the need for help with certain tasks is the first step in the process. The type of equipment required depends on the stage of the disease, the degree of disability, and the kind of task to be accomplished. Patients with rheumatoid arthritis, for instance, often find it difficult to perform tasks that require the joints to bear weight or oppose resistance. As a result, they tend to gain the most functional capability from products that provide joint support, increase leverage for lifting, and extend a range of motion.

Acquiring Assistive Devices

The best place to begin the process of acquiring assistive devices may be the doctor's office. A general practitioner or a rheumatologist can provide a referral to an occupational therapist. These medical professionals specialize in helping people with arthritis or other forms of disability accomplish daily tasks and live independently. They can evaluate a patient's home and work environments and recommend changes or adaptive equipment that may simplify many activities of daily living.

Many types of assistive devices and adaptive equipment can be purchased from hardware stores, medical supply companies, full-service pharmacies, or online retailers. Some stores provide training in the use of devices or offer help with the installation of equipment. Nonprofit organizations such as the Arthritis Foundation are another potential source of information about the range of devices available and the best places to get them. The U.S. Rehabilitation Services Administration (RSA) also supports Centers for Independent Living (CIL) in many communities across the country. These centers employ technology specialists who can recommend assistive devices to fit an individual's level of disability and specific needs. They also offer demonstrations on how to use assistive devices.

Types of Assistive Devices

Many different types of assistive devices are available to help people with arthritis perform the following daily activities:

- **Getting around.** Common devices that can help people with arthritis stand and walk more easily include orthotic shoe inserts, braces and splints, a cane or crutch, and extenders for chair legs.

- **Preparing food.** Assistive devices that can reduce joint strain in the kitchen include reach extenders, jar openers, lever-style faucets, large cabinet knobs, step stools, and labor-saving devices like electric can openers, food processors, dishwashers, and slow cookers.

- **Personal care.** Adaptive equipment to make bathing and grooming easier include handrails in the tub or shower, long-handled brushes or bath mitts, elevated toilet seats, and electric toothbrushes and razors.

- **Dressing.** Devices designed to assist people with arthritic limitations in getting dressed include sock pullers, zipper hooks, buttoning aids, and shoehorns.

- **Working.** Many types of workplace modifications and accommodations can help people with arthritis perform the functions of employment, including hands-free headsets, adjustable work tables, ergonomic workstation designs, and accessible restrooms.

- **Driving.** In addition to special car adaptations like steering wheel knobs, swivel seats, and wheelchair hoists, cars can be fitted with panoramic mirrors, seatbelt aids, and keyless entry and ignition systems to make driving easier for people with arthritis.

References

1. Arthritis Foundation. "Self-Help Arthritis Devices," n.d.

2. "Assistive Devices for Easier Living with RA," WebMD, 2014.

3. Brichford, Connie. "Assistive Devices for Rheumatoid Arthritis," Everyday Health, 2015.

Section 45.4

Driving When You Have Arthritis

This section includes text excerpted from "Driving
When You Have Arthritis," National Highway Traffic Safety
Administration (NHTSA), 2007. Reviewed April 2018.

You have been a safe driver for years. For you, driving means freedom and control. As you get older, changes in your physical and mental health can affect how safely you drive. Millions of people have arthritis. It causes pain, swelling, and stiffness in your body. If you have arthritis, talk with your family and healthcare provider about how it can affect your driving.

How Can Arthritis Affect the Way I Drive?

Arthritis can stop you from moving and bending your shoulders, hips, hands, head, and neck. This can limit your ability to:

- Get into and out of your car

- Hold and turn your steering wheel

- Turn on your ignition key

- Fasten your seat belt

- Move your head quickly and fully

- Look over your shoulder to check for cars in your blind spot

- Look left and right at intersections

- Make turns safely. Reverse your car into a parking space.

- Press the clutch pedal

- Press the brake and accelerator, especially in heavy traffic or driving during rush hours

- Look for oncoming traffic

Medicine for arthritis pain can make you sleepy. It may cause you to drift into another traffic lane, which can be dangerous for you and others.

What Should I Do if I Have Any of These Signs?

As soon as you notice one or more of these warning signs:

- Tell your family or someone you trust.

- See your healthcare provider.

- Find out about treatments that can help your joint pain, swelling, and stiffness, without making you sleepy.

What Can I Do When Arthritis Affects My Driving Safety?

It is important to understand how over time arthritis can change your driving safety. Your healthcare provider may suggest that you see a specialist to help you adjust to these changes. Two types of specialists can help you:

- A driver rehabilitation specialist can test how well you drive on and off the road.

- An occupational therapist with special training may be able to help in driving skills assessment and remediation. To find an occupational therapist, contact local hospitals and rehabilitation centers.

What Can I Do If I Have to Limit or Stop Driving?

If you have arthritis, you may still be able to drive safely. Work closely with your healthcare provider to manage your symptoms. Even if you have to limit or give up driving, you can stay active and do the things you like to do. First, plan ahead. Talk with family and friends about how you can shift from driver to passenger. Below are some ways to get where you want to go and see the people you want to see:

- Rides with family and friends

- Taxis, shuttle buses, or vans

- Public buses, trains, and subways

- Walking

- Paratransit services (special transportation services for people with disabilities) may help. Some offer door-to-door service.

Take someone with you. You may want to have a family member or friend go with you when you use public transportation or when you walk. Having someone with you can help you get where you want to go without confusion.

Find out about transportation services in your area. Many community-based volunteer programs offer free or low-cost transportation.

Chapter 46

Arthritis and Sexuality

One of the most common casualties of chronic illness is sexuality. Arthritis rarely affects reproductive organs, but physical symptoms such as functional disability and pain, common to arthritic disorders such as lupus, fibromyalgia, osteoarthritis, or rheumatoid arthritis, can greatly impact sexual function regardless of gender or age. While the severity of joint degeneration, fatigue, and degree of pain are the most important factors that have a direct bearing on intimacy issues and sexual expression, other factors, such as side effects of medication/surgery, and negative attitudes arising from poor sexual self-perception may also significantly impact sexual expression and enjoyment. These usually manifest differently in men and women. In men, arthritic disease may lead to erectile dysfunction (ED) and possible impotence, while women may experience vaginal dryness and a lowered sense of sexual desire and satisfaction. Also, as in the case of any chronic illness, living with arthritis is generally associated with depression and anxiety—and these, depending on the severity of pain and the loss of functional mobility, may often lead to a reactive loss of interest in sex.

Effect of Medication on Sexual Function

While most medications used to treat arthritis may have little effect on sexual functioning, instances of ED and erectile impotence

"Arthritis and Sexuality," © 2018 Omnigraphics. Reviewed April 2018.

have been reported with some disease-modifying anti-rheumatic drugs (DMARDs) such as methotrexate or hydroxychloroquine, which are used to control pain and swelling associated with arthritis and reduce damage to joints and long-term disability. Some antidepressant medications used to treat depression associated with arthritis are also known to cause problems with arousal, erection, and orgasm.

Sex after Joint Replacement

Joint replacement surgeries may often be rewarding in terms of sexual function, but care needs to be exercised before resuming any kind of normal activity, including sex. Depending on the extent of joint damage and type of surgery performed, the surgeon may advise rest during the initial period of diminished range of motion or flexibility following arthroplasty. After this period, patients are encouraged to resume normal activity of the joint within a "safe" range of motion. Typically, a newly replaced joint remains unstable for a period of time and patients are advised against forceful, extreme movements that can dislocate the new joint during sexual activity. Stretching and mild medication before sex may help relax muscles, but strong medication is not advised as it masks pain which can actually indicate a problem with recovery. As part of general postsurgery rehabilitation, the healthcare team may counsel patients on which sex positions to avoid so as to not exert pressure on the new joint.

Overcoming Barriers

Arthritis can adversely affect comfortable movements, regarded as important physical and psychosocial factors of sexual function. One of the first steps to overcoming barriers to sexual expression is learning to accept changes in sexual expression while gradually establishing a new paradigm that can help patients work around limitations set by disability and pain. Initiating a conversation on the subject with one's partner can go a long way toward addressing sexual problems associated with the disease. Healthcare providers also need to initiate discussion in this area, as such discussions can offer a platform that allows patients to acknowledge their fears; cope with loss of normal sexual function, and find ways to improve their sexual experience. A sex therapist may also assist patients in dealing with problems arising from sexual expressions associated with joint disease.

While sexuality may not be an issue at the time of diagnosis or during early onset of the disease, it may become particularly important as the disease progresses and relationships gravitate from part-ner-partner to partner-caregiver. Although most patients want to strive for normalcy in sexual expression and a return to their predis-ease status, it is important for them to accept their altered status with respect to their sexuality and to find creative ways to achieve sexual satisfaction despite their disability. Communicating with one's partner about their fears is the first step in overcoming potential barriers to sexual activity. In this regard, letting one's partner know if something is causing discomfiture, or if something is particularly pleasurable, may help take the strain off the relationship.

Maintaining Sexual Well-Being with Arthritis

- **Physical activity** is an important facet in improving physical and mental wellbeing for people with arthritis and can positively impact sexual expression by increasing muscle strength and tone to improve range of motion of the affected joints.

- **Planning ahead** to beat the symptoms. Engaging in sex soon after a relaxing massage or a warm shower may help make a patient's sexual experience less painful. It also helps to engage in sexual activity an hour after taking a painkiller. Women who experience vaginal dryness may find penetrative sex painful. Water-based gels offer lubrication and reduce pain associated with manual stimulation or penetration.

- **Thinking outside the box** by trying new positions that ease pressure on affected joints or by using props (pillows, furniture) can substantially reduce the discomfort associated with traditional sexual positions. Furthermore, penetrative sex does not have to be the only goal. Investing in physical and emotional intimacy may also help strengthen bonds and achieve sexual satisfaction.

- **Sex toys,** or devices used to facilitate sexual pleasure, are read-ily available online and can be particularly helpful for genital stimulation.

- **Sex counselors** can sometimes offer more benefits to patients having difficulties adjusting to limitations set by joint disease than a primary clinician can. Sex counselors can help in sexual rehabilitation by facilitating honest communication. They can offer advice related to the physical and functional aspects of sexual activity and thereby help partners develop a mutually rewarding sexual relationship despite disability.

References

1. "Sexual Function before and after Total Hip Replacement: Narrative Review," U.S. Library of Medicine (NLM), 2014.

2. "Will Arthritis Change Our Relationship?" Arthritis Research UK, 2018.

3. "Sex and Arthritis," American College of Rheumatology, 2017.

Chapter 47

Starting a Family: Pregnancy and Arthritis

Chapter Contents

Section 47.1—Pregnancy, Breastfeeding, and
        Bone Health.. 482
Section 47.2—Rheumatic Disease Management in
        Pregnant Women... 485

Section 47.1

Pregnancy, Breastfeeding, and Bone Health

This section includes text excerpted from "Pregnancy,
Breastfeeding and Bone Health," NationalNIH
Osteoporosis and Related Bone Diseases~
National Resource Center (NIH ORBD~NRC), May 2015.

Both pregnancy and breastfeeding cause changes in, and place extra demands on, women's bodies. Some of these may affect their bones. The good news is that most women do not experience bone problems during pregnancy and breastfeeding. And if their bones are affected during these times, the problem often is corrected easily. Nevertheless, taking care of one's bone health is especially important during pregnancy and breastfeeding, for the good health of both the mother and her baby.

Pregnancy and Bone Health

During pregnancy, the baby growing in its mother's womb needs plenty of calcium to develop its skeleton. This need is especially great during the last 3 months of pregnancy. If the mother doesn't get enough calcium, her baby will draw what it needs from the mother's bones. So, it is disconcerting that most women of childbearing years are not in the habit of getting enough calcium. Fortunately, pregnancy appears to help protect most women's calcium reserves in several ways:

- Pregnant women absorb calcium from food and supplements better than women who are not pregnant. This is especially true during the last half of pregnancy when the baby is growing quickly and has the greatest need for calcium.

- During pregnancy, women produce more estrogen, a hormone that protects bones.

- Any bone mass lost during pregnancy is typically restored within several months after the baby's delivery (or several months after breastfeeding is stopped).

Some studies suggest that pregnancy may be good for bone health overall. Some evidence suggests that the more times a woman has been pregnant (for at least 28 weeks), the greater her bone density and the lower her risk of fracture.

In some cases, women develop osteoporosis during pregnancy or breastfeeding, although this is rare. Osteoporosis is bone loss that is serious enough to result in fragile bones and increased risk of fracture.

In many cases, women who develop osteoporosis during pregnancy or breastfeeding will recover lost bone after childbirth or after they stop breastfeeding. It is less clear whether teenage mothers can recover lost bone and go on to optimize their bone mass.

Teen pregnancy and bone health. Teenage mothers may be at especially high risk for bone loss during pregnancy and for osteoporosis later in life. Unlike older women, teenage mothers are still building much of their own total bone mass. The unborn baby's need to develop its skeleton may compete with the young mother's need for calcium to build her own bones, compromising her ability to achieve optimal bone mass that will help protect her from osteoporosis later in life. To minimize any bone loss, pregnant teens should be especially careful to get enough calcium during pregnancy and breastfeeding.

Breastfeeding and Bone Health

Breastfeeding also affects a mother's bones. Studies have shown that women often lose 3–5 percent of their bone mass during breastfeeding, although they recover it rapidly after weaning. This bone loss may be caused by the growing baby's increased need for calcium, which is drawn from the mother's bones. The amount of calcium the mother needs depends on the amount of breast milk produced and how long breastfeeding continues. Women also may lose bone mass during breastfeeding because they're producing less estrogen, which is the hormone that protects bones. The good news is that, like bone lost during pregnancy, bone lost during breastfeeding is usually recovered within 6 months after breastfeeding ends.

Tips to Keep Bones Healthy during Pregnancy, Breastfeeding, and Beyond

Taking care of your bones is important throughout life, including before, during, and after pregnancy and breastfeeding. A balanced diet with adequate calcium, regular exercise, and a healthy lifestyle are good for mothers and their babies.

Calcium. Although this important mineral is important throughout your lifetime, your body's demand for calcium is greater during pregnancy and breastfeeding because both you and your baby need it. The

National Academy of Sciences (NAS) recommends that women who are pregnant or breastfeeding consume 1,000 mg (milligrams) of calcium each day. For pregnant teens, the recommended intake is even higher: 1,300 mg of calcium a day.

Good sources of calcium include:

- low-fat dairy products, such as milk, yogurt, cheese, and ice cream

- dark green, leafy vegetables, such as broccoli, collard greens, and bok choy

- canned sardines and salmon with bones

- tofu, almonds, and corn tortillas

- foods fortified with calcium, such as orange juice, cereals, and bread

In addition, your doctor probably will prescribe a vitamin and mineral supplement to take during pregnancy and breastfeeding to ensure that you get enough of this important mineral.

Exercise. Like muscles, bones respond to exercise by becoming stronger. Regular exercise, especially weight-bearing exercise that forces you to work against gravity, helps build and maintain strong bones. Examples of weight-bearing exercise include walking, climbing stairs, dancing, and weight training. Exercising during pregnancy can benefit your health in other ways, too. According to the American College of Obstetricians and Gynecologists (ACOG), being active during pregnancy can:

- help reduce backaches, constipation, bloating, and swelling

- help prevent or treat gestational diabetes (a type of diabetes that starts during pregnancy)

- increase energy

- improve mood

- improve posture

- promote muscle tone, strength, and endurance

- help you sleep better

- help you get back in shape after your baby is born

Before you begin or resume an exercise program, talk to your doctor about your plans.

Healthy lifestyle. Smoking is bad for your baby, bad for your bones, and bad for your heart and lungs. If you smoke, talk to your doctor about quitting. He or she can suggest resources to help you. Alcohol also is bad for pregnant and breastfeeding women and their babies, and excess alcohol is bad for bones. Be sure to follow your doctor's orders to avoid alcohol during this important time.

Section 47.2

Rheumatic Disease Management in Pregnant Women

"Rheumatic Disease Management in Pregnant Women,"
© 2015 Omnigraphics. Reviewed April 2018.

From conception to delivery, a woman's body goes through transformative changes during pregnancy. Some of these changes can impact the symptoms experienced by women with existing rheumatic diseases. Despite decades of research on the subject, doctors do not fully understand the relationship between pregnancy and arthritis symptoms, which has proven to be complex and sometimes contradictory.

For instance, studies have shown that a majority of women with rheumatoid arthritis find that their symptoms of pain and inflammation decrease considerably or even disappear completely during pregnancy. Yet about one-third of women with rheumatoid arthritis experience a flare in symptoms within a few weeks after giving birth. Research also suggests that women who have been pregnant have a 50 percent lower lifetime risk of developing rheumatoid arthritis.

Some of the common bodily changes associated with pregnancy—including weight gain, fluid retention, and increased elasticity of the joints—can cause problems for women with arthritis. These problems can be challenging to manage because many of the medications typically prescribed to treat arthritis are not considered safe for use during certain stages of pregnancy. On the whole, though, women with arthritis do not have more trouble conceiving or face significantly higher rates of pregnancy complications than the general population.

With proper obstetric care, most pregnant women with arthritis can expect successful outcomes.

The Ameliorating Effect of Pregnancy on Rheumatoid Arthritis

The first study to indicate that pregnancy led to spontaneous improvement in symptoms for women with existing rheumatoid arthritis was conducted in 1938. Although many later studies have confirmed this finding, doctors are still not sure exactly why pregnancy tends to ameliorate arthritis symptoms. Many experts believe that multiple pregnancy-related bodily changes combine to produce this beneficial effect on disease activity.

Changes to the immune system are one mechanism that may be involved. During pregnancy, a woman's immune response is naturally tamped down so that her body does not reject the growing fetus as a foreign invader. Researchers believe that this immunological adaptation also reduces the tendency for the immune system to overreact and attack the joints, as it does in rheumatoid arthritis and other autoimmune disorders.

A woman also undergoes many hormonal changes during pregnancy, as her body produces increased levels of estrogen, progesterone, and cortisol to support the baby. The surge in these hormones may suppress arthritis symptoms by increasing the production or action of anti-inflammatory proteins called cytokines. In addition, the growing fetus produces alpha-fetoprotein, which enters the mother's bloodstream through the placenta. This protein has been shown to suppress inflammation in the synovial fluid, which plays an important role in nourishing and lubricating joints.

The Postpartum Rheumatoid Arthritis Flare-Up

Although up to 70 percent of women with existing rheumatoid arthritis experience less pain and inflammation during pregnancy, many women find that their symptoms reappear or worsen within a few months of delivery. The exact cause of this flare-up in symptoms is unknown, but researchers suspect it may be related to postnatal changes in the immune system and hormone levels. One possible factor in the postpartum flare-up is an increase in the production of prolactin, a pituitary hormone that stimulates milk secretion and also has an inflammatory effect.

Treatment of Arthritis before and during Pregnancy

Since many of the medications commonly used to treat arthritis can have adverse effects on the developing fetus, women of childbearing age who have arthritis must be careful in choosing treatment options and planning pregnancies. Even though arthritis symptoms often improve during pregnancy, it can be challenging to keep disease activity under control while trying to become pregnant and during the postnatal period.

Prenatal counseling for women with rheumatoid arthritis should emphasize the importance of using contraception during therapy with disease-modifying antirheumatic drugs (DMARDs), especially methotrexate, leflunomide, and cyclophosphamide. Some of these medications take several months to leave the body, so women are encouraged to discontinue their use well before conception is planned. No pharmaceutical drugs can be considered absolutely safe during pregnancy, however, so patients should be educated about alternative methods of pain management, such as cold packs, moist heat, rest, and relaxation techniques.

Since women with arthritis do not have a significantly higher incidence of preterm birth, fetal growth restriction, or preeclampsia (pregnancy-induced high blood pressure), they generally do not require special obstetric monitoring during pregnancy. In addition to following the regular guidelines for healthy eating during pregnancy, patients with rheumatoid arthritis are advised to follow a low-fat, high-carbohydrate, high-fiber diet. Supplementary calcium, vitamin D, and fish oil are also recommended.

Pharmacotherapy in Pregnancy

Although treatment with pharmaceutical drugs can greatly reduce the symptoms of rheumatoid arthritis, some of the most commonly prescribed arthritis medications are not considered safe for use during pregnancy. While certain medications pose a mild risk to the developing fetus, however, others may cause serious harm and are, therefore, contraindicated in pregnancy. Women should always consult with their doctors to assess the risks and benefits of various drugs given their individual disease activity and severity of symptoms. Some general information about the pregnancy-related precautions pertaining to the main categories of drugs used to treat rheumatoid arthritis follows:

- **Corticosteroids.** Steroid medications are generally used to treat joint inflammation associated with rheumatoid arthritis.

Two of the most commonly used steroids, prednisone, and prednisolone mimic the action of natural corticosteroids produced by the adrenal glands. Although less than 10 percent of the maternal dosage crosses the placenta to the fetus, high doses may lead to adrenal insufficiency as well as increased risk of cleft palate in newborns.

- **Nonsteroidal anti-inflammatory drugs (NSAIDs).** Nonsteroidal anti-inflammatory drugs are generally considered safe for use in the first trimester of pregnancy. Use after 30 weeks of gestation, however, is associated with an increased risk of premature closure of a key blood vessel in the heart, potentially leading to cardiovascular dysfunction in the baby.

- **Disease-modifying antirheumatic drugs (DMARDs).** A few drugs in this category are considered relatively safe to use during pregnancy if necessary to control disease activity, including sulfasalazine, azathioprine, and hydroxychloroquine. Methotrexate and leflunomide, however, are contraindicated in pregnancy and carry a high risk of congenital abnormalities. Women are advised to discontinue use of both of these drugs well in advance of conception. Since both drugs can be passed to newborns through breast milk, they are also considered unsuitable for lactating mothers.

- **Biologics.** Little information is available concerning the effects of biologics such as abatacept and tocilizumab during pregnancy. As a result, doctors generally do not recommend their use by women who are pregnant or planning to become pregnant.

References

1. Dolhain, Radboud J.E.M. "Rheumatoid Arthritis and Pregnancy: Not Only for Rheumatologists Interested in Female Health Issues," Annals of the Rheumatic Diseases 69(2), 2010.

2. Dunkin, Mary Anne. "Rheumatoid Arthritis and Pregnancy," Arthritis Foundation, 2015.

3. Hazes, Johanna M.W., et al. "Rheumatoid Arthritis and Pregnancy: Evolution of Disease Activity and Pathophysiological Considerations for Drug Use," Rheumatology, September 1, 2011.

4. Pietrangelo, Ann. "Arthritis during Pregnancy: Symptoms, Treatments, and Remission," Healthline, 2014.

5. Temprano, Katherine E. "Rheumatoid Arthritis, and Pregnancy," Medscape, 2015.

Part Six

Additional Help and Information

Chapter 48

Glossary of Terms Related to Arthritis and Rheumatic Diseases

acupuncture: The use of fine needles inserted at specific points on the skin. Primarily used for pain relief, acupuncture may be a helpful component of an osteoarthritis treatment plan for some people.

acute pain: Acute pain often begins suddenly—after a fall or injury, for example—and lasts no longer than 6 weeks.

analgesics: Medications designed to relieve pain. Pure analgesics do not have an effect on inflammation.

ankylosing spondylitis: A form of arthritis that affects the spine, the sacroiliac joints, and sometimes the hips and shoulders. In severe cases, the joints of the spine fuse and the spine becomes rigid.

anterior cruciate ligament: A ligament in the knee that crosses from the underside of the femur to the top of the tibia. The ligament limits rotation and the forward movement of the tibia.

antinuclear antibody (ANA): A type of antibody directed against the nuclei of the body's cells. Because these antibodies can be found in

---

This glossary contains terms excerpted from documents produced by several sources deemed reliable.

the blood of children with lupus and some other rheumatic disorders, testing for them can be useful in diagnosis.

arthritis: Literally means joint inflammation but is often used to indicate a group of more than 100 rheumatic diseases. These diseases affect not only the joints but also other connective tissues of the body, including important supporting structures such as muscles, tendons, and ligaments, as well as the protective covering of internal organs.

arthrodesis: A surgical procedure that involves removing the joint and fusing the bones into one immobile unit, often using bone grafts from the person's own pelvis. Although the procedure limits movement, it can be useful for increasing stability and relieving pain in affected joints. The most commonly fused joints are the ankles and wrists and joints of the fingers and toes.

arthroscopic surgery: Repairing the interior of a joint by inserting a microscope-like device and surgical tools through small cuts rather than one, large surgical cut.

autoimmune disease: A disease in which the immune system, which is designed to protect the body from foreign invaders, mistakenly sees the body's own tissues as foreign and makes autoantibodies against them, leading to tissue destruction.

biologic response modifiers: Genetically engineered medications that help reduce inflammation and structural damage to the joints by interrupting the cascade of events that drive inflammation.

biologics: A relatively new class of medications that are genetically engineered to block a protein involved in the body's inflammatory response. Four biologics are approved by the U.S. Food and Drug Administration (FDA) for treating ankylosing spondylitis. They work by blocking a protein called tumor necrosis factor-alpha (TNF-a) that helps drive inflammation.

biomarkers: Physical signs or biological substances that indicate changes in bone or cartilage. Doctors believe they may one day be able to use biomarkers for diagnosing osteoarthritis before it causes noticeable joint damage and for monitoring the progression of the disease and its responsiveness to treatment.

biopsy: A procedure in which tissue is removed from the body and studied under a microscope. A biopsy of joint tissue may be used to diagnose some forms of arthritis.

bone spurs: Small growths of bone that can occur on the edges of a joint affected by osteoarthritis. These growths are also known as osteophytes.

bursa: A small sac of tissue located between a bone and other moving structures such as muscles, skin, or tendons. The bursa contains a lubricating fluid that allows these structures to glide smoothly.

bursitis: Inflammation of the bursae that cushion joints. Bursitis is a common cause of shoulder pain.

C-reactive protein: A protein produced by the body during the process of inflammation. A positive blood test for the protein indicates the presence of inflammation in the body. The test may be used in diagnosing rheumatoid arthritis and monitoring disease activity and the response of treatment.

cartilage: A hard but slippery coating on the end of each bone. The breakdown of joint cartilage is the primary feature of osteoarthritis.

chondroitin sulfate: A naturally existing substance in joint cartilage that is believed to draw fluid into the cartilage. Chondroitin is often taken in supplement form along with glucosamine as a treatment for osteoarthritis.

chronic pain: Chronic pain may begin either quickly or slowly; it generally lasts for 3 months or more.

collagen: A fabric-like material of fibrous threads that is a key component of the body's connective tissues. In scleroderma, either too much collagen is produced or it is produced in the wrong places, causing stiff and inflamed skin, blood vessels, and internal organs.

computed tomography (CT): An imaging technique that provides doctors with a three dimensional picture of the bone. It also shows "slices" of the bone, making the picture much clearer than X-rays.

connective tissue: Tissues such as skin, tendons, and cartilage that support and hold body parts together. The chief component of connective tissue is collagen.

corticosteroids: Powerful anti-inflammatory hormones made naturally in the body or synthetically for use as medicine. Corticosteroids may be taken by mouth or intravenously, or they may be injected into the affected joints to temporarily suppress the inflammation that causes arthritis-related swelling, warmth, loss of motion, and pain.

COX-2 inhibitors: A relatively new class of nonsteroidal anti-inflammatory drugs (NSAIDs) that are formulated to relieve pain and inflammation.

Crohn's disease: Inflammation of the small intestine or colon that causes diarrhea, cramps, and weight loss.

disease-modifying antirheumatic drugs (DMARDs): A class of medications used in the treatment of rheumatoid arthritis. DMARDs do more than ease the symptoms of rheumatoid arthritis like some other treatments. They often slow or stop the course of the disease to help prevent joint damage.

erythrocyte sedimentation rate (ESR or sed rate): A test that measures how quickly red blood cells fall to the bottom of a test tube of unclotted blood. Rapidly descending cells (an elevated sed rate) indicate inflammation in the body.

estrogen: The major sex hormone in women. Estrogen is known to play a role in regulation of bone growth. Research suggests that estrogen may also have a protective effect on cartilage.

fibromyalgia: A chronic syndrome that includes a history of widespread pain lasting more than 3 months and other general physical symptoms including fatigue, waking unrefreshed, and cognitive (memory or thought) problems.

flare: A period of heightened disease activity. In rheumatoid arthritis, a flare may be characterized by increased fatigue; fever; and painful, swollen, and tender joints.

gastroenterologist: A medical doctor who specializes in diagnosing and treating diseases of the digestive tract.

glucosamine: A substance that occurs naturally in the body, providing the building blocks to make and repair cartilage.

gout: A form of arthritis that is caused by a buildup of uric acid crystals in the joints, most commonly in the big toe.

hypothyroidism: A condition in which the thyroid gland (the gland that makes and stores hormones that regulate heart rate, blood pressure, body temperature, and the rate at which food is converted to energy) is underactive. Without treatment, this condition can result in fatigue, weight gain, other serious medical problems, and even death.

immune system: A complex network of specialized cells and organs that work together to defend the body against attacks by "foreign" invaders such as bacteria and viruses. In some rheumatic conditions, it appears that the immune system does not function properly and may even work against the body.

immunosuppressive drugs: Medicines that reduce the immune response, and therefore, may relieve some symptoms of Behçet's disease.

inflammation: The characteristic reaction of tissue to injury or disease. It is marked by four signs

joint: A junction where two bones meet. Most joints are composed of cartilage, joint space, the fibrous capsule, the synovium, and ligaments.

joint capsule: A tough membrane sac that encloses all the bones and other joint parts.

juvenile arthritis (JA): A term often used to describe arthritis in children.

juvenile idiopathic arthritis (JIA): A term for various types of chronic arthritis in children. Arthritis is an inflammation of the tissues lining the joints of the body. Juvenile idiopathic arthritis can cause swelling, pain, damage to the joints, and, in some cases, damage to other parts of the body. Juvenile idiopathic arthritis has replaced juvenile rheumatoid arthritis as the preferred term for the same condition.

juvenile rheumatoid arthritis (JRA): A term used to describe the most common types of arthritis in children. It is characterized by joint pain, swelling, tenderness, warmth, and stiffness that lasts for more than 6 weeks and cannot be explained by other causes. Previously, juvenile rheumatoid arthritis was the preferred term, but recently it has been replaced by juvenile idiopathic arthritis.

lateral collateral ligament: The ligament that runs along the outside of the knee joint. It provides stability to the outer (lateral) part of the knee.

ligaments: Tough bands of connective tissue that attach bones to each other, providing stability.

lumbar spine: The lower portion of the spine. The lumbar spine comprises five vertebrae.

lupus: A chronic inflammatory condition in which the immune system attacks the skin, joints, heart, lungs, blood, kidneys and brain. Also called systemic lupus erythematosus.

magnetic resonance imaging (MRI): A procedure that provides high resolution computerized images of internal body tissues. This procedure uses a strong magnet that passes a force through the body to create these images.

muscles: Bundles of specialized cells that contract and relax to produce movement when stimulated by nerves.

nonsteroidal anti-inflammatory drugs (NSAIDs): A class of medications that work to reduce pain, fever, and inflammation by blocking substances called prostaglandins. Some NSAIDs, such as ibuprofen (Motrin) and naproxen sodium (Aleve), are available over the counter (OTC), while many are available only with a doctor's prescription.

oligoarthritis: Refers to a form of juvenile idiopathic arthritis that affects four or fewer joints.

osteoarthritis: The most common form of arthritis. It is characterized by the breakdown of joint cartilage, leading to pain, stiffness, and disability.

osteophytes: Small growths of bone that can appear on the edges of a joint affected by osteoarthritis. These growths are also known as bone spurs.

osteoporosis: A condition in which the bones become porous and brittle and break easily.

osteotomy: A procedure that involves cutting and realigning bone, to shift the weight from a damaged and painful bone surface to a healthier one.

Paget disease: A bone disease that causes bones to grow larger and weaker than normal.

patella: A flat triangular bone located at the front of the knee joint. Also called the kneecap.

pericarditis: Inflammation of the pericardium, the membrane that surrounds the heart. Pericarditis is a feature of some rheumatic disorders, including systemic arthritis.

physiatrist: A medical doctor who specializes in nonsurgical treatment for injuries and illnesses that affect movement. Also called rehabilitation physician or rehabilitation medicine specialist.

pleuritis: Inflammation of the pleura, the membrane that covers the lungs and lines the inner chest wall. Pleuritis is a feature of some rheumatic disorders, including systemic arthritis.

polyarthritis: Refers to a form of juvenile idiopathic arthritis that affects five or more joints.

psoriasis: An autoimmune disease characterized by a red scaly rash that is often located over the surfaces of the elbows, knees, and scalp, and around or in the ears, navel, genitals, or buttocks. Approximately 10–15 percent of people with psoriasis develop an associated arthritis referred to as psoriatic arthritis.

purines: Found in the DNA and RNA within the nuclei of cells, purines are part of all human tissue and are found in many foods, especially those high in protein.

radius: The smaller of the two bones of the forearm. It is located on the thumb side of the arm.

Raynaud phenomenon: A condition in which the small blood vessels of the hands or feet contract in response to cold or anxiety. As the vessels contract, the hands or feet turn white and cold, then blue. As blood flow returns, they become red. Fingertip tissues may suffer damage, leading to ulcers, scars, or gangrene.

reactive arthritis: A form of arthritis that can develop after an intestinal or urinary tract infection. The disease causes pain and swelling around the joints and in the spine. People with the disease may also experience swelling of the eye and the reproductive and urinary tracts.

remission: A period when the symptoms of arthritis improve or disappear completely. Sometimes remission is permanent, but more often it is punctuated by flares of the disease.

rheumatic: An adjective used to describe a group of conditions characterized by inflammation or pain in the muscles, joints, and fibrous tissue. Rheumatic diseases or disorders can be related to autoimmunity or other causes.

rheumatic disorders: Disorders that affect the joints and soft tissues, causing pain, and sometimes inflammation, tissue damage, or disability

rheumatoid arthritis (RA): A form of arthritis in which the immune system attacks the tissues of the joints, leading to pain, inflammation, and eventually joint damage and malformation. It typically begins at a younger age than osteoarthritis does, causes swelling and redness in joints, and may make people feel sick, tired, and uncommonly feverish. Rheumatoid arthritis may also affect skin tissue, the lungs, the eyes, or the blood vessels.

rheumatoid factor: An antibody that is found often in the blood of adults with rheumatoid arthritis and once in a while in children with juvenile arthritis. For these children, testing for the antibody may be useful as a diagnostic tool.

rheumatologist: Doctors who diagnose and treat diseases of the bones, joints, muscles, and tendons, including arthritis and collagen diseases.

rotator cuff: A set of muscles and tendons that secures the arm to the shoulder blade and permits rotation of the arm.

sacroiliac joints: The joints where the spine and pelvis attach. The sacroiliac joints are often affected by types of arthritis referred to as spondyloarthropathies.

spinal stenosis: The narrowing of the spinal canal (through which the spinal cord runs), often by the overgrowth of bone caused by osteoarthritis of the spine.

stroke: Stoppage of blood flow to an area of the brain, causing permanent damage to nerve cells in that region. A stroke can occur either because an artery is clogged by a blood clot (called ischemic stroke) or an artery tears and bleeds into the brain. A stroke can cause symptoms such as loss of consciousness, problems with movement, and loss of speech.

synovial fluid: A fluid secreted by the synovium that lubricates the joint and keeps the cartilage smooth and healthy.

synovium: A thin membrane inside the joint capsule that secretes synovial fluid. In rheumatoid arthritis, the synovium is attacked by the immune system.

systemic: Refers to a disease that can affect the whole body, rather than just a specific organ or joints. For example, the juvenile idiopathic arthritis subtype systemic arthritis (formerly known as systemic juvenile rheumatoid arthritis) can affect the skin, blood vessels, bones, and membranes lining the chest wall, as well as the joints.

tendonitis: Inflammation or irritation of a tendon.

tendons: Tough, fibrous cords that connect muscles to bones.

tissue: A group of cells that act together to carry out a specific function in the body. Examples include muscle tissue, nervous system tissue (including the brain, spinal cord, and nerves), and connective tissue (including ligaments, tendons, bones, and fat). Organs are made up of tissues.

topical treatment: Medicine, such as a cream or rinse, which is put directly on the affected body part.

ulcerative colitis: Inflammation of the colon. Symptoms include stomach pain and diarrhea.

uric acid: A substance that results from the breakdown of purines, which are part of all human tissue and are found in many foods.

vertebrae: The individual bones that make up the spinal column.

X-ray: A procedure in which low-level radiation is passed through the body to produce a picture called a radiograph. X-rays of joints affected by osteoarthritis can show such things as cartilage loss, bone damage, and bone spurs.

Chapter 49

Directory of Organizations That Help People with Arthritis and Their Families

Government Agencies That Provide Information about Arthritis

Administration for Community Living (ACL)
330 C St. S.W.
Washington, DC 20001
Toll-Free: 800-677-1116
Phone: 202-401-4634
Website: www.acl.gov
E-mail: aclinfo@acl.hhs.gov

Agency for Healthcare Research and Quality (AHRQ)
Office of Communications and Knowledge Transfer
5600 Fishers Ln.
Seventh Fl.
Rockville, MD 20857
Phone: 301-427-1364
Website: www.ahrq.gov

Resources in this chapter were compiled from several sources deemed reliable; all contact information was verified and updated in April 2018.

Center for Nutrition Policy and Promotion (CNPP)
3101 Park Center Dr.
Alexandria, VA 22302-1594
Website: www.choosemyplate.gov

Centers for Disease Control and Prevention (CDC)
1600 Clifton Rd.
Atlanta, GA 30329-4027
Toll-Free: 800-CDC-INFO
(800-232-4636)
Toll-Free TTY: 888-232-6348
Website: www.cdc.gov
E-mail: cdcinfo@cdc.gov

Centers for Medicare and Medicaid Services (CMS)
7500 Security Blvd.
Baltimore, MD 21244
Toll-Free: 877-267-2323
Phone: 410-786-3000
Toll-Free TTY: 866-226-1819
TTY: 410-786-0727
Website: www.cms.gov

Division of Nutrition, Physical Activity, and Obesity (DNPAO)
Centers for Disease Control and Prevention (CDC)
Website: www.cdc.gov/nccdphp/dnpao

Eldercare Locator
U.S. Administration on Aging (AoA)
Toll-Free: 800-677-1116
Website: www.eldercare.gov
E-mail: eldercarelocator@n4a.org

Eunice Kennedy Shriver National Institute of Child Health and Human Development (NICHD)
P.O. Box 3006
Rockville, MD 20847
Toll-Free: 800-370-2943
Toll-Free TTY: 888-320-6942
Toll-Free Fax: 866-760-5947
Website: www.nichd.nih.gov
E-mail: NICHDInformation ResourceCenter@mail.nih.gov

Genetic and Rare Diseases Information Center (GARD)
P.O. Box 8126
Gaithersburg, MD 20898-8126
Toll-Free: 888-205-2311
Phone: 301-251-4925
Toll-Free TTY: 888-205-3223
Fax: 301-251-4911
Website: rarediseases.info.nih.gov

Healthfinder®
National Health Information Center (NHIC)
200 Independence Ave. S.W.
Washington, DC 20201
Website: www.healthfinder.gov
E-mail: healthfinder@hhs.gov

Lister Hill National Center for Biomedical Communications (LHNCBC)
U.S. National Library of Medicine (NLM)
Bldg. 38A, Seventh Fl.
8600 Rockville Pike
Bethesda, MD 20894
Toll-Free: 888-346-3656
Phone: 301-496-4441
Fax: 301-402-0118
Website: www.lhncbc.nlm.nih.gov
E-mail: nlmlhclhcques@mail.nih.gov

National Aeronautics and Space Administration (NASA)
300 E. St. S.W.
Ste. 5R30
Washington, DC 20546
Phone: 202-358-0001
Fax: 202-358-4338
Website: www.nasa.gov

National Center for Chronic Disease Prevention and Health Promotion (NCCDPHP)
Centers for Disease Control and Prevention (CDC)
Website: www.cdc.gov/chronicdisease

National Center for Complementary and Integrative Health (NCCIH)
National Institutes of Health (NIH)
9000 Rockville Pike
Bethesda, MD 20892
Toll-Free: 888-644-6226
Toll-Free TTY: 866-464-3615
Website: nccih.nih.gov

National Center for Emerging and Zoonotic Infectious Diseases (NCEZID)
Centers for Disease Control and Prevention (CDC)
Website: www.cdc.gov/ncezid

National Center for Health Statistics (NCHS)
Centers for Disease Control and Prevention (CDC)
Website: www.cdc.gov/nchs/index.htm

National Center for Injury Prevention and Control (NCIPC)
Centers for Disease Control and Prevention (CDC)
Website: www.cdc.gov/injury

National Eye Institute (NEI)
Information Office
31 Center Dr. MSC 2510
Bethesda, MD 20892-2510
Phone: 301-496-5248
Website: nei.nih.gov
E-mail: 2020@nei.nih.gov

National Heart, Lung, and Blood Institute (NHLBI)
NHLBI Center for Health Information
P.O. Box 30105
Bethesda, MD 20824-0105
Phone: 301-592-8573
Website: www.nhlbi.nih.gov/about/contact/health-information-and-clinical-trials
E-mail: nhlbiinfo@nhlbi.nih.gov

National Highway Traffic Safety Administration (NHTSA)
1200 New Jersey Ave. S.E.
W. Bldg.
Washington, DC 20590
Toll-Free: 888-327-4236
Phone: 202-366-4000
Toll-Free TTY: 800- 424-9153
Website: www.nhtsa.gov

National Institute of Allergy and Infectious Diseases (NIAID)
Office of Communications and Government Relations
5601 Fishers Ln. MSC 9806
Bethesda, MD 20892-9806
Toll-Free: 866-284-4107
Phone: 301-496-5717
Toll-Free TDD: 800-877-8339
Fax: 301-402-3573
Website: www.niaid.nih.gov
E-mail: ocpostoffice@niaid.nih.gov

National Institute of Arthritis and Musculoskeletal and Skin Diseases (NIAMS)
NIAMS Information Clearinghouse
Bethesda, MD 20892-3675
Toll-Free: 877-22-NIAMS (877-226-4267)
Phone: 301-495-4484
TTY: 301-565-2966
Fax: 301-718-6366
Website: www.niams.nih.gov
E-mail: NIAMSinfo@mail.nih.gov

National Institute of Dental and Craniofacial Research (NIDCR)
National Oral Health Information Clearinghouse (NOHIC)
Toll-Free: 866-232-4528
Website: www.nidcr.nih.gov
E-mail: nidcrinfo@mail.nih.gov

National Institute of Diabetes and Digestive and Kidney Diseases (NIDDK)
Health Information Center
Toll-Free: 800-860-8747
Toll-Free TTY: 866-569-1162
Website: www.niddk.nih.gov
E-mail: healthinfo@niddk.nih.gov

National Institute of Mental Health (NIMH)
Science Writing, Press, and
Dissemination Branch
6001 Executive Blvd.
Rm. 6200 MSC 9663
Bethesda, MD 20892-9663
Toll-Free: 866-615-6464
Toll-Free TTY: 866-415-8051
TTY: 301-443-8431
Fax: 301-443-4279
Website: www.nimh.nih.gov
E-mail: nimhinfo@nih.gov

National Institute of Neurological Disorders and Stroke (NINDS)
NIH Neurological Institute
P.O. Box 5801
Bethesda, MD 20824
Toll-Free: 800-352-9424
Phone: 301-496-5751
Website: www.ninds.nih.gov

National Institute on Aging (NIA)
Bldg. 31 Rm. 5C27
31 Center Dr. MSC 2292
Bethesda, MD 20892
Toll-Free: 800-222-2225
Toll-Free TTY: 800-222-4225
Website: www.nia.nih.gov
E-mail: niaic@nia.nih.gov

National Institutes of Health (NIH)
9000 Rockville Pike
Bethesda, MD 20892
Phone: 301-496-4000
TTY 301-402-9612
Website: www.nih.gov
E-mail: NIHinfo@od.nih.gov

NIH News in Health
NIH Office of Communications
and Public Liaison (OCPL)
Bldg. 31 Rm. 5B64
Bethesda, MD 20892-2094
Phone: 301-451-8224
Website: newsinhealth.nih.gov
E-mail: nihnewsinhealth@
od.nih.gov

NIH Osteoporosis and Related Bone Diseases ~ National Resource Center
Toll-Free: 800-624-BONE
(800-624-2663)
Phone: 202-223-0344
TTY: 202-466-4315
Fax: 202-293-2356
Website: www.bones.nih.gov
E-mail: NIHBoneInfo@mail.nih.
gov

Occupational Safety and Health Administration (OSHA)
U.S. Department of Labor (DOL)
200 Constitution Ave. N.W.
Washington, DC 20210
Toll-Free: 800-321-OSHA
(800-321-6742)
Website: www.osha.gov

Office of Dietary Supplements (ODS)
National Institutes of Health (NIH)
6100 Executive Blvd.
Rm. 3B01 MSC 7517
Bethesda, MD 20892-7517
Phone: 301-435-2920
Fax: 301-480-1845
Website: www.ods.od.nih.gov
E-mail: ods@nih.gov

Office of Disease Prevention (ODP)
National Institutes of Health (NIH)
6100 Executive Blvd.
Rm. 2B03 MSC 7523
Bethesda, MD 20892-7523
Phone: 301-827-5561
Fax: 301-480-7660
Website: www.prevention.nih.gov

Office of Disease Prevention and Health Promotion (ODPHP)
U.S. Department of Health and Human Services (HHS)
Tower Bldg. 1101 Wootton Pkwy Ste. LL100
Rockville, MD 20852
Phone: 240-453-8280
Fax: 240-453-8281
Website: www.health.gov
E-mail: odphpinfo@hhs.gov

Office of Research on Women's Health (ORWH)
6707 Democracy Blvd.
Bethesda, MD 20817
Phone: 301-402-1770
Fax: 301-402-0005
Website: orwh.od.nih.gov

Office on Women's Health (OWH)
U.S. Department of Health and Human Services (HHS)
S.W. Rm. 712E
200 Independence Ave.
Washington, DC 20201
Toll-Free: 800-994-9662
Website: www.womenshealth.gov

U.S. Department of Health and Human Services (HHS)
Hubert H. Humphrey Bldg.
Washington, DC 20201
Toll-Free: 877-696-6775
Website: www.hhs.gov

U.S. Department of Veterans Affairs (VA)
810 Vermont Ave. N.W.
Washington, DC 20420
Toll-Free: 877-222-VETS (877-222-8387)
Website: www.va.gov

U.S. Food and Drug Administration (FDA)
10903 New Hampshire Ave.
Silver Spring, MD 20993
Toll-Free: 888-INFO-FDA (888-463-6332)
Website: www.fda.gov

U.S. National Library of Medicine (NLM)
8600 Rockville Pike
Bethesda, MD 20894
Toll-Free: 888-FIND-NLM (888-346-3656)
Phone: 301-594-5983
Website: www.nlm.nih.gov

Private Agencies That Provide Information about Arthritis

Aging Life Care Association (ALCA)
3275 W. Ina Rd.
Ste. 130
Tucson, AZ 85741-2198
Phone: 520-881-8008
Fax: 520-325-7925
Website: www.aginglifecare.org

Alliance for Lupus Research (ALR)
275 Madison Ave.
10th Fl.
New York, NY 10016
Toll-Free: 800-867-1743
Website: www.lupusresearch.org
E-mail: info@lupusresearch.org

American Academy of Dermatology (AAD)
P.O. Box 1968
Des Plaines, IL 60017
Toll-Free: 888-462-DERM
(888-462-3376)
Phone: 847-240-1280
Fax: 847-240-1859
Website: www.aad.org

American Academy of Ophthalmology (AAO)
P.O. Box 7424
San Francisco, CA 94120-7424
Fax: 415-561-8533
Website: www.aao.org
E-mail: SupportAAD@aad.org

American Academy of Orthopaedic Surgeons (AAOS)
9400 W. Higgins Rd.
Rosemont, IL 60018
Phone: 847-823-7186
Fax: 847-823-8125
Website: www.aaos.org
Email: customerservice@aaos.org

American Association for Dental Research (AADR)
1619 Duke St.
Alexandria, VA 22314-3406
Phone: 703-548-0066
Fax: 703-548-1883
Website: www.iadr.org/AADR

American Autoimmune Related Diseases Association (AARDA)
2100 Gratiot Ave.
Eastpointe, MI 48021
United States
Phone: 586-776-3900
Website: www.aarda.org
E-mail: aarda@aarda.org

American Behcet's Disease Association (ABDA)
P.O. Box 80576
Rochester, MI 48308
Website: www.behcets.com
E-mail: webmaster@behcets.com

American College of Rheumatology (ACR)
2200 Lake Blvd. N.E.
Atlanta, GA 30319
Phone: 404-633-3777
Fax: 404-633-1870
Website: www.rheumatology.org
E-mail: foundation@
rheumatology.org

American Council on Exercise (ACE)
4851 Paramount Dr.
San Diego, CA 92123
Toll-Free: 888-825-3636
Website: www.acefitness.org
E-mail: support@acefitness.org

American Dental Association (ADA)
211 E. Chicago Ave.
Chicago, IL 60611-2678
Phone: 312-440-2500
Website: www.ada.org
E-mail: International-Member@
ada.org

American Geriatrics Society (AGS)
40 Fulton St.
18th Fl.
New York, NY 10038
Phone: 212-308-1414
Fax: 212-832-8646
Website: www.
americangeriatrics.org
E-mail: info.amger@
americangeriatrics.org

American Orthopedic Society for Sports Medicine (AOSSM)
9400 W. Higgins Rd.
Ste. 300
Rosemont, IL 60018
Toll-Free: 877-321-3500
Phone: 847-292-4900
Fax: 847-292-4905
Website: www.sportsmed.org

American Physical Therapy Association (APTA)
1111 N. Fairfax St.
Alexandria, VA 22314-1488
Toll-Free: 800-999-2782
Phone: 703-684-APTA
(703-684-2782)
Fax: 703-684-7343
Website: www.apta.org

American Shoulder and Elbow Surgeons (ASES)
9400 W. Higgins Rd.
Ste. 500
Rosemont, IL 60018
Phone: 847-698-1629
Fax: 847-268-9499
Website: www.ases-assn.org
E-mail: ases@aaos.org

American Skin Association (ASA)
6 E. 43rd St.
28th Fl.
New York, NY 10017
Phone: 212-889-4858
Website: www.americanskin.org
E-mail: info@americanskin.org

American Society for Bone and Mineral Research (ASBMR)
2025 M St. N.W.
Ste. 800
Washington, DC 20036-3309
Phone: 202-367-1161
Fax: 202-367-2161
Website: www.asbmr.org
E-mail: asbmr@asbmr.org

Arthritis Foundation
1355 Peachtree St. N.E.
Ste. 600
Atlanta, GA 30309
Phone: 404-872-7100
Website: www.arthritis.org

Dermatology Foundation
1560 Sherman Ave.
Ste. 500
Evanston, IL 60201-4808
Phone: 847-328-2256
Fax: 847-328-0509
Website: www.
dermatologyfoundation.org

Family Caregiver Alliance (FCA)
National Center on Caregiving (NCC)
285 Montgomery St.
Ste. 950
San Francisco, CA 94104
Toll-Free: 800-445-8106
Phone: 415-434-3388
Website: www.caregiver.org
E-mail: info@caregiver.org

Fibromyalgia Network
P.O. Box 31750
Tucson, AZ 85751-1750
Phone: 520-290-5508
Fax: 520-290-5550
Website: fmnetnews.iraherman.
com/about-us/contact
E-mail: inquiry@fmnetnews.com

Fibrous Dysplasia Foundation (FDF)
2885 Sanford Ave. S.W. #40754
Grandville, MI 49418
Website: www.fibrousdysplasia.
org
E-mail: info@fibrousdysplasia.
org

Hip Society
9400 W. Higgins Rd.
Ste. 500
Rosemont, IL 60018
Phone: 847-698-1638
Fax: 847-268-9745
Website: www.hipsoc.org
E-mail: hip@aaos.org

Juvenile Arthritis Association (JAA)
8549 Wilshire Blvd.
Ste. 103
Beverly Hills, CA 90211
Website: www.juvenilearthritis.
org
E-mail: info@juvenilearthritis.org

LeadingAge
2519 Connecticut Ave. N.W.
Washington, DC 20008
Phone: 202-783-2242
Website: www.leadingage.org
E-mail: info@LeadingAge.org

Low-Income Home Energy Assistance Program (LIHEAP)
Office of Community Services, Division of Energy Assistance
330 C St. S.W.
Mary E. Switzer Bldg. Fifth Fl. W.
Washington, DC 20201
Toll-Free: 866-674-6327
Phone: 202-401-9351
Toll-Free Fax: 866-367-6228
Website: www.liheap.ncat.org/referral.htm

Lupus Foundation of America (LFA)
2121 K St. N.W.
Ste. 200
Washington, DC 20037
Toll-Free: 800-558-0121
Phone: 202-349-1155
Fax: 202-349-1156
Website: www.lupus.org
E-mail: info@lupus.org

MAGIC Foundation
4200 Cantera Dr.
Ste. 106
Warrenville, IL 60555
Toll-Free: 800-362-4423
Phone: 630-836-8200
Fax: 630-836-8181
Website: www.magicfoundation.org
E-mail: contactus@magicfoundation.org

Mental Health America (MHA)
500 Montgomery St.
Ste. 820
Alexandria, VA 22314
Toll-Free: 800-969-6642
Phone: 703-684-7722
Fax: 703-684-5968
Website: www.mentalhealthamerica.net

Muscular Dystrophy Association (MDA)
222 S. Riverside Plaza
Ste. 1500
Chicago, IL 60606
Toll-Free: 800-572-1717
Website: www.mda.org
E-mail: mda@mdausa.org

National Adult Day Services Association (NADSA)
11350 Random Hills Rd.
Ste. 800
Fairfax, VA 22030
Toll-Free: 877-745-1440
Website: www.nadsa.org
E-mail: info@nadsa.org

National Alliance for Caregiving (NAFC)
4720 Montgomery Ln.
Ste. 205
Bethesda, MD 20814
Phone: 301-718-8444
Fax: 301-951-9067
Website: www.caregiving.org
E-mail: info@caregiving.org

National Fibromyalgia Association (NFA)
3857 Birch St.
Ste. 312
Newport Beach, CA 92660
Website: www.fmaware.org
E-mail: nfa@fmaware.org

National Fibromyalgia Partnership (NFP)
P.O. Box 2355
Centreville, VA 20122
Website: www.fmpartnership.org

National Organization for Rare Disorders, Inc. (NORD)
55 Kenosia Ave.
Danbury, CT 06810
Toll-Free: 800-999-NORD
(800-999-6673)
Phone: 203-744-0100
Fax: 203-263-9938
Website: www.rarediseases.org
E-mail: orphan@rarediseases.org

National Psoriasis Foundation (NPF)
6600 S.W. 92nd Ave.
Ste. 300
Portland, OR 97223-7195
Toll-Free: 800-723-9166
Phone: 503-244-7404
Fax: 503-245-0626
Website: www.psoriasis.org
E-mail: getinfo@psoriasis.org

National Resource Center on Supportive Housing and Home Modification (NRCSHHM)
Andrus Gerontology Center
3715 McClintock Ave.
Los Angeles, CA 90089
Phone: 213-740-1364
Fax: 213-740-7069
Website: www.homemods.org
E-mail: homemods@usc.edu

North American Spine Society (NASS)
300 New Jersey Ave. N.W.
Washington, DC 20001
Phone: 630-230-3671
Website: www.spine.org

Osteogenesis Imperfecta Foundation (OI)
804 W. Diamond Ave.
Ste. 210
Gaithersburg, MD 20878
Toll-Free: 844-889-7579
Phone: 301-947-0083
Fax: 301-947-0456
Website: www.oif.org
E-mail: bonelink@oif.org

Rebuilding Together
999 N. Capitol St. N.E.
Ste. 701
Washington, DC 20002
Toll-Free: 800-473-4229
Website: rebuildingtogether.org
E-mail: info@reBldg.together.org

Scleroderma Foundation (SF)
300 Rosewood Dr.
Ste. 105
Danvers, MA 01923
Toll-Free: 800-722-4673
Fax: 978-463-5809
Website: www.scleroderma.org
E-mail: sfinfo@scleroderma.org

Sjögren's Syndrome Foundation
10701 Parkridge Blvd.
Ste. 170
Reston, VA 20191
Toll-Free: 800-475-6473
Phone: 301-530-4420
Fax: 301-530-4415
Website: www.sjogrens.org

Spondylitis Association of America (SAA)
16360 Roscoe Blvd.
Ste. 100
Van Nuys, CA 91406
Toll-Free: 800-777-8189
Phone: 818-892-1616
Website: www.spondylitis.org
E-mail: info@spondylitis.org

St. Jude Children's Research Hospital
262 Danny Thomas Place
Memphis, TN 38105
Toll-Free TTY: 901-595-1040
Website: www.stjude.org

YMCA of the USA
101 N. Wacker Dr.
Chicago, IL 60606
Toll-Free: 800-872-9622
Phone: 312-977-0031
Website: www.ymca.net
E-mail: fullfiment@ymca.net

Patient Assistance Programs for Rheumatology-Related Drugs

Abatacept (Orencia®)
The ORENCIA® (abatacept) On Call™ Patient Support
Bristol-Myers Squibb
345 Park Ave.
New York, NY 10154
Toll-Free: 800-ORENCIA (800-673-6242)
Website: www.orencia.bmscustomerconnect.com

Adalimumab (Humira®)
AbbVie Patient Assistance Foundation
Website: www.abbviepaf.org

Belimumab (Benlysta®)
BENLYSTA Gateway
BENLYSTA® Patient Assistance Program (PAP)
Toll-Free: 877-423-6597
Website: www.benlysta.com/financial/index.html

Calcium (Nalfon®)
Xspire Pharma Fenoprofen
P.O. Box 1724
Madison, MS 39110
Phone: 601-990-9497
Fax: 601-510-9318
Website: www.xspirerx.com
E-mail: customerservice@
xspirerx.com

Celecoxib (Celebrex®)
Pfizer RxPathways
235 E. 42nd St.
New York, NY 10017
Toll-Free: 844-989-PATH
(844-989-7284)
Phone: 212-733-2323
Website: www.pfizerrxpathways.
com

Colcrys®
Takeda Patient Assistance
Program
Deerfield, IL 60015
Toll-Free: 800-830-9159
Phone: 224-554-6500
Website: www.takeda.us/
responsibility/patient_
assistance_program.aspx

Denosumab (Prolia®)
The Safety Net Foundation
P.O. Box 18769
Louisville, KY 40261-7821
Toll-Free: 888-762-6436
Toll-Free Fax: 866-549-7239
Website: www.
safetynetfoundation.com

*Hydroxychloroquine
(Plaquenil®)*
Sanofi Patient Connection™
55 Corporate Dr.
Bridgewater, NJ 08807
Toll-Free: 800-981-2491
Website: www.sanofi.us

Infliximab (Remicade®)
Johnson & Johnson Patient
Assistance Foundation, Inc.
P.O. Box 221857
Charlotte, NC 28222-1857
Toll-Free: 800-652-6227
Toll-Free Fax: 888-526-5168
Website: www.jjpaf.org

Leflunomide (Arava®)
Rx Outreach
P.O. Box 66536
St. Louis, MO 63166-6536
Toll-Free: 888-RXO-1234
(888-796-1234)
Toll-Free Fax: 800-875-6591
Website: www.rxoutreach.org
E-mail: questions@rxoutreach.
org

Meloxicam (Mobic®)
Boehringer Ingelheim Cares
Foundation, Inc.
900 Ridgebury Rd.
P.O. Box 368
Ridgefield, CT 06877-0368
Toll-Free: 800-243-0127
Toll-Free TTY: 800-246-6196
Website: www.mobictablet.com/
home

Milnacipran HCl (Savella®)
Teva Pharma, Inc.
5 Basel St. Petach Tikva
Israel, 49131
Phone: 972-3-9267267
Fax: 972-3-9234050
Website: www.tevapharm.com

Raloxifene (Evista®)
Lilly Cares Patient Assistance
Program
P.O. Box 230999
Centreville, VA 20120
Toll-Free: 855-LLY-TRUE
(855-559-8783)
Fax: 703-310-2534
Website: www.lillytruassist.com

Rituximab (Rituxan®)
Genentech® Access to Care
Foundation (GATCF)
1 DNA Way, MS #858a
South San Francisco, CA
94080-4990
Toll-Free: 866-4ACCESS
(866-422-2377)
Website: www.genentech-access.
com/patients
E-mail: info@genentech-access.
com

Sodium Hyaluronate
(Hyalgan®)
HYALGAN® Reimbursement
and Patient Assistance
P.O. Box 219
Gloucester, MA 01931
Toll-Free: 800-503-6897
Phone: 978-281-6666
Fax: 206-260-8850
Website: www.needymeds.org

Teriparatide (Forteo®)
Forteo Patient Assistance
Program
P.O. Box 4668
Trenton, NJ 08650-9108
Toll-Free: 866-4-FORTEO
(866-436-7836)
Toll-Free Fax: 866-436-7830
Website: www.forteo.com

Prescription Drug Assistance Programs

Medicare Part D Prescription
Drug Plans
Medicare Contact Center
Operations
P.O. Box 1270
Lawrence, KS 66044
Toll-Free: 800-633-4227
Toll-Free TTY: 877-486-2048
Website: www.medicare.gov

National Alliance on Mental
Illness (NAMI)
3803 N. Fairfax Dr.
Ste.100
Arlington, VA 22203
Toll-Free: 800-950-6264
Phone: 703-524-7600
Website: www.nami.org

NeedyMeds
P.O. Box 219
Gloucester, MA 01931
Toll-Free: 800-503-6897
Fax: 206-260-8850
Website: www.needymeds.org
E-mail: info@needy.org

Partnership for Prescription Assistance (PPA)
Toll-Free: 888-4PPA-NOW
(888-477-2669)
Website: www.pparx.org

Index

Index

Page numbers followed by 'n' indicate a footnote. Page numbers in *italics* indicate a table or illustration.

A

AAOS *see* American Academy of Orthopaedic Surgeons
abatacept
  disease-modifying antirheumatic drugs (DMARDs) 304
  juvenile arthritis 103
  patient assistance program 514
  pregnancy 490
  tabulated *316*
acetaminophen
  bone spurs 116
  dietary supplement 425
  hip arthritis 50
  knee arthritis 56
  osteoarthritis 308
  Paget disease 240
  rheumatic diseases 26
  tabulated *378*
Achilles tendonitis, defined 122
AC joint *see* acromioclavicular joint
acromioclavicular joint (AC joint), shoulder arthritis 43
acupuncture
  carpal tunnel syndrome 128

acupuncture, *continued*
  childhood arthritis 93
  defined 495
  fibromyalgia 136
  overview 437–8
  Paget disease 238
  spinal stenosis 70
"Acupuncture: In Depth" (NCCIH) 437n
acute pain
  chronic pain 375
  defined 495
  heat and cold therapies 324
adalimumab
  disease-modifying antirheumatic drugs (DMARDs) 304
  juvenile arthritis 103
  tabulated *316*
Administration for Community Living (ACL), contact 503
administrative controls, ergonomics 272
age factor
  bone growth 4
  bone spurs 115
  calcium requirement 15
  childhood arthritis 87
  fibromyalgia 132
  knee arthritis 55
  lupus 169

age factor, *continued*
  osteoarthritis 49
  osteoporosis 193
  rheumatoid arthritis 73
acromion, depicted *43*
acromioclavicular, depicted *43*
Agency for Healthcare Research and
  Quality (AHRQ)
  contact 503
  publications
      managing osteoarthritis
        pain 307n
      rheumatoid arthritis
        medicines 315n
"Aging in Place: Growing Old at
  Home" (NIA) 460n
Aging Life Care Association (ALCA),
  contact 509
AHRQ *see* Agency for Healthcare
  Research and Quality
alcohol use
  bones 11
  fibromyalgia 136
  gout 146
  Lyme disease 158
  osteoporosis 194
  scleroderma 260
  surgery 334
Alliance for Lupus Research (ALR),
  contact 509
American Academy of Dermatology
  (AAD), contact 509
American Academy of Ophthalmology
  (AAO), contact 509
American Academy of
  Orthopaedic Surgeons (AAOS),
  contact 509
American Association for Dental
  Research (AADR), contact 509
American Autoimmune Related
  Diseases Association (AARDA),
  contact 509
American Behcet's Disease
  Association (ABDA), contact 509
American College of Rheumatology
  (ACR), contact 510
American Council on Exercise (ACE),
  contact 510
American Dental Association (ADA),
  contact 510

American Geriatrics Society (AGS),
  contact 510
American Orthopedic Society
  for Sports Medicine (AOSSM),
  contact 510
American Physical Therapy
  Association (APTA), contact 510
American Shoulder and Elbow
  Surgeons (ASES), contact 510
American Skin Association (ASA),
  contact 510
American Society for Bone and
  Mineral Research (ASBMR),
  contact 511
ANA *see* antinuclear antibodies
anakinra
  disease-modifying antirheumatic
    drugs (DMARDs) 317
  rheumatoid arthritis 304
analgesics
  defined 493
  fibromyalgia 142
  osteoarthritis 205
  rheumatoid arthritis 303
anemia
  arthritis 205
  gout 147
  lupus 176
  rheumatoid arthritis 74
  systemic lupus erythematosus 165
ANKH gene, chondrocalcinosis 2 150
ankle arthritis, overview 56–60
ankylosing spondylitis
  defined 493
  juvenile arthritis 96
  overview 105–8
  secondary osteoporosis 222
"Ankylosing Spondylitis" (NIAMS) 105n
anterior cruciate ligament (ACL)
  arthritis 55
  defined 493
  depicted *53*, *64*
  knee replacement 345
anticoagulants (heparin)
  ginger 420
  lupus 178
  osteoporosis 199
anti-cyclic citrullinated peptide (anti-
  CCP) antibody test, wrist arthritis 46

antimalarials, systemic lupus
erythematosus 166
antinuclear antibody (ANA)
defined 493
described 90
lupus 177
Aralen (chloroquine), lupus 178
Arava (leflunomide), rheumatoid
arthritis 316
arthritis
arthroscopy 331
assistive devices 470
Behçet disease 111
bone fusion surgery 334
bone spurs 118
bursitis 120
carpal tunnel syndrome 127
children 82
comorbidities 276
complementary and alternative
medicine 433
driving 473
fibromyalgia 132
foot 56
healthy eating 449
hip 48
HIV 280
hot and cold therapies 324
inflammatory bowel disease 282
joints 79
knee 52
lupus 173
Lyme disease 154
magnets 439
massage therapy 440
mental health 455
osteoporosis 204
overview 23–8
Paget disease 232
physical activity 396
polymyositis 183
psoriasis 255
risk factors overview 35–41
self management 372
sexuality 477
shoulder 42
shoulder replacement 357
sleep deprivation 381
statistics 29

arthritis, *continued*
steroid injections 326
vision loss 95
water aerobics 395
weight management 382
wrist 44
see also osteoarthritis; reactive
arthritis; rheumatoid arthritis
arthritis and diabetes, described 278
arthritis and heart disease,
described 277
"Arthritis and Human
Immunodeficiency Virus"
(Omnigraphics) 280n
arthritis and obesity, described 278
"Arthritis and Rheumatic Diseases"
(NIAMS) 23n
"Arthritis and Sexuality"
(Omnigraphics) 477n
"Arthritis—At a Glance Reports"
(CDC) 36n
Arthritis Foundation, contact 511
"Arthritis—Frequently Asked
Questions (FAQs)" (CDC) 322n
"Arthritis Mechanisms May Vary by
Joint" (NIH) 79n
"Arthritis—National Statistics"
(CDC) 29n
arthritis of shoulder, overview 42–4
arthritis of the foot and ankle,
overview 56–60
"Arthritis of the Foot and Ankle"
(Omnigraphics) 56n
arthritis of the hip, overview 48–52
"Arthritis of the Hip" (Omnigraphics) 48n
arthritis of the knee, overview 52–6
arthritis of the wrist, overview 44–8
"Arthritis of the Wrist"
(Omnigraphics) 44n
"Arthritis—Osteoarthritis" (CDC) 64n
"Arthritis—Physical Activity for
Arthritis" (CDC) 396n
"Arthritis—Rheumatoid Arthritis"
(CDC) 72n
"Arthritis—Risk Factor" (CDC) 36n
arthrodesis
defined 494
described 59
overview 363–7

arthroplasty
  foot arthritis 60
  hip replacement 350
  joint replacement 478
  shoulder 44
arthroscopic surgery, defined 494
"Arthroscopic Surgery"
  (Omnigraphics) 330n
arthroscopy
  foot arthritis 59
  knee arthritis 55
  overview 330–3
  shoulder arthritis 43
articular cartilage, depicted *53*
Aspercreme, tabulated *310*
aspirin
  ankylosing spondylitis 107
  bursitis 119
  carpal tunnel syndrome 128
  gout 147
  juvenile arthritis 102
  knee arthritis 56
  osteoarthritis 311
  Paget disease 240
  rheumatoid arthritis 303
  shoulder arthritis 44
  tendonitis 122
assistive devices
  arthritis 470
  hip arthritis 51
  polymyositis 183
"Assistive Devices"
  (Omnigraphics) 470n
"Association of Painful
  Musculoskeletal Conditions and
  Migraine Headache With Mental
  and Sleep Disorders Among Adults
  With Disabilities, Spain, 2007–2008"
  (CDC) 455n
autoantibodies
  autoimmune disorders 88
  lupus 177
autoimmune diseases
  defined 494
  dermatomyositis 182
  gout 147
  lupus 171
  thunder god vine 421

autoimmune disorder
  childhood arthritis 88
  juvenile arthritis 102
  rheumatoid arthritis 39
  wrist arthritis 45
autoinflammation, childhood
  arthritis 88
autoinflammatory disorders,
  childhood arthritis 88
azathioprine
  Behçet disease 111
  dermatomyositis 182
  pregnancy 488
Azulfidine (sulfasalazine), tabulated *316*

B

baby formula, bone growth 15
balanced diet
  gout 452
  muscles 5
  osteoporosis 194
  Paget disease 243
balneotherapy (hydrotherapy)
  chronic pain 435
  fibromyalgia 141
Behçet disease, overview 109–12
"Behçet disease" (GARD) 109n
"Behçet's Disease" (NIAMS) 109n
Belimumab (Benlysta®), patient
  assistance program 514
"The Benefits of Flaxseed"
  (USDA) 417n
bicep muscle, depicted *43*
biceps tendonitis, defined 121
biofeedback
  chronic pain management 379
  fibromyalgia 141
biologic response modifiers (biologics)
  defined 494
  juvenile arthritis 93
  overview 101–4
  pregnancy 488
  rheumatic diseases 27
  rheumatoid arthritis 303
  wrist arthritis 47
biomarkers
  defined 494
  weight management 386

biopsy, defined 494
bisphosphonates
  lupus 171
  osteoporosis 200
  Paget disease of bone 235
blood clots, Behçet disease 110
blood pressure
  fall prevention 196
  osteoarthritis 312
  scleroderma 261
BMD *see* bone mineral density
body mass index (BMI)
  hip replacement 351
  massage therapy 441
  osteoarthritis 49
  weight management 385
body size, osteoporosis 190
bone density
  bone fragility 470
  osteoporosis 170
  physical activity 84
bone density test, osteoporosis 229
bone formation, osteoporosis 188
bone fractures, osteoporosis 296
bone fusion surgery, overview 333–9
"Bone Fusion Surgery"
  (Omnigraphics) 333n
bone mineral density (BMD)
  bone fragility 469
  glucocorticoid medications 222
  osteoporosis management 170
bone pain, Paget disease 232
bone resorption, defined 188
bone spurs
  arthroscopy 59
  defined 494
  depicted *64*
  osteoarthritis 49
  overview 114–8
"Bone Spurs" (Omnigraphics) 114n
bones
  ankylosing spondylitis 105
  chondrocalcinosis 2 150
  osteoporosis 204
  overview 6–8
  Paget disease 237
Borrelia burgdorferi, Lyme
  disease 154
Bouchard nodes, osteoarthritis 65

breastfeeding, arthritis 481
broken bones *see* bone fractures
bull's eye rash, Lyme disease 155
bunions, foot and ankle arthritis 58
bursa
  defined 495
  depicted *118*
bursitis
  defined 495
  overview 118–21
"Bursitis" (NIAMS) 118n

C

C-reactive protein
  arthritis of the wrist 46
  defined 495
  rheumatoid arthritis (RA) 302
calcinosis, dermatomyositis 182
calcitonin
  lupus and osteoporosis 171
  osteoporosis treatment 200, 214
  Paget disease of bone 235
calcium
  bone health 11
  chondrocalcinosis 2 150
  juvenile arthritis 83
  osteoporosis 195, 201
  osteoporosis management
    strategies 170
  patient assistance program 515
  pregnancy and arthritis 483
"Calcium and Vitamin D: Important
  at Every Age" (NIH) 220n
calcium pyrophosphate
  deposition disease or CPPD,
  chondrocalcinosis 2 150
calcium pyrophosphate
  dihydrate (CPP) crystals,
  chondrocalcinosis 2 152
calcium supplement
  bone health 12
  osteoporosis 217
capsaicin
  chronic pain management 378
  osteoarthritis medicines 310
carpal tunnel release, described 128
carpal tunnel syndrome (CTS),
  overview 125–9

"Carpal Tunnel Syndrome Fact Sheet"
(NINDS) 125n
cartilage
  arthritis of the knee 55
  arthritis of the wrist 45
  chondrocalcinosis 2 150
  glucosamine and chondroitin 410
  joint surgeries 357
  knee osteoarthritis 326
  osteoarthritis (OA) 64
  Paget disease and osteoarthritis 237
cataracts, rheumatoid arthritis and
  vision loss 95
"Cat's Claw" (NCCIH) 413n
CDC *see* Centers for Disease Control
  and Prevention
celecoxib
  osteoarthritis medicines 309, 410
  patient assistance program 515
cell turnover, psoriasis 251
cells
  arthritis mechanisms 80
  osteoporosis in aging 227
Center for Nutrition Policy and
  Promotion (CNPP), contact 504
Centers for Disease Control and
  Prevention (CDC)
  contact 504
  publications
    arthritis 36n
    arthritis and mental
      health 455n
    arthritis and swimming 406n
    arthritis at work 271n
    arthritis risk factors 36n
    arthritis self-management 455n
    arthritis statistics 29n
    arthritis treatment 322n
    comorbidities 276n
    inflammatory bowel
      disease 282n
    joint pain 445n
    managing arthritis 371n
    musculoskeletal conditions 455n
    opioid overdose 375n
    osteoarthritis 64n
    physical activity for
      arthritis 396n
    rheumatoid arthritis 72n, 299n

Centers for Medicare & Medicaid
  Services (CMS), contact 504
cervical, depicted *73*
childhood arthritis, overview 82–103
children
  childhood arthritis 85
  Lyme disease 154
  see also juvenile idiopathic arthritis
chiropractic
  bone spurs 117
  CAM 434
  carpal tunnel syndrome 128
  spinal stenosis 70
chiropractic adjustments, bone
  spurs 117
chlorambucil, Behçet disease 111
chloroquine, lupus 178
cholesterol
  arthritis-related to other
    disorders 277
  flaxseed and flaxseed oil 417
  healthy eating and arthritis 451
  lupus 167
  rheumatoid arthritis (RA) 75
chondrocalcinosis 2, overview 149–52
"Chondrocalcinosis 2" (GARD) 149n
chondroitin
  dietary supplements 9, 425
  overview 410–3
  tabulated *310*
chondroitin sulfate, defined 495
chronic fatigue syndrome,
  fibromyalgia 135
"Chronic Illness & Mental Health"
  (NIMH) 455n
chronic lung disease (CLD), bone
  health 21
chronic pain
  arthritis and mental health 456
  arthritis and sleep deprivation 383
  CAM 435
  defined 495
  overview 375–9
  rheumatoid arthritis 299
"Chronic Pain" (NIH) 375n
chronic pain management
  overview 375–9
  see also chronic pain
clavicle, depicted *43*

claw foot, arthritis of the foot and
 ankle 58
cognitive behavioral therapy (CBT)
 arthritis and mental health 457
 chronic pain management 379
colchicine
 Behçet disease 111
 gout 148
Colcrys®, patient assistance
 program 515
cold therapy, arthritis and other
 rheumatic diseases 447
collagen
 defined 495
 myositis 82
 scleroderma 25, 259
collapsed vertebrae, osteoporosis 187
"Complementary, Alternative, or
 Integrative Health: What's in a
 Name?" (NCCIH) 432n
"Complementary Health
 Approaches for Chronic Pain"
 (NCCIH) 435n
computed tomography (CT),
 defined 495
"Comorbidities" (CDC) 276n
comorbidity
 arthritis and mental health 456
 arthritis and sleep deprivation 381
 overview 276–80
connective tissue
 childhood arthritis 90
 defined 495
 glucosamine and chondroitin 410
 menisci 54
 Sjögren syndrome 265
corticosteroids
 arthritis and rheumatic diseases 27
 arthritis of shoulder 44
 arthritis treatment 327
 Behçet disease 111
 chondrocalcinosis 2 152
 dermatomyositis 182
 gout 148
 juvenile arthritis 93
 lupus 178
 pregnancy and arthritis 487
 systemic lupus erythematosus 166
cortisol, pregnancy and arthritis 486

cortisone
 juvenile rheumatoid arthritis and
  vision loss 98
 osteoporosis 189
 shoulder replacement surgery 358
cost of arthritis, statistics 31
counselors
 arthritis and sexuality 479
 fibromyalgia 135
COX-inhibitors, defined 495
cramping, spinal stenosis 69
C-reactive protein
 arthritis of the wrist 46
 rheumatoid arthritis 302
Crohn's disease
 defined 496
 inflammatory bowel disease
  (IBD) 282
 osteoporosis 189
CTS *see* carpal tunnel syndrome
Cushing disease, bone health 21
cutaneous lupus erythematosus
 (CLE), described 172
cyclooxygenase-2 (COX-2) inhibitors,
 childhood arthritis 91
cyclophosphamide
 Behçet disease 111
 dermatomyositis 182
 pregnancy and arthritis 487
cyclosporine
 ankylosing spondylitis
 Behçet disease 111
 dermatomyositis 182
 gout 147
 osteoporosis 191
cytokines
 healthy eating and arthritis 449
 juvenile arthritis 102
 pregnancy and arthritis 486
 weight management and arthritis 392

D

deer ticks, Lyme disease
degenerative joint disease *see*
 osteoarthritis
denosumab
 osteoporosis 214
 patient assistance program 515

dentists
  scleroderma 260
  Sjögren syndrome 269
Department of Health and Human
  Services (DHHS; HHS) *see* U.S.
  Department of Health and Human
  Services
depression
  arthritis and mental health 456
  arthritis and sleep deprivation 383
  lupus 165
  osteoporosis 212
  rheumatoid arthritis 74
  yoga 400
dermatologists
  psoriasis 252
  reactive arthritis 161
  scleroderma 258
  systemic lupus erythematosus 167
Dermatology Foundation, contact 511
dermatomyositis
  childhood arthritis 91
  myositis 181
"Dermatomyositis Information Page"
  (NINDS) 181n
dexamethasone, osteoporosis 193
DHHS *see* U.S. Department of Health
  and Human Services
diabetes
  arthritis 278, 372
  arthritis risk factors 36
  arthrodesis 366
  bursitis 118
  carpal tunnel syndrome 127
  healthy eating and arthritis 450
  lupus 174
  osteoporosis 212
  psoriasis 250
  rheumatoid arthritis 75
  tendonitis 122
diclofenac, tabulated *309*
dietary supplements
  bone health 9
  osteoporosis in aging 228
  overview 425–6
digestive problems, scleroderma 260
disability and limitation, statistics 32
discoid lupus erythematosus,
  described 172

disease-modifying antirheumatic
  drugs (DMARDs)
  ankylosing spondylitis 107
  childhood arthritis 92
  defined 496
  pregnancy and arthritis 488
  rheumatoid arthritis 303
  tabulated *316*
disk, surgical procedures used to treat
  arthritis 334
dislocation
  joint replacements 344
  joint surgeries 355
Division of Nutrition, Physical
  Activity, and Obesity (DNPAO),
  contact 504
DMARD *see* disease-modifying
  antirheumatic drugs
"Driving When You Have Arthritis"
  (NHTSA) 473n
drug-induced lupus, described 172
dry cough, Sjögren syndrome 264
dry eyes
  lupus 176
  rheumatoid arthritis 74
  rheumatoid arthritis and
    osteoporosis 207
  Sjögren syndrome 264
dry mouth
  fibromyalgia 138
  lupus 176
  scleroderma 260
dry skin
  Sjögren syndrome 264
  tabulated *310*
dual-energy X-ray absorptiometry
  (DXA)
  bone fragility 470
  diagnosing osteoporosis 192
DXA *see* dual-energy X-ray
  absorptiometry

E

Eldercare Locator, contact 504
electromyography (EMG), carpal
  tunnel syndrome 127
employment
  assistive devices for arthritis
    patients 472

employment, *continued*
  mental health 455
  rheumatoid arthritis
    complications 76
Enbrel (etanercept)
  juvenile arthritis 103
  rheumatoid arthritis medicines 317
  tabulated *316*
endocrine disorders, osteoporosis 19
endocrinologists
  osteoporosis 194, 295
  Paget disease of bone 235
  systemic lupus erythematosus 167
engineering controls, work-related
  arthritis and ergonomics 272
enthesitis-related JIA
  juvenile arthritis 87
  juvenile idiopathic arthritis 100
environmental factors
  juvenile idiopathic arthritis 37
  osteoporosis 188
  Paget disease of bone 19, 232
  psoriatic arthritis 39
  rheumatoid arthritis 39, 75
  Sjögren syndrome 265
  systemic lupus erythematosus 165
epigenetic markers, arthritis
  mechanisms 80
ergonomics
  carpal tunnel syndrome 129
  work-related arthritis 274
erythema migrans (EM), Lyme
  disease 154
erythrocyte sedimentation rate (ESR
  or sed rate)
  arthritis of the wrist 46
  childhood arthritis 90
  defined 496
  rheumatoid arthritis 302
erythrodermic psoriasis, described 251
ESR *see* erythrocyte sedimentation
  rate
estrogen
  bone density 219
  breastfeeding and bone health 483
  defined 496
  hypogonadism 222
  lupus 171
  osteoporosis 170, 189

etanercept
  disease-modifying antirheumatic
    drugs (DMARDs) 303
  juvenile arthritis 103
  rheumatoid arthritis medicines 317
  tabulated *316*
Eunice Kennedy Shriver National
  Institute of Child Health and
  Human Development (NICHD),
  contact 504
"Evening Primrose Oil"
  (NCCIH) 415n
exercise
  ankylosing spondylitis 107
  arthritis and rheumatic diseases 26
  arthritis of hip 50
  arthritis of the foot and ankle 59
  arthritis of the knee 56
  arthritis of the wrist 46
  arthritis self-management
    program 458
  bone fragility 469
  bone health 484
  bursitis 119
  carpal tunnel syndrome 129
  chronic neck pain 405
  dietary supplements 425
  falls 17
  fibromyalgia 404
  gout 149
  heat and cold therapies for
    arthritis 324
  injuries 6
  joint replacement surgery 342
  managing arthritis 323
  myositis 181
  osteoarthritis 66
  osteoporosis management strategies
    170, 203
  Paget disease of bone 236
  pain management 66
  physical therapy 93
  reactive arthritis 161
  rheumatoid arthritis 79
  scleroderma 259
  tendonitis 122
  water aerobics 406
  weight management and
    arthritis 389

extraglandular involvement, Sjögren
syndrome 267
eye problems, juvenile idiopathic
arthritis 100

F

"Facts a New Patient Needs to Know
about Paget's Disease of Bone"
(NIH) 241n
fall prevention, osteoporosis 196, 229
falls
avoiding falls 464
bone fragility 467
breaking bones 17
fall prevention 196
geriatricians 296
osteoporosis 187, 215
seniors 16
family history
childhood arthritis 89
gout 146
inflammatory bowel disease 284
juvenile idiopathic arthritis 99
lupus 169
osteoarthritis 393
osteoporosis 191, 204
psoriatic arthritis 254
risk of depression 456
Family Caregiver Alliance (FCA),
contact 511
fatigue
arthritis and sexuality 477
fibromyalgia 132
lupus 174
Lyme disease 155
myositis 181
osteoporosis management
strategies 170
rheumatoid arthritis 72, 207
Sjögren syndrome 265
sleep deprivation 383
systemic lupus erythematosus 166
tai chi and qi gong 404
turmeric 423
FDA *see* U.S. Food and Drug
Administration
feet
ankylosing spondylitis 105

feet, *continued*
approved drugs 138
arthritis and rheumatic
diseases 24
arthritis of the foot and ankle 57
avoiding falls 465
childhood arthritis 85
fibromyalgia 133
healthy diet 8
osteoporosis 203
prevention of falls and fractures 468
psoriasis 251
Raynaud phenomenon 259
rheumatoid arthritis 74
see also arthritis of the foot and
ankle
femur
depicted *53, 346*
hip joint 48
hip replacement 350
knee joint 54
osteoarthritis 56
fibromyalgia
arthritis and rheumatic diseases 23
arthritis and sexuality 477
complementary health
approaches 435
defined 496
magnets 439
overview 131–43
tabulated *378*
tai chi and qi gong 403
"Fibromyalgia" (OWH) 132n
Fibromyalgia Network, contact 511
Fibrous Dysplasia Foundation (FDF),
contact 511
flares
antimalarial drugs 178
defined 496
lupus 175
pustular psoriasis 251
rheumatoid arthritis 74
systemic lupus erythematosus 164
flat feet, arthritis of the foot and
ankle 58
flaxseed oil, overview 417–8
fluoride
osteoarthritis 69
Sjögren syndrome 269

"Focusing on Fibromyalgia—A
Puzzling and Painful Condition"
(NIH) 132n
Food and Drug Administration
(FDA) *see* U.S. Food and Drug
Administration
"For People With Osteoporosis: How
to Find a Doctor" (NIH) 295n
fracture
arthritis of the foot and ankle 57
avoiding fractures 464
bone fragility 470
bone health 82
carpal tunnel syndrome 126
healthy bones 9
lupus 168
osteoporosis 186, 192, 219
posttraumatic arthritis 357
fragility fracture, osteoporosis 229
fusion
arthrodesis 364
bone grafts 365
bone morphogenetic proteins 336
carpal bones 47
intra-articular arthrodesis 365
postoperative protocol and physical
therapy 366

G

gastroenterologist
ankylosing spondylitis 108
defined 496
genes
ankylosing spondylitis 105
arthritis and rheumatic diseases 26
arthritis mechanisms 80
chondrocalcinosis 2 151
fibromyalgia 133
juvenile idiopathic arthritis 38
lupus 180
psoriasis 250
rheumatoid arthritis 39
risk factors for arthritis 37
Genetic and Rare Diseases
Information Center (GARD)
contact 504
publications
Behçet disease 109n
chondrocalcinosis 2 149n

Genetics Home Reference (GHR)
publications
juvenile idiopathic arthritis
37n, 99n
psoriatic arthritis 37n
rheumatoid arthritis 37n
genital sores, Behçet disease 110
giant cell arteritis
overview 247–8
polymyalgia rheumatica 25
"Giant Cell Arteritis"
(NIAMS) 245n
"Ginger" (NCCIH) 419n
glenohumeral joint, depicted *43*
glucocorticoids
bone loss 199
osteoporosis 189
steroid medications 222
weak bones 21
glucosamine
analgesics 308
defined 496
dietary supplements 9
osteoarthritis 425
overview 410–3
tabulated *310*
"Glucosamine and Chondroitin for
Osteoarthritis" (NCCIH) 410n
Golfer's elbow, tendonitis 121
golimumab, rheumatoid arthritis 304
gonococcal arthritis, infectious
arthritis 24
gout
arthritis and rheumatic diseases 24
bursitis 118
chondrocalcinosis 2 150
defined 496
dietary management 452
overview 146–9
tendonitis 122
work-related arthritis 271
"Gout" (NIAMS) 146n
"Gripped by Gout—Avoiding the Ache
and Agony" (NIH) 146n
guided imagery
fibromyalgia 143
mind and body practices 434
guttate psoriasis, types of
psoriasis 251

gynecologists
  osteoporosis 194
  reactive arthritis 161

H

hair loss
  systemic lupus erythematosus 165
  thunder god vine 422
hammertoe, arthritis of the foot and
  ankle 58
hamstring muscles, arthritis of the
  knee 54
"Handout on Health: Osteoporosis"
  (NIH) 186n
hands
  bursitis 120
  carpal tunnel syndrome 126
  childhood arthritis 85
  fall prevention 197
  falls and fractures prevention 467
  fibromyalgia 133
  glucosamine and chondroitin 410
  osteoarthritis 65
  rheumatoid arthritis 207
  scleroderma 259
  steroid injections and knee
    osteoarthritis 326
hard bone, osteoporosis 227
headaches
  acupuncture 437
  fibromyalgia 133
  giant cell arteritis 247
  lupus 165
  Paget disease of bone 233
  polymyalgia rheumatica 25
  tabulated *242*
Healthfinder®, contact 504
"Healthy Bones Matter" (NIAMS) 4n
"Healthy Eating and Arthritis"
  (Omnigraphics) 449n
"Healthy Joints Matter" (NIAMS) 4n
"Healthy Muscles Matter"
  (NIAMS) 4n
"Healthy Swimming—Health
  Benefits of Water-Based Exercise"
  (CDC) 406n
healthy weight
  ankylosing spondylitis 107

healthy weight, *continued*
  arthritis diet 450
  bone loss 11
  exercise 323
  gout 149
  healthy diet 9
  managing arthritis 373
  osteoarthritis 67
  rheumatoid arthritis 77
hearing loss
  Paget disease of bone 233
  tabulated *242*
heart-healthy diet, gout 149
heart problems
  lupus 174
  Lyme disease 155
  osteoarthritis medicines 312
  scleroderma 261
  tabulated *309*
"Heat and Cold Therapies for
  Arthritis" (Omnigraphics) 324n
heat therapy
  arthritis and other rheumatic
    diseases 447
  bone spurs 116
  myositis 181
  polymyositis 183
Heberden nodes, osteoarthritis 65
"Help Members of Your Community
  Thrive" (CDC) 455n
hematologists, systemic lupus
  erythematosus 167
heparin
  osteoporosis 191
  treating lupus 178
HHS *see* U.S. Department of Health
  and Human Services
high blood pressure
  gout 147
  kidney problems 173
  lupus 167
  medicines and dryness 270
  nonsteroidal anti-inflammatory
    drugs 92
  pain management 138
  pregnancy 487
  psoriasis 250
  scleroderma 261
  sodium 450
  yoga 400

hip arthritis, overview 48–52
hip fracture
    fall prevention 197
    force and direction of a fall 466
    healthy bones 10
    osteoporosis 187, 219
hip replacement surgery
    overview 350–6
    see also total hip replacement
"Hip Replacement Surgery"
    (NIAMS) 350n
Hip Society, contact 511
hips
    ankylosing spondylitis 105
    arthritis of the foot and ankle 58
    bone spurs 114
    bursitis 119
    chondrocalcinosis 2 150
    fibromyalgia 139
    glucosamine and chondroitin 410
    joint replacement surgery 341
    osteoarthritis 24, 65
    overweight 324
    painful joints 78
    steroid injections and knee
        osteoarthritis 326
Hispanics, arthritis and rheumatic
    diseases 24
"A History of Lyme Disease,
    Symptoms, Diagnosis,
    Treatment and Prevention"
    (NIAID) 154n
HLA-B27, ankylosing spondylitis 27
hormonal changes
    fibromyalgia 134
    rheumatoid arthritis 486
hormones
    gout 148
    hypogonadism 222
    lupus 175
    osteoarthritis 425
    osteoporosis 296
    rheumatoid arthritis 78
    systemic lupus erythematosus 165
hormone therapy
    estrogen 200
    lupus 171
    osteoporosis 214
hospitalizations, osteoarthritis 32

hot and cold packs, arthritis of the
    wrist 46
"How to Choose a Doctor You Can
    Talk To" (NIA) 290n
human immunodeficiency virus (HIV)
    overview 280–2
    polymyositis 183
human leukocyte antigen (HLA)
    complex, juvenile idiopathic
    arthritis 38, 101
human parathyroid hormone
    osteoporosis 215
    parathyroid hormone 200
Humira (adalimumab), juvenile
    arthritis 103
hydrocodone
    arthritis and rheumatic diseases 26
    opioids and pain management 376
hydrotherapy
    therapy fibromyalgia 141
    water-based exercise and chronic
        illness 406
hydroxychloroquine
    disease-modifying antirheumatic
        drugs (DMARDs) 303
    rheumatoid arthritis medicines 317
    sexual function 478
    tabulated *316*
hypercalciuria
    osteoporosis 223
    secondary osteoporosis 221
hyperthyroidism, weak bones 20
hyperuricemia, dietary management
    of gout 452
hypogonadism
    described 222
    secondary osteoporosis 221
hypothyroidism
    defined 496
    fibromyalgia 140
    gout 147

I

ibuprofen
    ankylosing spondylitis 107
    bone spurs 116
    bursitis 119
    carpal tunnel syndrome 128

ibuprofen, *continued*
  chondrocalcinosis 2 152
  hip arthritis 50
  juvenile arthritis 102
  lupus 177
  nonsteroidal anti-inflammatory
    drugs 26
  osteoarthritis 56
  Paget disease 240
  polymyalgia rheumatica 247
  shoulder arthritis 44
  side effects 311
  systemic lupus erythematosus 166
  tabulated *309*
  tendonitis 122
idiopathic *see* juvenile idiopathic
  arthritis
immobilization
  arthrodesis 366
  secondary osteoporosis 224
immune system
  antinuclear antibody test 177
  Behçet disease 110
  cat's claw 413
  corticosteroids 178
  cyclosporine 147
  defined 496
  disease-modifying antirheumatic
    drugs (DMARDs) 27
  human immunodeficiency virus 280
  inflammatory bowel disease 284
  juvenile idiopathic arthritis 38, 99
  lupus 171
  psoriasis 251
  reactive arthritis 160
  rheumatoid arthritis 7, 72
  scleroderma 258
  Sjögren syndrome 263
  systemic lupus erythematosus
    25, 164
immunosuppressive drugs
  Behçet disease 111
  defined 497
  secondary osteoporosis 221
impingement, bone spurs 115
infectious arthritis
  overview 161–2
  rheumatic diseases 24
  see also septic arthritis

"Infectious Arthritis" (NIH) 161n
inflammation
  anti-inflammatory drugs 98
  arthritis diet 450
  arthritis of the foot and ankle 57
  biologics 47
  bone spurs 116
  corticosteroids 92
  enthesitis-related arthritis 100
  erythrocyte sedimentation
    rate 302
  excess body fat 449
  fish oil supplements 305
  inflammatory bowel disease 282
  juvenile idiopathic arthritis 37
  lupus 166
  lupus nephritis 174
  Lyme disease 155
  myositis 181
  nonsteroidal anti-inflammatory
    drugs 91
  polymyalgia rheumatica 245
  psoriatic arthritis 38, 281
  reactive arthritis 159
  rheumatic diseases 23
  rheumatoid arthritis 39
  slit lamp examination 97
  steroids 47
  synovial fluid 45
  synovitis 330
  thermotherapy 324
  thunder god vine 421
  turmeric 423
  ulcerative colitis 283
  uric acid 452
  uveitis 94
inflammatory bowel disease (IBD)
  enthesitis 87
  omega-3 fatty acids 417
  overview 282–85
inflammatory myopathies
  dermatomyositis 182
  polymyositis 183
infliximab
  biologic response modifiers 304
  eye disease 112
  patient assistance program 515
  rheumatoid arthritis 317
  tabulated *316*

"Information for Patients about
Paget's Disease of Bone" (NIH) 232n
interleukin-1 (IL-1), biologic agents 93
internists
   described 296
   fibromyalgia 140
   osteoporosis 194
   psoriasis 252
   scleroderma 258
   Sjögren syndrome 267
inverse psoriasis, psoriasis type 251
intervertebral disk, depicted *68*

J

janus kinase inhibitors, arthritis and
   rheumatic diseases medications 27
JIA *see* juvenile idiopathic arthritis
joint
   arthritis 36
   arthroplasty 60
   bone spur 114
   defined 497
   depicted *64*
   described 52
   disease-modifying antirheumatic
      drugs (DMARDs) 27
   fibromyalgia 132
   gout 146
   juvenile arthritis 85
   juvenile idiopathic arthritis 37, 99
   osteoarthritis 49
   psoriatic arthritis 38
   rheumatoid arthritis 57
   synovium 73
   tendonitis 121
   uveitis 94
joint capsule
   defined 497
   enthesis 87
   hip joint 48
"Joint Fusion Surgery (Arthrodesis)"
   (Omnigraphics) 363n
joint replacement surgery,
   overview 341–4
"Joint Replacement Surgery"
   (NIAMS) 341n
JRA *see* juvenile rheumatoid arthritis
Jumper's knee, tendonitis types 121

juvenile arthritis (JA)
   defined 497
   described 102
   overview 85–94
"Juvenile Arthritis" (NIAMS) 85n
Juvenile Arthritis Association (JAA),
   contact 511
"Juvenile Arthritis: Discoveries Lead
   to Newer Treatments" (FDA) 101n
juvenile idiopathic arthritis (JIA),
   defined 497
"Juvenile Idiopathic Arthritis" (GHR)
   37n, 99n
juvenile rheumatoid arthritis (JRA)
   defined 497
   described 37
   vision problem 94
"Juvenile Rheumatoid Arthritis and
   Vision Loss" (Omnigraphics) 94n

K

Kelley-Seegmiller syndrome (KSS),
   uric acid 147
kidney problems
   lupus 168
   scleroderma 261
"Kids and Their Bones: A Guide for
   Parents" (NIH) 82n
kids' bones, overview 82–5
Kienböck disease, osteoarthritis 45
Kineret (anakinra), tabulated *316*
"Knee Injuries and Disorders"
   (NIH) 345n
"Knee Problems" (NIAMS) 52n
"Knee Replacement" (NIH) 345n
knee replacement surgery
   described 346
   Paget disease-related arthritis 240
knees
   arthritis 55
   bursitis 119
   chondrocalcinosis 2 150
   dermatomyositis 182
   described 52
   glucosamine 411
   knee osteoarthritis 326
   osteoarthritis 65
   psoriasis 251
   rheumatoid arthritis 299

L

lateral collateral ligament
  defined 497
  depicted *53, 64, 346*
  ligaments 55
LeadingAge, contact 511
leflunomide
  disease-modifying antirheumatic
    drugs (DMARDs) 303
  patient assistance program 515
  pregnancy 488
  side effects 319
  tabulated *316*
Lesch-Nyhan syndrome (LNS),
  excessive uric acid 147
levodopa, gout 147
ligaments
  ankylosing spondylitis 105
  bones 6
  defined 497
  described 54
  enthesis 87
  physical therapy 50
  polymyalgia rheumatica 25
  rheumatic diseases 23
light therapy, psoriasis treatment 252
Lister Hill National Center for
  Biomedical Communications
  (LHNCBC), contact 505
liver problems, neonatal lupus 173
"Living with Fibromyalgia, Drugs
  Approved to Manage Pain"
  (FDA) 137n
"Living with Severe Joint Pain"
  (CDC) 445n
long bones, Paget disease 234
"Long-term Benefit of Steroid
  Injections for Knee Osteoarthritis
  Challenged" (NIAMS) 326
loss of feeling, spinal stenosis 69
Low-Income Home Energy Assistance
  Program (LIHEAP), contact 512
lumbar spine
  back pain 391
  defined 497
  depicted *73*
lung problems, systemic
  scleroderma 261

lupus
  defined 497
  described 168
  osteoporosis 169
  sexual function 477
  thunder god vine 421
  see systemic lupus erythematosus
"Lupus" (OWH) 171n
lupus and osteoporosis, described 168
Lupus Foundation of America (LFA),
  contact 512
Lyme disease
  arthritis 154
  infectious arthritis 24
lyrica and cymbalta, pain medicines 137

M

MAGIC Foundation, contact 512
magnetic jewelry, alternative
  therapies for arthritis 93
magnetic resonance imaging (MRI)
  bone fusion surgery 333
  defined 497
  inflammatory bowel disease 285
  rheumatoid arthritis 302
  shoulder replacement surgery 361
"Magnets for Pain" (NCCIH) 439n
"Managing Arthritis" (CDC) 371n
"Managing Osteoarthritis Pain
  with Medicines—A Review of the
  Research for Adults" (AHRQ) 307n
massage
  alternative therapies for arthritis 93
  fibromyalgia 136
massage therapy, overview 440–2
medial collateral ligament, knee 54
median nerve, carpal tunnel
  syndrome 125
medical devices, safety 440
medical history
  ankylosing spondylitis 106
  arthritis of the foot or ankle 58
  bursitis 119
  glaucoma 95
  juvenile arthritis 89
  osteoarthritis 66
  spinal stenosis 77
  spinal stenosis 70

Medicare Part D Prescription Drug
Plans, contact 516
medications
arthritis and rheumatic diseases 26
arthritis of the wrist 47
bone spurs 116
chondrocalcinosis 2 152
depression 457
fibromyalgia 379
giant cell arteritis 248
gout 147
hip arthritis 50
juvenile arthritis 91
lupus 166
myositis 181
osteoarthritis 379
osteoporosis 171, 199
pain management 338, 376
rheumatoid arthritis 222
shoulder arthritis 44
tabulated *378*
uveitis 94
weight loss 388
meloxicam (Mobic®), patient
assistance program 515
menisci
joint fusion surgery 363
knee joint 54
meniscus, depicted *53*, *346*
menopause
bone loss 211
carpal tunnel syndrome 126
gout 146
hypogonadism 222
osteoporosis 169
Mental Health America (MHA),
contact 512
methotrexate
Behçet disease 111
dermatomyositis 182
disease-modifying antirheumatic
drugs (DMARDs) 92
juvenile arthritis 102
osteoporosis 199
rheumatoid arthritis 317, 487
side effect 319, 478
tabulated *316*
uveitis 98
microfractures, Paget disease 239

milnacipran HCl (Savella®), patient
assistance program 516
"Mind and Body Practices for
Fibromyalgia: What the Science
Says" (NCCIH) 141n
mind and body therapy,
fibromyalgia 141
"Mind and Body Therapy for
Fibromyalgia" (HHS) 141n
mouth sores
Behçet disease 110
lupus 176
methotrexate 319
reactive arthritis 159
MRI *see* magnetic resonance imaging
multiple sclerosis (MS), thunder god
vine 421
Muscular Dystrophy Association
(MDA), contact 512
muscle strain, muscle injury 6
muscles
arthritis of the knee 55
arthroscopy 59
bursitis 118
defined 498
exercise 79
facts 5
fibromyalgia 140
groups 54
inflammation 181
physical activity 8
physical therapy 50
polymyalgia rheumatica 25
nonsteroidal anti-inflammatory
drugs 178
rheumatic diseases 23
shoulder bones 42
yoga 117
myofascial release therapy,
fibromyalgia 136
myositis
HIV-related rheumatic diseases 281
overview 181–4
"Myositis" (NIH) 181n

N

nabumetone, nonsteroidal anti-
inflammatory drugs (NSAIDs) 312

naproxen
  ankylosing spondylitis 107
  bone spurs 116
  bursitis 119
  juvenile arthritis 91
  lupus 166
  osteoarthritis 309
  Paget disease 240
  tendonitis 122
National Adult Day Services
  Association (NADSA), contact 512
National Aeronautics and Space
  Administration (NASA), contact
National Alliance for Caregiving
  (NAFC), contact 512
National Alliance on Mental Illness
  (NAMI), contact 517
National Center for Chronic Disease
  Prevention and Health Promotion
  (NCCDPHP), contact 505
National Center for Complementary
  and Integrative Health (NCCIH)
  contact 505
  publications
      acupuncture 437n
      CAM for chronic pain 435n
      cat's claw 413n
      complementary and alternative
        medicine 432n
      evening primrose oil 415n
      ginger 419n
      glucosamine and
        chondroitin 410n
      magnets for pain 439n
      mind and body practices for
        fibromyalgia 141n
      supplements for
        osteoarthritis 425n
      tai chi and qi gong 403n
      thunder god vine 421n
      turmeric 423n
      yoga 399n
National Center for Emerging
  and Zoonotic Infectious Diseases
  (NCEZID), contact 505
National Center for Health Statistics
  (NCHS), contact 505
National Center for Injury Prevention
  and Control (NCIPC), contact 505

National Eye Institute (NEI),
  contact 505
National Fibromyalgia Association
  (NFA), contact 513
National Fibromyalgia Partnership
  (NFP), contact 513
National Heart, Lung, and Blood
  Institute (NHLBI), contact 506
National Highway Traffic Safety
  Administration (NHTSA)
  contact 506
  publication
      arthritis and automobile
        driving 473n
National Institute on Aging (NIA)
  publications
      aging and arthritis 460n
      choosing a doctor 290n
      osteoarthritis 64n
      tips for patients 293n
National Institute of Allergy and
  Infectious Diseases (NIAID)
  contact 506
  publication
      Lyme disease 154n
National Institute of Arthritis and
  Musculoskeletal and Skin Diseases
  (NIAMS)
  contact 506
  publications
      ankylosing spondylitis 105n
      arthritis and rheumatic
        diseases 23n
      Behçet disease 109n
      bursitis 118n
      giant cell arteritis 245n
      gout 146n
      healthy bones 4n
      hip replacement surgery 350n
      joint replacement surgery 341n
      joints 4n
      juvenile arthritis 85n
      knee problems 52n
      muscles 4n
      polymyalgia rheumatica 245n
      psoriasis 250n
      psoriatic arthritis 253n
      rabies 445n
      reactive arthritis 159n

National Institute of Arthritis and
Musculoskeletal and Skin Diseases
(NIAMS)
publications, *continued*
rheumatoid arthritis 72n
rheumatoid arthritis and
osteoporosis 207n
rheumatoid arthritis
treatment 299n
scleroderma 257n
shoulder arthritis 42n
shoulder problems 42n
Sjögren syndrome 263n
spinal stenosis 68n
steroid injections and knee
osteoarthritis 326n
systemic lupus erythematosus
(lupus) 164n
tendonitis 121n
National Institute of Dental and
Craniofacial Research (NIDCR),
contact 506
National Institute of Diabetes and
Digestive and Kidney Diseases
(NIDDK), contact 506
National Institute of Mental Health
(NIMH)
contact 507
publication
chronic illness and mental
health 455n
National Institute of Neurological
Disorders and Stroke (NINDS)
contact 507
publications
carpal tunnel syndrome 125n
myositis 181n
National Institute on Aging (NIA),
contact 507
National Institutes of Health (NIH)
contact 507
publications
arthritis mechanisms 79n
bone health and
osteoporosis 9n
calcium and vitamin D 220n
chronic pain 375n
fall prevention 464n
fibromyalgia 132n

National Institutes of Health (NIH)
publications, *continued*
find a doctor 295n
gout 146n
infectious arthritis 161n
kids and their bones 82n
knee injuries and
disorders 345n
knee replacement 345n
lupus and osteoporosis 168n
mind and body therapy 141n
myositis 181n
osteoporosis 186n
osteoporosis and arthritis 204n
osteoporosis in men 220n
Paget disease 232n, 241n, 236n
pain and Paget disease of
bone 239n
painful joints 77n
pregnancy, breastfeeding, and
bone health 482n
National Organization for Rare
Disorders, Inc. (NORD), contact 513
National Psoriasis Foundation (NPF),
contact 513
National Resource Center on
Supportive Housing and Home
Modification (NRCSHHM),
contact 513
NeedyMeds, contact 516
neonatal lupus, described 173
nerve problems, evening primrose
oil 416
nerve roots, depicted *68*
nervous system
chronic pain 375
Lyme disease 155
muscle control 210
Pagetic bone 234
spinal stenosis 70
neurologists
osteoarthritis 70
Paget disease 235
spinal stenosis 70
neurotransmitters, fibromyalgia 134
NHIS *see* National Health Interview
Study
NIA *see* National Institute on Aging
niacin, gout 147

NIAMS *see* National Institute of Arthritis and Musculoskeletal and Skin Diseases

NIH *see* National Institutes of Health

NIH News in Health, contact 507

NIH Osteoporosis and Related Bone Diseases ~ National Resource Center, contact 507

NINDS *see* National Institute of Neurological Disorders and Stroke

NLM *see* U.S. National Library of Medicine

nonsteroidal anti-inflammatory drugs (NSAIDs)
  ankylosing spondylitis 107
  bone spurs 116
  carpal tunnel syndrome 128
  chondrocalcinosis 2 152
  defined 498
  gout 148
  hip arthritis 50
  juvenile arthritis 91
  lupus 178
  osteoarthritis 56
  pain management 338
  polymyalgia rheumatica 247
  pregnancy 488
  reactive arthritis 160
  rheumatic diseases 26
  rheumatoid arthritis 78
  shoulder arthritis 44
  Sjögren syndrome 267
  systemic lupus erythematosus 166
  wrist arthritis 47

North American Spine Society (NASS), contact 513

NSAIDs *see* nonsteroidal anti-inflammatory drugs

numbness
  bone spurs 115
  carpal tunnel syndrome 125
  fibromyalgia 133
  nerve damage 332
  osteoarthritis 66
  Sjögren syndrome 265
  spinal stenosis 69

nutritional supplements
  Paget disease 238
  systemic lupus erythematosus 167

O

obesity
  arthritis 30
  exercise 396
  osteoarthritis 37
  physical inactivity 279
  psoriasis 250
  rheumatoid arthritis 75

Occupational Safety and Health Administration (OSHA), contact 507

occupational therapists, polymyositis 183

Office of Dietary Supplements (ODS)
  contact 507
  publication
    omega-3 fatty acids 427n

Office of Disease Prevention (ODP), contact 508

Office of Disease Prevention and Health Promotion (ODPHP), contact 508

Office of Research on Women's Health (ORWH), contact 508

Office on Women's Health (OWH)
  contact 508
  publications
    fibromyalgia 132n
    lupus 171n
    osteoporosis 210n

oligoarthritis
  defined 498
  described 99

"Omega-3 Fatty Acids" (ODS) 427n

Omnigraphics
  publications
    arthritis and HIV 280n
    arthritis and sexuality 477n
    arthroscopic surgery 330n
    assistive devices 470n
    bone fusion surgery 333n
    bone spurs 114n
    foot and ankle arthritis 56n
    healthy eating and arthritis 449n
    heat and cold therapies 324n
    hip arthritis 48n
    joint fusion surgery 363n
    juvenile rheumatoid arthritis and vision loss 94n

Omnigraphics
  publications, *continued*
    rheumatic disease
      management 487n
    shoulder replacement 356n
    wrist arthritis 44n
ophthalmologists, reactive
  arthritis 161
"Opioid Overdose" (CDC) 375n
opioids
  bone fusion surgery 338
  pain management 375
Orencia (abatacept), juvenile
  arthritis 103
orthopedic surgeons
  described 296
  spinal stenosis 70
osteoarthritis (OA)
  acupuncture 437
  bone spurs 114
  botulinum toxin
  defined 498
  described 7
  dietary supplements 425
  electromagnets 439
  foot and ankle 56
  ginger 419
  glucosamine and chondroitin 410
  hip joint 49
  knees 55
  medicine 307
  overview 64–7
  Paget disease 236
  sleep disturbance 381
  statistics 29
"Osteoarthritis" (NIA) 64n
osteoblasts, described 188
osteoclasts, described 188
osteogenesis imperfecta (OI)
  genetic abnormalities 19
  osteoporosis in men 222
Osteogenesis Imperfecta Foundation
  (OI), contact 513
osteomalacia, bones 19
osteophytes
  bone spurs 115
  defined 498
  osteoarthritis 49

osteoporosis
  defined 498
  described 268
  falls and fractures 464
  lupus 169
  medical specialists 296
  overview 186–229
  pregnancy 483
"Osteoporosis" (OWH) 210n
"Osteoporosis and Arthritis: Two
  Common but Different Conditions"
  (NIH) 204n
"Osteoporosis in Aging" (HHS) 227n
"Osteoporosis in Men" (NIH) 220n
osteotomy
  defined 498
  joint replacement surgery 342
  Paget disease 235
otolaryngologists, Paget disease 235
overweight
  arthritis 323
  gout 149
  osteoarthritis 308
  rheumatoid arthritis 300
oxycodone, rheumatoid arthritis 26

P

Paget disease
  defined 498
  osteoarthritis 69
  overview 231–45
"Paget's Disease of Bone and
  Osteoarthritis: Different Yet
  Related" (NIH) 236n
"Pain and Paget's Disease of Bone"
  (NIH) 239n
pain management
  complementary and alternative
    medicine 432
  described 338
  osteoporosis 206
  pregnancy and arthritis 487
  rheumatoid arthritis 305
  see also chronic pain management
pain relievers
  carpal tunnel syndrome 128
  chondrocalcinosis 2 150
  rheumatic diseases 26
  rheumatoid arthritis 303

"Painful Joints?" (NIH) 77n
parathyroid hormone,
  osteoporosis 200
Partnership for Prescription
  Assistance (PPA), contact 517
patella
  defined 498
  depicted *53, 346*
patellar tendon, depicted *53, 346*
pericarditis
  childhood arthritis 86
  defined 498
personal protective equipment (PPE),
  work-related arthritis 273
parvovirus arthritis, rheumatic
  diseases 24
Phalen maneuver, carpal tunnel
  syndrome 127
physiatrists
  defined 498
  described 296
  osteoporosis 194
  reactive arthritis 161
physical examination
  arthritis of the hip 50
  arthritis of the knee 55
  arthritis of the shoulder 43
  arthritis of the wrist 45
  arthroscopy 330
  bone spurs 116
  bursitis 119
  carpal tunnel syndrome 126
  fibromyalgia 140
  osteoarthritis 66
  rheumatoid arthritis 301
  shoulder replacement surgery 361
  tendonitis 122
physical therapy
  arthritis of the hip 50
  arthritis of the knee 56
  arthritis of the shoulder 44
  bone spurs 116
  childhood arthritis 93
  chondrocalcinosis 2
  dermatomyositis 182
  fibromyalgia 136
  osteoporosis 205
  shoulder replacement surgery 362
  tendonitis 123

physicians
  acupuncture 438
  inflammatory bowel disease 285
  Lyme disease 154
  Paget disease 240
"Pilot Study with 25 Veterans Yields
  Promising Results on Swedish
  Massage for Knee Pain" (VA) 440n
Plaquenil (hydroxychloroquine)
  lupus 178
  rheumatoid arthritis 316
pleuritis
  childhood arthritis 86
  defined 498
polyarthritis, defined 498
polymyalgia rheumatica
  described 25
  overview 245–8
"Polymyalgia Rheumatica"
  (NIAMS) 245n
polymyositis
  defined 25
  myositis 181
  Sjögren syndrome 264
"Polymyositis Information Page"
  (NINDS) 181n
posterior cruciate ligament (PCL)
  arthritis of the knee 55
  depicted *53, 64, 346*
posttraumatic arthritis, feet 56
prednisone
  carpal tunnel syndrome 128
  childhood arthritis 92
  giant cell arteritis (GCA) 248
  gout 148
  lupus 178
  rheumatoid arthritis medicines 316
"Pregnancy, Breastfeeding and Bone
  Health" (NIH) 482n
premature heart disease, rheumatoid
  arthritis 75
"Preventing Falls and Related
  Fractures" (NIH) 464n
progestin, osteoporosis 200
prostaglandins, childhood arthritis 91
pseudogout, chondrocalcinosis 2 150
psoriasis
  arthritis and rheumatic disease 25
  childhood arthritis 87

psoriasis, *continued*
  defined 499
  gout 147
  human immunodeficiency virus 281
  juvenile idiopathic arthritis 100
  juvenile rheumatoid arthritis and
      vision loss 96
  overview 251–5
  see also psoriatic arthritis
psoriatic arthritis
  defined 25
  genetics risk factor for arthritis 38
  overview 253–5
  psoriasis 250
puberty, osteoporosis 190
pulmonologists, scleroderma 258
purines
  arthritis and other rheumatic
      diseases 447
  defined 499
  gout 146

Q

  healthy eating and arthritis 452
qi gong
  complementary health approaches
      for chronic pain 435
  fibromyalgia 137
  mind and body therapy 141
  overview 403–5
quadriceps muscles, arthritis of the
    knee 54
quadriceps tendons, depicted *53, 346*

R

"Rabies" (NIAMS) 445n
radius, defined 499
raloxifene (Evista®), patient
    assistance program 516
Raynaud phenomenon
  defined 499
  scleroderma 259
reactive arthritis
  defined 499
  human immunodeficiency virus 281
  overview 159–61
"Reactive Arthritis" (NIAMS) 159n

Rebuilding Together, contact 513
rehabilitation
  ankylosing spondylitis 108
  arthritis and sexuality 478
  childhood arthritis 93
  described 362
  hip replacement surgery 354
  osteoporosis 194
relaxation therapy, rheumatic
    diseases 447
Remicade (infliximab), rheumatoid
    arthritis 317
remission
  defined 499
  lupus 175
  rheumatoid arthritis 74
  systemic lupus erythematosus 164
renal insufficiency, gout 147
rheumatoid arthritis (RA)
  arthritis and sexuality 477
  assistive devices for arthritis
      patients 471
  carpal tunnel syndrome 126
  childhood arthritis 89
  chronic pain 435
  defined 499
  described 39
  fibromyalgia 133
  foot arthritis 56
  juvenile idiopathic arthritis 99
  lupus 173
  Lyme disease 154
  omega-3 fatty acids 429
  osteoporosis 189
  overview 72–80
  pregnancy 486
  rheumatic diseases 23
  shoulder arthritis 43
  shoulder replacement surgery 358
  statistics 29
  work-related arthritis 271
"Rheumatoid Arthritis" (GHR) 37n
"Rheumatoid Arthritis" (NIAMS) 72n
"Rheumatoid Arthritis (RA)"
    (CDC) 299n
"Rheumatoid Arthritis Medicines"
    (AHRQ) 315n
"Rheumatoid Arthritis—Treatment"
    (NIAMS) 299n

"Rheumatic Disease Management
in Pregnant Women"
(Omnigraphics) 485n
rheumatic diseases
comorbidities 276
human immunodeficiency virus 281
juvenile arthritis 85
overview 23–7
pregnancy 485
Sjögren syndrome 263
rheumatic disorders, defined 499
rheumatologists
bursitis 120
fibromyalgia 140
osteoarthritis 70
osteoporosis 194
Paget disease 235
reactive arthritis 161
scleroderma 258
tendonitis 123
Rheumatrex (methotrexate),
rheumatoid arthritis 317
rituximab (Rituxan®), patient
assistance program 516
rotator cuff
bone spurs 114
defined 500
shoulder pain 42
shoulder replacement 357
tendonitis 121
rotator cuff disease *see* bursitis;
tendonitis
rotator cuff tendonitis
defined 121
depicted *43*

S

sacroiliac joints
childhood arthritis 87
defined 500
sacrum, depicted *73*
S-adenosyl-L-methionine (SAMe),
described 426
salivary glands, Sjögren syndrome 265
SAMe *see* S-adenosyl-L-methionine
scapula
arthritis of shoulder 44
depicted *43*

scleroderma
described 25
overview 257–61
Sjögren syndrome 264
"Scleroderma" (NIAMS) 257n
Scleroderma Foundation (SF),
contact 514
sedatives, osteoporosis 196
sed rate *see* erythrocyte sedimentation
rate
"Self-Management Education"
(CDC) 455n
septic arthritis
human immunodeficiency virus 281
overview 161–2
sex hormone deficiencies,
osteoporosis 190
"Shoulder Problems" (NIAMS) 42n
shoulder joint, depicted *43*
"Shoulder Replacement"
(Omnigraphics) 356n
"6 Things You Should Know
about Dietary Supplements for
Osteoarthritis" (NCCIH) 425n
Sjögren syndrome, overview 263–70
"Sjögren's Syndrome" (NIAMS) 263n
Sjögren's Syndrome Foundation,
contact 514
skeletal muscle
polymyositis 183
weight management and
arthritis 386
skin problems
psoriasis 252
scleroderma 259
systemic lupus erythematosus 167
skin sores
Behçet disease 110
reactive arthritis 160
scleroderma 259
SLE *see* systemic lupus erythematosus
sleep deprivation, arthritis 381
"Sleep Disturbance in Osteoarthritis:
Linkages with Pain, Disability, and
Depressive Symptoms" (HHS) 381n
smoking
bone fusion surgery 334
complementary and alternative
medicine 433

smoking, *continued*
  juvenile arthritis 84
  lupus 175
  osteoporosis 191
  pregnancy 485
  rheumatoid arthritis 75
smooth muscle, described 6
sodium hyaluronate (Hyalgan®),
  patient assistance program 516
spinal cord, depicted *68*
spinal stenosis
  bone fusion surgery 334
  bone spurs 115
  defined 500
  overview 68–70
"Spinal Stenosis" (NIAMS) 68n
Spondylitis Association of America
  (SAA), contact 514
spondyloarthropathies, rheumatic
  diseases 24
spongy bone, osteoporosis in
  aging 227
sports injuries, knee replacement 345
sprain
  carpal tunnel syndrome 126
  foot arthritis 57
  wrist arthritis 45
statistics, arthritis overview 29–33
steroids
  pregnancy 488
  rheumatoid arthritis 316
  shoulder replacement 357
  wrist arthritis 47
stretching exercises
  bone spurs 116
  carpal tunnel syndrome 129
  scleroderma 258
  yoga 401
stroke
  defined 500
  flaxseed and flaxseed oil 418
  giant cell arteritis 247
  lupus 174
  osteoarthritis 67
  osteoporosis 212
  yoga 400
stiffness of the joint
  osteoarthritis 65
  rheumatoid arthritis 39

St. Jude Children's Research Hospital,
  contact 514
stomach bleeding, tabulated *309*
subacute cutaneous lupus
  erythematosus, defined 172
sulfasalazine
  pregnancy 488
  rheumatoid arthritis 303
  tabulated *316*
  thunder god vine 421
Sulfazine (sulfasalazine), rheumatoid
  arthritis 317
support groups
  fibromyalgia 135
  psoriasis 253
"The Surgeon General's Report on
  Bone Health and Osteoporosis:
  What It Means to You" (NIH) 9n
surgical procedures
  arthritis 330
  foot arthritis 59
  hip replacement 350
  irritable bowel syndrome 285
  shoulder replacement 359
  wrist arthritis 46
Swedish massage, described 441
swimming
  chronic pain 379
  foot arthritis 59
  hip replacement 356
  managing arthritis 373
  mental health 406
  osteoarthritis 67
  osteoporosis 203
  rheumatic diseases 446
  rheumatoid arthritis 76
  scleroderma 260
synovial fluid
  arthroscopy 331
  chondrocalcinosis 2 151
  defined 500
  depicted *64*
  foot arthritis 57
  hip arthritis 48
  pregnancy 486
  rheumatic diseases 26
  wrist arthritis 45
synovial membrane
  arthroscopy 330

synovial membrane, *continued*
  depicted *64*
  hip arthritis 48
  shoulder replacement 357
synovitis, arthroscopy 330
synovium
  defined 500
  foot arthritis 57
  knee arthritis 55
  rheumatic diseases 24
  rheumatoid arthritis 73
systemic lupus erythematosus (SLE)
  described 172
  human immunodeficiency virus 281
  overview 164–7
  rheumatic diseases 25
  Sjögren syndrome 264
"Systemic Lupus Erythematosus
  (Lupus)" (NIAMS) 164n
systemic, defined 500

T

t-score
  aging 228
  diagnosing osteoporosis 192
tai chi
  bone health 17
  complementary and alternative
    medicine 434
  osteoporosis prevention 219
  overview 403–5
  see also qi gong
"Tai Chi and Qi Gong: In Depth"
  (NCCIH) 403n
"Talking with Medical Specialists:
  Tips for Patients" (NIA) 293n
taping, bone spurs treatment 116
tendonitis
  arthritis and rheumatic diseases 25
  overview 121–4
  see also tendons
"Tendonitis" (NIAMS) 121n
tendons
  ankylosing spondylitis 105
  arthritis and rheumatic diseases 25
  bone spurs 114
  carpal tunnel syndrome 125
  childhood arthritis 85

tendons, *continued*
  depicted *64*
  knee replacement 345
  muscles 6
  osteoporosis 296
  shoulder pain 42
  shoulder replacement 357
  tendonitis 122
  see also tendonitis
tennis elbow, tendonitis 121
teriparatide
  osteoporosis treatment 215
  patient assistance program 516
testosterone replacement therapy
  (TRT), osteoporosis 222
Theragen, osteoarthritis
  medicines 308
thoracic, depicted *73*
thunder god vine
  overview 421–2
  rheumatoid arthritis 436
tibia, joints affected by arthritis 54
tick bite, Lyme disease 154
tingling
  arthroscopic surgery 332
  carpal tunnel syndrome 126
  fibromyalgia 133
  Sjögren syndrome 265
  yoga 401
tissue
  arthritis and ergonomics 272
  carpal tunnel syndrome 129
  genetic risk factor for arthritis 38
  hip replacement 352
  joint fusion surgery 365
  joint replacement surgery 342
  kids bone health 82
  knee arthritis 53
  osteoporosis and arthritis 204
  Paget disease of bone and
    osteoarthritis 236
  rheumatoid arthritis 299
  shoulder arthritis 42
  Sjögren syndrome 265
  steroid injections and knee
    osteoarthritis 327
  weight management 386
tobacco use, osteoporosis 191
topical treatment, psoriasis 252

total hip replacement, hip arthritis 51
total joint replacement, overview of
    arthritis and rheumatic diseases 27
total knee replacement
    complementary health
        approaches 436
    overview 345–7
trauma
    arthroscopic surgery 331
    bone spurs 115
    bursitis 119
    fibromyalgia 133
    joint fusion surgery 364
    rheumatoid arthritis and vision
        loss 96
    shoulder replacement 358
Trexall (methotrexate)
    arthritis and sexuality 478
    childhood arthritis 92
    dermatomyositis 182
    rheumatoid arthritis medicines 317
tumor necrosis factor (TNF)
    Behçet disease 111
    childhood arthritis 93
    weight management and arthritis 392
turmeric, overview 423–4

U

UC *see* ulcerative colitis
ulcerative colitis
    arthritis and inflammatory bowel
        disease 282
    childhood arthritis 96
    defined 501
underweight, bone health 11
undifferentiated arthritis
    childhood arthritis 90
    juvenile idiopathic arthritis 100
uric acid
    defined 501
    gout 146
    healthy eating and arthritis 452
    HIV-related rheumatic diseases 282
urologists, reactive arthritis 161
U.S. Department of Agriculture
    (USDA)
    publication
        flaxseed 417n

U.S. Department of Health and
    Human Services (HHS)
    contact 508
    publications
        arthritis and sleep
            deprivation 381n
        osteoporosis in aging 227n
        weight management and
            arthritis 385n
U.S. Department of Veterans Affairs
    (VA)
    contact 508
    publication
        massage therapy and knee
            pain 440n
U.S. Food and Drug Administration
    (FDA)
    contact 508
    publications
        juvenile arthritis 101n
        fibromyalgia 137n
U.S. National Library of Medicine
    (NLM), contact 508
uveitis, juvenile rheumatoid arthritis
    and vision loss 94

V

vaginal dryness
    arthritis and sexuality 477
    osteoporosis 200
    Sjögren syndrome 264
vertebrae
    bone fusion surgery 333
    defined 501
    depicted *68*
    osteoporosis 187, 222
vertebral fractures, osteoporosis 187
Vicodin (Hydrocodone), chronic pain
    management 376
vision loss
    Behçet disease 109
    effects of omega-3s 429
    giant cell arteritis 247
    overview 94–8
vitamin D
    bone fragility 469
    bone health 5
    childhood arthritis 83

vitamin D, *continued*
  described 14
  fibromyalgia 142
  osteoporosis management 170
  Paget disease 235
  rheumatoid arthritis 305, 320
vitamin supplements
  joint replacement surgery 342
  see also dietary supplements
voltaren (Diclofenac), tabulated *309*

W

warfarin
  glucosamine and chondroitin 412
  lupus treatment 178
  osteoarthritis medicines 311
water aerobics
  exercise and arthritis 397
  fibromyalgia 379
  overview 406–7
  treating and managing
    arthritis 323
wear and tear
  arthritis of foot and ankle 57
  arthritis of hip joint 49
  arthritis of shoulder 43
  arthroscopic surgery 331
  bone fusion surgery 337
  bone health 8
  bone spurs 115
  joint surgeries 360
  Paget disease 234
weight management
  arthritis of the foot and ankle 58
  overview 385–93
  work-related arthritis and
    ergonomics 272
"Weight Loss and Obesity in the
  Treatment and Prevention of
  Osteoarthritis" (HHS) 385n
"What Is Inflammatory Bowel Disease
  (IBD)?" (CDC) 282n
"What People with Lupus Need to
  Know about Osteoporosis"
  (NIH) 168n

"What People With Rheumatoid
  Arthritis Need to Know About
  Osteoporosis" (NIAMS) 207n
"Who Needs a Knee Replacement?"
  (NIH) 345n
work-related arthritis, overview 271–4
"Work-Related Musculoskeletal
  Disorders and Ergonomics"
  (CDC) 271n

X

X-rays
  arthritis treatment 322
  arthroscopic surgery 330
  bone fusion surgery 334
  bone health 18
  bursitis 119
  carpal tunnel syndrome 127
  childhood arthritis 90
  chondrocalcinosis 150
  defined 501
  osteoartritis 66
  osteoporosis 191
  Paget disease 233
  psoriatic arthritis 254
  reactive arthritis 160
  rheumatoid arthritis 302
  tendonitis 122

Y

YMCA of the USA, contact 514
yoga
  complementary and alternative
    medicine 433
  exercise and arthritis 398
  fibromyalgia treatment 136
  overview 399–403
  preventing osteoporosis 219
"Yoga: In Depth" (NCCIH) 399n

Z

Zipsor, tabulated *309*
Zostrix, tabulated *310*